Textbook of

Mental Health Nursing

Textbook of
Mental Health Nursing

D Elakkuvana Bhaskara Raj
MSc (N) MSc (Psy) MPhil (Psy) PGDHM
Associate Professor and Head of the Department
Padmashree Institute of Nursing
Bengaluru, Karnataka, India

JAYPEE

JAYPEE BROTHERS MEDICAL PUBLISHERS (P) LTD

New Delhi • London

(JAYPEE) **Jaypee Brothers Medical Publishers (P) Ltd**

Headquarters
EMCA House
23/23-B, Ansari Road, Daryaganj
New Delhi 110 002, India
Landline: +91-11-23272143, +91-11-23272703
+91-11-23282021, +91-11-23245672
E-mail: jaypee@jaypeebrothers.com

Corporate Office
Jaypee Brothers Medical Publishers (P) Ltd.
4838/24, Ansari Road, Daryaganj
New Delhi 110 002, India
Phone: +91-11-43574357
Fax: +91-11-43574314
E-mail: jaypee@jaypeebrothers.com

Overseas Offices
J.P. Medical Ltd 83 Victoria
Street, London SW1H 0HW
(UK) Phone:
+44-2031708910 Email:
info@jpmedpub.com

EU GPSR Authorised Representative
Logos Europe, 9 rue Nicolas Poussin
17000, La Rochelle, France
Phone: +33 (0) 6 67 93 73 78
E-mail: Contact@logoseurope.eu

Inquiries for bulk sales may be solicited at: jaypee@jaypeebrothers.com

Textbook of Mental Health Nursing

First Edition: 2021, *Reprint:* **2025**

ISBN 978-93-5025-167-6

Printed in India

Dedicated to

My Beloved Parents, Brothers, Sister
and
My wife Mrs Nima,
who encouraged me to go for it on my own

I would also like to thank
My friend GK Venkataraman
for his constant support and
encouragement throughout the years

Preface

The role of a psychiatric nurse has undergone rapid and dynamic changes in recent years. The present day practising nurses also require a concise, ready reference source for better understanding of mental illnesses and mental health problems, in order to take proper care of their patients.

The chapters in this book are organized in logical sequence based on practical view. The text deals with the history of mental health care, legal aspects, classification of mental disorders, communication and therapeutic relationship, various mental disorders with nursing care and community psychiatry.

Appendices provide an easy and practical guide to important short answers and NANDA diagnosis.

The book is written in a simple style and easy-to-understand language at the level of standard patient care. It is benefited to BSc and MSc (Nursing) students.

I have made sincere and hard effort to bring out this book in an understandable and applicable manner for health care professionals to practise psychiatric nursing. Your constructive criticisms and valuable suggestions for improvement are welcomed.

D Elakkuvana Bhaskara Raj

Acknowledgments

I would like to express a deep sense of gratitude to "Almighty" who is continuously giving the moral and guidance required in all my deeds.

I like to acknowledge and thank all my family members especially my brothers Sri Rama, Bharatha Vijay Kumar and sister Girija Rani who lend their supports in accomplishing this task.

I would like to express my gratitude to my wife Mrs Nima, who gave continuous cooperation and valued assistance in bringing out this book.

I would also like to thank all the staff of M/s Jaypee Brothers Medical Publishers (P) Ltd., New Delhi, in particular Mr Vasudev H, Author Co-ordinator and Mr Kumar, Sales Representative, Bengaluru branch for their moral support in bring out this book.

Contents

1 Mental Health: Mental Illness Concepts

INTRODUCTION

The World Health Organization defines "Health" as a "State of complete physical, mental, social and spiritual wellbeing, not merely the absence of disease or infirmity".

HS Hayman defines health as "a state of feeling sound in body, mind and spirit with a sense of reserve power".

All definitions say that a healthy individual is not only physically healthy but is also mentally healthy. Mental health is an integral part/component of the total health.

Definition of Mental Health

1. Mental health is a happy blending of intellectual, emotional, physical, social and spiritual qualities of a person.
2. Meninger defined mental health as the adjustment of human being to the world and to each other with the maximum of effectiveness and happiness. The chief characteristics of mental health is the adjustment.
3. The American Psychiatric Association (APA) (2003) defines mental health as the successful performance of mental functions shown by productive activities, fulfilling relationships with other people and the ability to adapt to change and to cope with adversity.
4. Robinson (1983) defined mental health as a dynamic state in which thought, feeling and behavior that is age-appropriate and congruent with the local and cultural norms is demonstrated.

The Criteria for Mental Health

Maria Jaboda (1958) has identified a list of 6 indicators that she suggests are a reflection of mental health.

1. A positive attitude towards self.
2. Growth, development and the ability to achieve self-actualization (according to age).
3. Integration.
4. Autonomy.
5. Perception of reality.
6. Environmental mastery.

According to Maslow (1970), believed that mental health individuals possessed the following characteristics:

1. An appropriate perception of reality.
2. The ability to accept oneself, others and human nature.
3. The ability to manifest spontaneity.
4. The capacity for focusing concentration on problem solving.
5. A need for detachment and desire for privacy .
6. Independence, autonomy.
7. An intensity of emotional reaction.
8. An identification of humankind.
9. Satisfactory interpersonal relationships.
10. Strong sense of ethics.
11. Creativity.

Factors Influencing Mental Health

1. **Nutrition:** Balanced nutrition is important for the growth and development of an individual. Vitamin deficiencies enhance personality problems. A sick person may have problems of adjustment on account of feelings of integrity.
2. **Play:** When the children given the chance to play in their peer group, their mental health will be promoted.
3. **Perinatal care:** If women are not properly ready for facing the consequences, if they have not accepted motherhood adequately and if their married life has not been too happy, there is a risk of their developing psychopathological reactions.

4. **Happy home/parenting:** A Good home is that where there is a harmonious relationship between parents, where parents understand the needs and interests of their children and where there is an atmosphere of happiness and freedom, contributes greatly to the mental health of every member.

   A mother gives affections and security to her children contributes to their mental health, whereas mother who is nervous, tense or self-centered, overprotective, disciplinary practices with children are laying the foundations of ill health.
5. **Good community services:** Healthy community services provide healthy atmosphere to the society. It promote mental health, prevent mental illness and rehabilitative chronic mental illness.
6. **Adequate school:** School is a positive factor in the development of sound mental health. It provides a curriculum, enriched by activities, meeting the needs and interests of people.
7. **Early prevention:** Prevention is better than cure. Early prevention equals to health promotion. Early stage of life provides good personal care, treatment for the particular diseases like fever, neurological disease, etc. It prevent severe mental illness.
8. **Treatment of physical illness:** Persons suffering from serious physical defects may have problems of adjustment on account of inferiority feeling which they have not been able to deal with adequately. An individual with a feeling of physical wellbeing ordinarily enjoys a good disposition and is enthusiastic and intellectually alert.
9. **Lifestyle:** The individual who follows a hygienic regimen, pertaining to food, drink, elimination, bathing, physical activity, work, sleep, rest, relaxation, prevention of disease and correction of defects is more likely to have good mental health.
10. **Right man for right job:** According to the qualification and also the technical training of the person he has to be placed in his working environment otherwise he developed frustration and mental stress which results in mental illness/adjustment problems.
11. **Marital relationships:** Healthy marital relationships will promote mental health. Good interactions among husband and

wife, good understanding among them will promote mental health.

12. **Intercaste and interreligious marriages:** It promotes the extend of their love and affection towards both the family members more than they will be free from their community fixations.
13. **Guidance and counseling:** In order to promote the mental health of the individuals, they can be given the guidance and counseling in the colleges and schools. Consultation at a critical period of growth and development may have a lasting effect on the student's attitude towards mental health and illness.
14. **Interpersonal relationship with society:** Social environment provide the knowledge, the skills, interest, attitudes, habits, values and goals. So, social functioning promote mental health.
    Other factors influencing a person's mental health are:
    - Individual factors.
    - Interpersonal factors.
    - Sociocultural factors.

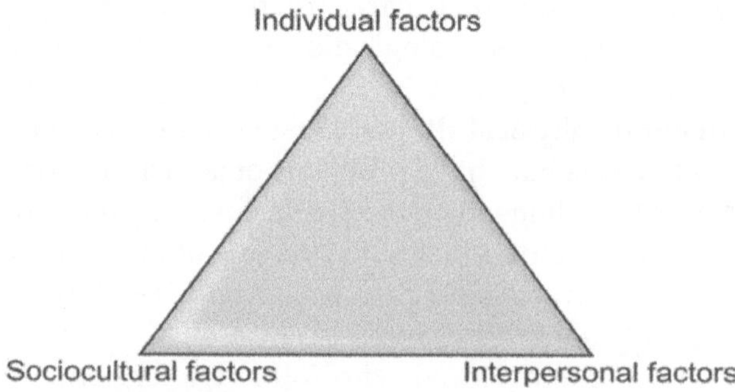

Individual factors are:

1. Biological make-up.
2. Sense of harmony in life.
3. Vitality.
4. Ability to find meaning in life.
5. Emotional negligence.
6. Spirituality.

Interpersonal factors:
1. Effective communication.
2. Ability to help others.
3. Intimacy and a balance of separateness.

Sociocultural factors:
1. Sense of community.
2. Access to adequate resources.
3. Intolerance of violence.

Characteristics of Mentally Healthy Individual

1. Has ability to make adjustment.
2. He solves his problems.
3. Has sense of personal worth, feels worth and important.
4. Has a philosophy of living.
5. Develops a capacity to tolerate frustrations.
6. Shows emotional maturity.
7. Enjoyment of play, leisure and spare time activities.
8. A well adjusted person or a mentally healthy person can get along with other people.
9. Finds satisfaction and fulfillment in exercising and expanding his potential.
10. He feels secure in a group and shows understanding of other people's problems and motives.
11. The person shows emotional maturity in his behavior.
12. The person has a variety of interests and generally lives a well-balanced life of work, rest and recreation.
13. The person is able to think for himself and can make his/her own decisions.
14. Ability to accept criticism or blame.

MENTAL ILLNESS

Definitions

1. **In the DSM-IV-TR (American Psychiatric Association 2000),** mental illness or mental disorder is defined as:

A clinically significant behavior of psychological syndrome or pattern that occurs in a person and that is associated with present distress (e.g. a painful symptom) or disability (e.g. impairment in one or more important areas of functioning), or with a significantly increased risk of suffering death, pain, disability or an important loss of freedom and is not merely an expectable and culturally sanctioned response to a particular event (e.g. the death of a loved one).

Factors Affecting Mental Health or the Factors Contributing to Mental Illness

There are various theories that explain the cause of mental illness, but none is accented as definitely causing mental illness. The various categories of affecting mental illness:

1. Biological factors.
2. Psychological factors.
3. Sociocultural factors.

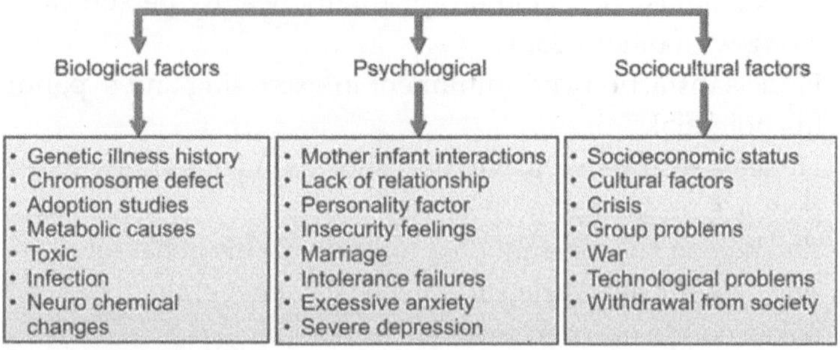

Other factors are:

1. Individual factors:
   - Biologic makeup, anxiety, worries and fears.
   - Sense of disharmony in life.
2. Interpersonal factors:
   - Ineffective communication.
   - Excessive dependency.
   - Withdrawal from relationship.
   - Loss of emotional control.

3. Sociocultural factors:
   - Lack of resource.
   - Poverty and discrimination-racism, classism and sexism.
   - Homelessness.

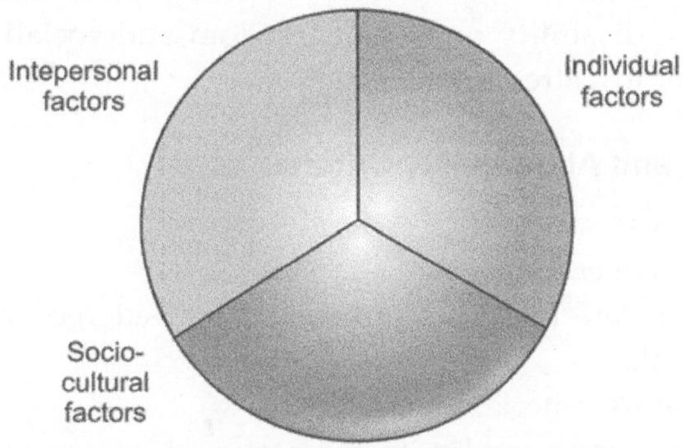

Mental Hygiene

Mental hygiene deals with the ways of maintaining mental health as well as doing away with mental illness. It is also concerned with investigation of the loss of mental health and the taxing advocacy or measure for its preservation which studies the laws and means of achieving mental health.

CONCEPT OF NORMALITY AND ABNORMALITY

The term "normal" seems to be derived from the word "norma" which means a "carpenter" square or rule. A norm therefore became a rule, pattern or standard.

The term "abnormal" with its prefix "ab" (away from) thus came to signify the deviance or variation from the normal.

PSYCHIATRY

Definition

1. Psychiatric disorder is defined as a disturbance of (i) cognition (though) or (ii) conation (action) or (iii) affect on any disequilibrium between the three.

—Niraj Ahuja (1994)

2. According to DSM – IV,

   A mental disorder should be a manifestation of behavioral, psychological and/or biological dysfunction in that person.

   So, psychiatric disorder is defined as clinically significant psychological or behavioral syndrome that causes significant distress, disability or loss of freedom and socially deviant behavior to a stressful life event.

Normality and Abnormality Criteria

It is of 2 types.

- Descriptive criteria:
  They indicate the types of behavior considered normal and abnormal.
- Explanatory criteria:
  These are concerned with the assumed process underlying abnormal behavior, that is, with the way in which abnormal behavior differs from normal behavior.

A) Descriptive Criteria

Statistical criteria   Non-statistical criteria

i) Statistical criteria: According to this criteria, 'average' is normal. A person is abnormal when he or she deviates from the 'average'. e.g. Average height and weight

Criteria of statistical view.

1. Any deviation from the average.
2. All deviant from one another in some dimensions.
3. It is based on quantity and quality of individual.

ii) *Non-statistical Criteria*:

1. **Ethical (or) moral criteria:** For being taken as normal, the behavior should be appropriate and desirable from the view point or ethics or normality.

2. **Criteria for social conformity:** Those who conform to societal norms are considered normal and those who do not care for them are labeled abnormal.
3. **Criterion of ideal or perfection:** Normal behavior is equated with perfect or ideal behavior. Others are called abnormal behavior.
4. **Legal criterion:** A law abiding citizen is normal but the one who violates the law is labeled abnormal.

B) Explanatory Criteria

i) Pathological criterion (medical)
ii) Psychological criterion
iii) Adjustment criterion

i) **Pathological or medical criterion:** It is based upon a behavior depends on functioning of the nervous system. In this way, all abnormal people are affected with some mental illness or disease.
ii) **Psychological criterion:** Psychological functioning, whether defective or normal—is deciding factor of abnormal/normal behavior → Higher mental functioning—According to environment.
iii) **Adjustment criterion:** A person is said to be normal or abnormal to extent he feels adjusted or maladjusted with his self and his environment. The normal people always integrate or adjust their needs, motive, interest and other cognitive aspects with those but abnormal people are not integrated.

Concepts of Mental Health or Normality

There are several models for understanding what is "normality".

Models

1. *Medical model*: Normal mental health is conceptualized as absence of disease or psychopathology.

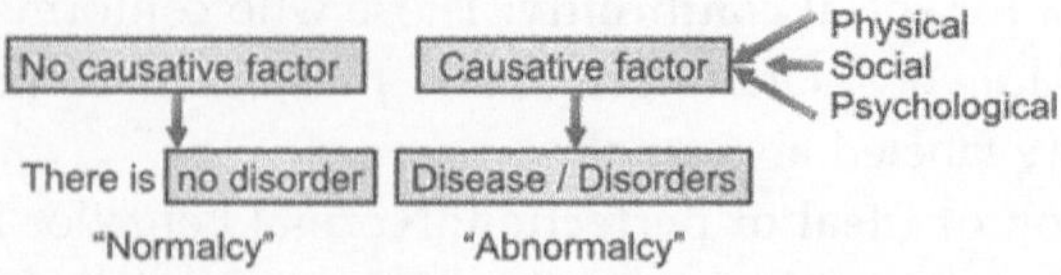

2. *Statistical model*: Statistically normal mental health falls within 2 standard deviation (SD) of the normal distribution curve.
3. *Utopian model*: In this model, the focus in defining normality is on "Optimal Functioning".

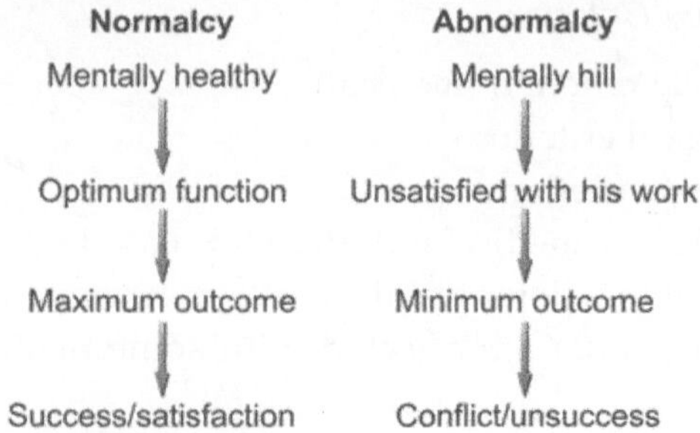

4. **Subjective model (Individual)**: Here says that absence of disability or distress or help—seeking behavior thereof, i.e. individual is not affected by any disturbance through causes.
5. **Social model:** Normalcy believes that normal person is expected to behave in a socially permissive behavior.
6. **Process model:** Normalcy is a dynamic and changing process rather than as a static concept. Along with this combined with any other model mentioned here.
7. **Continuum model:** Normality and abnormality as falling at the two ends of a continuum, rather than being disparate entities.

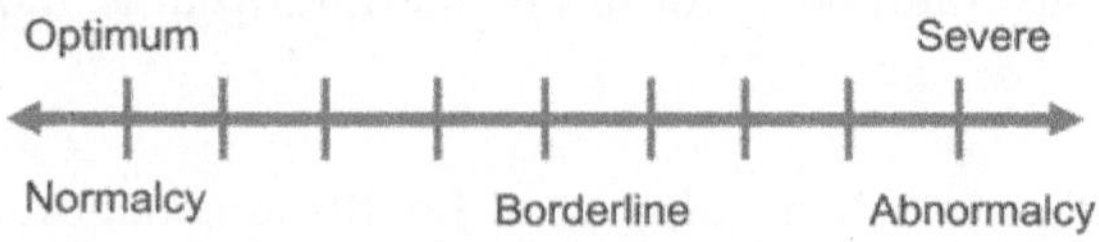

Other Concepts of Normalcy

1. Reality orientation
2. Self-awareness and self-knowledge

3. Self-esteem and self-acceptance
4. Ability to exercise voluntary control over behavior,
5. Ability to form affectionate relationships,
6. Pursuance of productive, goal—directive activities.

Characteristics of Normalcy

1. *Sociability*: Here, an individual who conforms to the traditions, modes of accepted behavior, forms and function which prevail in the social environment is called norm.
2. *Healthy, Security and Balance*: Mental health is a normal state of wellbeing, that is a positive but relative quality life. The normal individuals make conscious or unconscious efforts to maintain that social, economic, physical and psychological health as well as security.
3. *Balance and fulfillment of needs*: The quality of the normal being, his complete fulfillment of needs, which makes for balance and strength that retain a balanced outlook.

Characteristics of Abnormalcy

Abnormal means "away from the normal". The terms used in abnormality will include:
1. Abnormal as deviation from societal norms.
2. Abnormal as maladaptive.
3. Abnormal behavior.
4. maladaptive behavior.
5. Emotional disturbance.
6. Behavioral problems.

2 Role of Psychiatric Nurse

EXPANDED AND EXTENDED ROLE

Introduction

Psychiatric mental health nurses work in a variety of hospital and community settings. During recent years in the development of health services in the world, much emphasis has been placed on the "expanding role" of the nurse. Psychiatric nursing is a specialty area within the discipline of nursing. Traditionally, the role of the nurses was to provide care and comforts as they carried out specific nursing function, but changes in nursing of the day have expanded the role to include increased emphasis on health promotion and illness prevention, as well as concern for the client as a whole. Tremendous changes has happened in all specialities of nursing including psychiatric nursing. The role shift of psychiatric nursing and mental health care are influenced by factors like economics, financing of health care, information technology, managed behavioral health care, the psychobiologic shift, accountability in practice and mental health research.

Development of Psychiatric Nursing Roles

"A role is a set of expected and actual behaviors associated with a position in a social structure"—Hardy and Hardy (1988).

A role is "the sum total of expected behaviors, the behaviors expected from a person who occupies a particular position and status in a social pattern". The role of psychiatric nurse expanded after World War II. The discovery of psychiatric nursing theory and practice by Hildegard Peplau gave impetus to the advanced practice in psychiatric nursing. Many of the nursing roles are taken up by other new professionals, like activity therapists. But new roles are emerging for psychiatric nursing. Some of the new roles for psychiatric nurses in US are entrepreneur, manager, clinician, educator and researcher. Depending on the state laws, nurses are practicing psychotherapy and prescribing medicines to uncomplicated patients in US.

Traditional Roles of Nursing

Contemporary nursing requires that the nurse possess knowledge and skills in different areas.

- Caregiver, communicator, educator/teacher, manager, advocate, leader, counselor, researcher, career development.

Expanded and Extended Roles of Nurse

Expanded role of nurse is the one that the nurse assumes by virtue of education and experiences. It goes beyond the traditional nursing roles with additional responsibilities.

- Clinician, nurse researcher, nurse administrator/manager, nurse educator, advanced practice nurse (APN), nurse practitioner, clinical nurse specialist (CNS), school health nurse, critical care nurse, family nurse practitioner, trauma nurse specialist.

The concept of extended roles means to reach out. The role of the nurse needs change along with that of other health professional which means that the knowledge and skills of nurse needs to be broadened. Extended nursing facilities are that agency which provides variety of services for the patient of all age groups which may be a part of hospital or institution or a separate institution may be proprietary or nonproprietary.

- Nurse entrepreneurs, nurse anesthetist, nurse informatics, palliative care nurse/hospice care nurse, nurse oncologist, nurse prescriber, infection control nurse, nurse endoscopist

Expanded and Extended Roles of Psychiatric Nurse

The expansion of nursing role can be perceived in two ways:

First, the expansion is within the realm of medical knowledge and associated skills are required for the treatment and care of those who are ill, both acute and chronic. This role shares most of the characteristics of the replacement function, as the expansion is based on increasing the medical knowledge and skills of the nurse so that her understanding of the pathological processes, diagnosis, and treatment closely parallels that of the medical person. Although the medical aspects are favored in expanding the role in the direction of replacement, nursing has attempted to attend also to the psychological and social components which prevail in each particular illness situation like in psychiatric nursing.

Second, the expanded role for nursing is being enacted in primary care settings where emphasis is on the development and maintenance of family health. It is an expansion of nursing into areas of need which are unmet and unfulfilled at this time; it is also an expansion of the core of what nursing basically is.

Expanded care role largely involves:

1. The elements of normal nursing roles like
   - Psychiatric assessment
   - Patient and career education
   - Basic psychotherapeutic practices
2. Advanced practice roles
   - Psychiatric diagnoses
   - Prescribing single emergency doses
   - Modifying doses of wide ranging psychotropic medication
   - Autonomy in admission and discharge.

The various roles of psychiatric nurses are as listed below:

1. Primary nurse/RN or novice

   Primary nurse is responsible for the individual client's nursing care, whether in t he community or in hospital. In UK, the term psychiatric nurse has now largely been replaced with mental health nurse. In US, at the basic level psychiatric-mental health nurses are registered nurses (RNs) with baccalaureate degree who demonstrate skills beyond the beginning RN or novice to the specialty. These nurses are nationally certified by the American Nurses Credentialing Center (ANCC) within the speciality.

2. Ward manager/sister

   The ward sister has the central responsibility for integrating and strengthening interprofessinal relationships and communication.

3. Psychiatric/Mental Health Clinical Nurse Specialists (PMHCNS)

   The Psychiatric Mental Health Clinical Nurse Specialist is an Advanced Practice Registered Nurse who specializes in psychiatric nursing care issues of children, adolescents and adults who have mental health and substance abuse disorders. The nurse is an expert in providing nursing care in a specialty area of work, for example child and adolescent psychiatry or HIV and AIDS counseling, based on authoritative knowledge and expert skills.

4. Mental health nurse practitioner (MHNP)

   Mental Health Nurse Practitioner, also known as Psychiatric Nurse Practitioner, works in a primary care facility, outpatient mental health clinic or in a hospital or community health center. MHNPs evaluate and provide care for patients who have psychiatric disorders, medical mental conditions or substance abuse problems. They are licensed to provide emergency psychiatric services, psychosocial and physical assessment of their patients, treatment plans, and to continually manage patient care. They may also serve as consultants or as educators for families and staff; however, the MHNP has a greater focus on psychiatric diagnosis, including the differential diagnosis of medical disorders with psychiatric symptoms, and on medication treatment for psychiatric disorders. The role of the nurse practitioner has been described as the apex of nursing practice. Such a statement has significant implications for the professional status of nursing in its own right.

5. Nurse Therapist
   First develop in Maudsley Hospital in London, where nurse trained in psychotherapy techniques. The nurse specialist is recognized as a trained and skilled independent practitioner, who diagnoses, prescribes and caries out treatment for clients in hospital and community settings. The nurse therapist may be private practice nurse.
6. Nurse Manager
   Nurse manager work less directly with clients, but has the responsibility to provide nursing leadership to ensure that an appropriate therapeutic milieu is maintained. A key responsibility is the support and development of nurses representing nursing views to senior managers. Nurse manager plays an important role in negotiating and allocating nursing resources within clinical directorates.
7. Nurse Researcher
   The role of nurse has expanded with increase in complexity of skills required. Investigates problems to improve nursing care and to further define and expand the scope of nursing practice. Nurse researcher may be employed in an academic setting, hospital, or independent professional/community service agency. Minimum educational requirement-doctoral degree, with master in nursing.
8. Nurse Educator/Health Educator
   Nurse educators work in educational institutions, staff development dept. of healthcare agencies, client education dept(teach the disabled/ill and their families about care to provide at home). Nurse educator need experience in clinical practice to provide with practical skills and theoretical knowledge. Require graduate degree in nursing and an additional education in the educational process, many hold doctorate/advanced degree in nursing, education, administration, etc.
9. Community Mental Health Nurse (CMHN)
   Deinstitutionalization in the 1960s gave birth to the community mental health services and community mental health nurses.

The focus of community mental health programs are primary, secondary and tertiary prevention of mental illness. The community mental health nurse provides psychiatric home care. Nursing services for the patient with active psychiatric illness includes comprehensive assessment, performing venipuncture for medication or liver function monitoring, providing psychoeducation and conducting psychotherapy. They may also specialize in areas such as drug and alcohol rehabilitation, or child and adolescent mental health.

10. Psychiatric consultation-liaison nurse/liaison mental health nurse.
    Nurses practicing in this subspecialty are in an advanced practice role. In addition to direct care of patients/families, psychiatric consultation-liaison nurses (PCLN) also function in consultative, collaborative and educative relationships with nurses and other health care providers to enhance their knowledge and skills in addressing the biopsychosocial aspects of care. PCLNs may practice in many settings: Hospitals, rehabilitation facilities, long-term care facilities, home care and clinics. The psychiatric nurse liaison provided consultation to nurses and attending physicians who were providing care to patients with a medical/psychiatric illnesses.
11. Forensic Psychiatric Nurses
    The word forensic pertains to legal proceedings. When forensics is applied in the context of health care it refers specifically to that area of law applied in the criminal justice system. Forensic psychiatric nursing is a relatively new branch of nursing under the broader term of mental health care. Forensic nursing is "the application of the forensic aspects of health care combined with the biopsychosocial education of the registered nurse in the scientific investigation and treatment of trauma and/or death of victims and perpetrators of violence, criminal activity and traumatic accidents" (Lynch, 1991). Forensic nurse is "a nurse who provides care of victims of traumatic injuries and catastrophic accidents, assessment and treatment of perpetrators of crime and violence and the families of both".

The people whom forensic psychiatric nurses care for have been charged with an offense under criminal law and are thus ensconced in the criminal justice system and may be pre- or post-sentencing.

Subspecialties of Forensic Nursing

1. Clinical forensic nursing
   "The application of the forensic aspects of health care in the scientific investigation and treatment of trauma and or death or related medicolegal issues to living patients or those whose death is pronounced upon arrival or during trauma treatment" (Lynch, 1991).
2. Forensic correctional nursing
   "The provision of biopsychosocial nursing care to individuals who have been charged or convicted of a crime" (Kent-Wilkinson, 1995).
3. Forensic ER nursing
   "The awareness and provision of forensic aspects of care provided to all patients by nurses who practice in emergency rooms" (Kent-Wilkinson and McCracken, 2002).
4. Forensic geriatric nursing
   "The application of nursing knowledge to the provision of care and concern to aging individuals with regards to any legal or human rights issues of abuse and/or neglect or exploitation" (Kent-Wilkinson, 1997).
5. Forensic legal nurse consulting
   Registered nurses who use their clinical knowledge and expertise to assist attorneys with their cases in any context where law and medicine overlap. They fit under the broad umbrella of forensic nursing and are the one group of forensic nurses whose expertise is used primarily in civil, rather than in criminal cases.
6. Forensic mental health nursing
   The application of nursing knowledge and provision of psychiatric rehabilitative care to individuals who have interfaced in some way with the criminal justice system and as

a result of that interface, have been judicially designated mentally ill and in need of psychiatric evaluation and/or treatment.

7. Forensic investigator nursing (death or medical examiner nurse). The application of nursing knowledge in the investigation of any medicolegal death. Medicolegal deaths include any unexpected or violent death. Wherever the cause of death is unclear or even remotely suspicious, the medical examiner must investigate.
8. Forensic examiner nursing
   Provide an incisive examination and evaluation of trauma, related to sexual assault and other types of impersonal violence. Serves as an liaison between the health care institution, legal agencies and court of law.
9. Sexual assault nursing (clinician or examiner)
   A registered nurse who has been specially trained to provide comprehensive care to sexual assault survivors. She is usually certified by her local institution after completing a training program of approximately 40 hours. Demonstrated competence in conducting a comprehensive evidential examination is also required.
10. Geropsychiatric nursing
    Geriatric psychiatric services are a specialty in mental health care in US and some European countries. There are specific curriculum based certification courses in this speciality.
11. Nurse case manager
    Case management or management of care on a case-by-case basis. The client is assigned to a case manager, the person who coordinates all types of care needed by the client. The approach is designed to decrease fragmented care from a variety of sources. Eliminate unneeded overlap of services, provide care in the least restrictive environment, decreases cost for the insurers.
12. Child and adolescent psychiatric nurses
    Members range from the psychiatric staff nurse generalist in the secure adolescent unit to the advanced practice, clinical

Nurse specialist providing psychotherapy, consultation and psychopharmacological intervention in various settings including inpatient, outpatient, schools and community mental health centers to the doctorally prepared PhD and DNS teaching in university settings or conducting research. They have separate certification exams under American Nurses Credentialing Center (ANCC).

Role of Psychiatric Nurses—Indian Context

- History reveals, as early in fourth century AD, during the period of Emperor Ashoka, hospitals with 15 beds for mentally ill with two male and two female nurses.
- The role of the nurses was to administer herbal medication to psychiatric patients in addition to meeting their basic needs.
- In India, the role of psychiatric nurse is largely confined to institutional care.
- There are developments in the form of community mental health care role and nurse educator role.
- Nurses with experience in mental health care or having special training in psychiatry with diploma or masters degree work in community mental health programs.

BIBLIOGRAPHY

1. Allen FM. Comparative Theories of the Expanded Role in Nursing and Implications for Nursing Practice: A Working Paper. Canadian Journal of Nursing Research 1999;30(4):83-9.
2. Kent-Wilkinson A. Forensic Files: Forensic Specialties Kent-Wilkinson A. Forensic Files: Forensic Specialties 2002.
3. Lynch, 1991; IAFN - International Association of Forensic Nursing, 1993.
4. Shea CA, Pelletier LR, Poster, EC, Stuart GW, Verhey MP. Advanced Practice Nursing in Psychiatric and Mental Health Care. APNA. Mosby: St Louis Missouri, 1999.
5. Stephen E, Brenda H, Elizabeth M. Mental health nurse practitioner: Expanded or advanced? International Journal of Mental Health Nursing 2005(14)3: 181-6(6).

3 Historical Development of Psychiatry and Psychiatric Nursing

INTRODUCTION

With the introduction of understanding of the human behavior during the later part of the 19th century, it led to a change towards the mentally ill patients. Subsequently, in the third decade of the 20th century introduction of the physical form of treatment is followed.

By the fourth decade, pharmacology for the mentally ill was introduced. So, the mentally ill started getting better care.

HISTORY OF PSYCHIATRY IN INDIA

Till about 17th century all abnormal behavior was believed to be act of the "devil", i.e. "Against God", "Mentally ill" were considered evil and described as witches. Gradually over the passing time, mental illness was considered as deviant behavior and mentally ill were considered socially unacceptable and put in jails along with other criminals. In the modern era, there was a shift from "evil to ill". Mentally ill were called as "mad" or "insane" and were placed in special places called as "asylums". However, gradually these asylums became the place for human exploitation. Phillipe Pinel was the first psychiatrist to free these mentally ill from asylum. Clifford Beers work "The mind that found itself" brought in light the treatment meted out to these people in asylums, resulting in a strong reaction to the plights of mentally ill. This uproar resulted in starting of "mental-hygiene" movement.

In the 20th century, the work of Freud and BF Skinner and JB Watson gave a scientific combination of biological and social theories to explain the etiology of mental illness.

Systems of Psychological Medicine in India

Ayurveda

Mental disorders are represented in Ancient India in various types of literature. The etiogenesis of these disorders was thought to be endogenous because of provoked humors like vatonmad, Pittonmad and Kaphonmand. Exogenously the causes were attributed to sudden fear or association with ill influence of certain mythological gods or demon, Charak Samhita designated Psychiatry as "Bhuta Vidya".

The description of personality is to be in terms of Sathvik, Rajasik and Tamasik representing intellectual and moral, emotional and passionatic and impulsive, respectively and Tamsik is more or less near mental subnormality or angry. Treatment of mental disorders mainly included psychotherapy, physiotherapy, shock, drug treatment, hypnotism and religious discourses by Sages. Psychotherapy used to be in the form of talismans, charms, prayers and sleeping in temples with rituals. The indigenous manner of giving shock to the patient was terrorizing them by snakes, lions, elephant or men dressed as bandits. Then use of 10 to 100 years old medicated ghee, Drugs Cordifolia, horse radish (shigru) with asafetida and rock salt, centella asiatica (brahmi) with catechu and honey and powder of roots of serpentine were widely used.

Unani System

Najamuddin Muhammad (1222 AD), an indian physician, described seven types of mental disorders viz. Sauda-a-Tabee (Schizophrenia); Muree Sauda (depression); Ishk (delusion of love); Nisyan (Organic mental disorder); Haziyan (paranoid state); Malikholia-a-maraki (delirium). Psychotherapy was known as Ilaj-I-Nafsani in Unani Medicine.

Siddha System

"Siddhi" means achievement and Siddhas are men who have achieved results in medicine, as well as yoga and tapas. The great saga "Agastya", one of the 18 Siddhas has contributed greatly to the Siddha system of medicine of the South. He formulated a treatise on mental diseases called as "Agastiyar Kirigai Nool", in which 18 psychiatric disorders with appropriate treatment methods are described.

Revolution in Psychiatry

The history of psychiatry had witnessed 3 major revolutions that have given its present status. First revolution occurred when it was believed that sin and witchcraft are responsible for mental illness and mentally ill were chained in jails and asylums. They were considered as outcaste from society. Second revolution was the advent of psychoanalysis that explained the etiology of psychiatric disorders. Third revolution was the development of community psychiatry that resulted in the integration of mental health care in the community. Fourth revolution was the development of Psychopharmacology. It is current revolution in psychiatry.

Mental Illness to Mental Health: Indian Perspective

Indian culture has always given a great importance to spiritual life. Wig (1990 :73) stated that religious texts in India have stressed the search for the spiritual meaning of life and detachment from material thing.

One of the earliest Indian Psychiatrists to explain the importance of health was Govindaswamy in 1948. He gave 3 objectives of mental health - regaining of the health of mentally ill person; prevention of mental illness in a vulnerable individual; and protection and development at all levels, of human society, of secure, affectionate and satisfying human relationships and in the reduction of hostile tensions in persons and groups (Govindaswamy, 1970).

According to one aspect, put forward by Govindaswamy (1970) selfishness on the psychological side and starvation on the physical side are responsible for the disorganization of individual and society. The second aspect stressed the importance of culture to understand the personality functioning. Carstairs and Kapur (1976) and Chakraborty (1990) found the relation between social stress, modernization and occurrence of mental disorder. The third aspect is the use of traditional concepts of therapy, e.g. Yoga by Patanjali and fourth aspect is importance of family in therapy .

Institutionalization of Mentally ill in India

During the reigns of King Ashoka, many hospitals were established for mentally ill. A temple of Lord Venkateswara at Thirumukkudal, Chingleput District, Tamil Nadu, contains inscription on the walls belonging to Chola period. The inscription mentioned a hospital and a school. The hospital was named as Sri Veera Cholaeswara hospital and contained 15 beds.

Maulana Fazulur-Lah Hakim, an indian physician was in charge of the first Indian mental asylum, i. e. Mandu Hospital opened by Mahmood Khilji (1436-1469) at Dhar, MP First lunatic Asylum, Bombay Asylum, was built in modern India in approximately 1750 AD at the cost of 125/–, no traces of it is present today. In 1794, a private lunatic asylum was opened at Kilpauk, Madras. The central mental hospital, Yerwada, Pune was opened in 1889. First asylum for insane soldiers was started at Monghyr, Bihar and was known as Monghyr Asylum (1795).

Maxell Jones in 1953 introduced the concept of therapeutic community resulting in the improvement in the Mental Hospital conditions. Subsequently, other facilities such as occupational therapy, recreational facilities, outdoor games and picnics were started in mental hospitals . Lt. Col. Berkley Hill Was the pioneer in starting occupational therapy at the European Mental Hospital, Kanke, Ranchi, in 1935. However, in spite of all these facilities, the adjustment of the mentally ill patients was poor in these hospitals (Bhattacharya and Chatterjee 1978).

National Institute of Mental Health and Neurosciences

On the recommendation of Bhore Committee (in 1946), All India Institute of Mental Health was set up in 1954, which became the National Institute of Mental Health and Neurosciences in 1974 at Bengaluru (formerly Bangalore).

An expert committee of WHO in 1974, made several important recommendations, urging its members to consider mental disorder as a high priority problem. The recommendations included: to undertake pilot projects to assess existing mental health care program in a defined populations and training program for health workers and to devise a manual for the same (Isac 1986).

Hence, first community Mental Health unit (CMHU) was started with the Dept. of Psychiatry at NIMHANS in 1975. For short term training of primary care personal, a Rural Mental Health Center was inaugurated in Dec'1976 at Sakalwara, 15 km from Bangalore. Mental Health clinic was opened in a General Hospital in Bangalore to involve General Practitioners in Mental Health, Seminars and orientation programs for General Practitioners and school teachers were conducted. The first training program for Primary Health Care was started in 1978-79. During 1978-1984 Indian Council of Medical Research funded and conducted a multicenter collaborative project on "severe mental morbidity" in Bangalore, Baroda, Calcutta and Patiala. Various training programs for psychiatrists, Clinical Psychologists, Psychiatric Social Workers, Psychiatric nurses and Primary Care doctors were conducted at Sakalwara unit between 1981-82 (Ministry of health and family welfare, 1989).

National Mental Health Program (NMHP)

Due to results obtained by all these research efforts, NMHP was launched in 1982. Certain studies were undertaken under NMHP to integrate mental health with PHC. These included : Raipur Rani Project (1975-1981), Sakalwara project (1975), ICMR project, Jaipur Project (1982-84) and Bellary Project .

The specific vulnerable population, children, disaster population, tribal population, the elderly population and homeless mentally ill, is included for mental health care planning.

General Hospital Psychiatric Units (GHPU)

Till early sixties, Mental Hospitals were the only place available for the treatment of mentally ill. However, as compared to the number of mental ill patients, the services available were very less. Hence General Hospital Psychiatric Units were started to deal with the increasing number of patients.

The first GHPU was started in RG Kar Medical College and Hospital, Calcutta in 1933 and GMC RJJ group of Hospitals Bombay in 1938. (Khanna et al 1974). The number has gradually increased since then. Gradually, GHPU started the PG training centers at Delhi, Chandigarh, Lucknow, Bombay, Madurai, etc. resulting in development of District Psychiatrist unit.

Community Psychiatry

Mental Health Camps In India

The first psychiatric mental health camp in India was organised in 1972, at Bagalkot, a taluka town of Mysore. Earlier some service centers were organized by members of team of Kripamayee Nursing Home, Miraj. Following this, Indian Psychiatric Society also started taking active interest in mental health camp organization and various health camps were arranged in different parts of India (such as Nandi, Ghosh, Sarkar, Banerjee in 1978, Luktuke in 1976).

Voluntary Health Sector (VHS) in Mental Health

There have been strong mass media movement all over India in last decade where various issues related to mental health are brought in public domain. The social movements in relation to Darubandi are doing commendable work and are very well known. Other organization like SCARF (Chennai), Richmond fellowship foundation (Bangalore), Cadbum are also helping people in rehabilitation and integrating them in the society.

In these various organizations, active efforts have been taken to improve quality of care of patients and rehabilitate them in society. Various self help groups such as Alcohol Anonymous, Narcotic Anonymous, have been organized by people. The major effort of VHS is evident in the area of suicide and deaddiction where various kind of activities are being carried out to help people in crisis, e.g. Sanjeevani in Delhi, Sneha in Madras, Prerna in Mumbai.

Psychiatric Social Work

The establishment of Mental Health Organization under the directorate of health services was first recommended in 1946 by the health survey and development committee of the government of India. The first Psychiatric Social worker was appointed in the Child Guidance Clinic started in 1937 by Sir Dorabji Tata Graduate School of social work (now Known as Tata Institute of Social Sciences) in Mumbai. Banerjee was the pioneer of Psychiatric Social Work training in India; Institute of training in America appointed her the leader of Department of Medical and Psychiatric Social Work established in 1948. The other Social Workers and psychiatrists who gave a major boost to Psychiatric Social Work in India were Vidyasagar, Sarada Menon, UB Kashyap, BD Bhatia, PB Buckshey.

Gradually training for social work started in various centers such as National Institute of Neuropsychiatry in Bangalore (now known as NIMHANS), Indian Council of Mental Hygiene (Institute of Psychiatry and Mental hygiene).

Mental Health Act

Lunatic Asylum Act, Act 36 of 1856 was modified to form Indian Lunacy Act, Act 4 of 1912. The enactment of act resulted in opening of new asylums and improvement in the condition of asylums. The name lunatic asylum was changed to mental hospital in 1920. In 1946, the Bhore Committee recommended changes in Indian Lunacy Act 1912, as it had become outdated. Indian Psychiatric Society formed in January 1947 quickly acted on the recommendation and a committee consisted of Dr J Roy, Major R B Davis, Dr Hasib was formed. It was finally enacted on 22nd May, 1987.

Special Issues

Drug Dependence : Alcohol

In Rig Veda, 2 types of beverages are described:

Soma Juice: According to vedic hymns, soma was a mushroom and a cannabis like substance (Sethi 1979) and "Sura" – a drink that was obtained from fermented barley after distillation. In Atharva veda "Sura" was mentioned as a reward for performance of sacrifices. In the sutra period (800-300 BC) besides sura, many other drinks were widely prevalent, e.g.: Kilala – a drink prepared from Brown Sugar, wines imported from Afghanistan were commonly known as "Kapisayani".

Consumption of alcholic drink was looked down upon by Buddha and Lord Mahavira, use of alcohol was prohibited among Muslims and owing to this, ban on use of alcohol was first excised during Moghul period. However, use of alcohol on religious grounds was allowed to the "Tantrik" section of saktas among Hindus.

According to Charak, moderate drinking was pleasing, digestive, nourishing and providing intelligence, but excessive drinking causes "various elements".

Ala-u-din khilji tried to control the manufacture and sale of alcohol. His successors Mubarak Shah and Akbar followed him.

Other Drugs

The use of cannabis in Indian culture is reported more than 2000 years ago. Cannabis was known to increase concentration during meditation, hence was used by Hindu saints, its use was widespread in religious places like Hardwar, Varanasi, Puri, etc. use of cannabis is also mentioned in "Atharva Veda". Opium use became popular during Moghul period.

Gradually in the modern era, there was a gradual increase in the drug abuse and the associated complications and antisocial activities. Due to this various laws, Opium Act 1857, Opium Act 1878, Dangerous Drugs Act, 1930, Certain provisions of Cr. PC 1973, were enacted to deal with drug abuse.

Alternative patterns of care of mental health in community have developed which include GHPU at district level, Home Care Program, Foster Care, Partial Hospitalization, etc.

Psychotherapy

Psychotherapy in Ancient India dates back to the times of Pandavas. In "Bhagvad Geeta" there is an incidence of counseling in the battle-field given by Lord Krishna to Arjuna. Guru-Chela relationship is another example of psychotherapy in Ancient India. Neki (1973, 1974) examined the Guru-Chela relationship as therapeutic paradigm.

Dr Girinder Shekhar Bose founded the Indian Psychoanalytical Association in 1922 in Calcutta. A training institute of psychoanalysis to train young psychoanalysts was started. Satyananda was another analyst who was greatly influenced by Melanie Klein and had received his personal analysis from Berkley Hill. AV Vasavada was the only Jungian analyst in India. Dr NS Vahia contributed in the research on the role of Yoga in promotion of mental health.

Research

Various aspect of research work was carried out in India during the period 1947-1972. Wig and Akhtar in 1974 reviewed the research work and found that focus was on mental health and illness in India. Lots of work was done on the phenomenology and natural history eg General Paresis of Insane, relationship between leprosy and mental illness, Indian adaptation of psychological tests and construction of Intelligence tests to suit Indian needs. Remarkable work was done in the fields of epidemiology, phenomenology and treatment of mental illnesses. However, there was no up to date laboratory research and hardly any attention was paid to psychotherapy education.

ICMR contributed greatly in the research work in the form of "strategies for research on mental health"(ICMR 1981).

Continuing Medical Education (CME)

On the 35th anniversary of the Indian Psychiatric Society, in 1983, Dr LP Shah in Mumbai started the first of the series of Continuing Medical Education. The first mid-term CME was held in1990. Since then Indian Psychiatric Society and West Zone conduct annual and mid-term CME every year on various novel issues .

PSYCHIATRIC ASSOCIATIONS IN INDIA

Indian Psychiatric Society (IPS)

Berkeley hill in 1929, founded the Indian Association for mental hygiene. In 1935, the Indian division of the royal Medico-Psychological Association was formed due to the efforts of Dr. Banarasi Das. In 1946, Dr Nagendra Nath De consulted Major RB Davis of the Hospital for Mental disease, Kanke, Ranchi and Brigadier TA Munro, Advisor in Psychiatry to the Indian Army and decided to revive the association. Due to their efforts the Indian Psychiatric Society was inaugurated at Delhi on 7th January 1947. The rules and regulations were framed by the eminent Psychiatrist such as Dhunjibhoy, Rosie, Kenton, Llyodo, Dr Masani, Shah, Johnson, Govindaswamy and Kak Dr NN De presided over the first annual meeting of association on 2nd january 1948 at Patna. Since then annual meetings are held at different places.

Indian Journal of Psychiatry

It was started in 1949 as Indian Journal of Neurology and Psychiatry, was edited by Dr Nagendra nath De. After 6 issues publication was stopped in 1954. It was renamed as Indian Journal of Psychiatry in 1958 and Lt. Col. Bardhan, a pathologist was appointed as its editor

The other specific associations which were formed by psychiatrist in India are also very active such as Indian Association of Social Psychiatry and Indian Association of suicide in 1996.

Present Scenerio of Psychiatric Services in India

National Mental Health Program was implemented to provide services to rural as well as urban population. However even today 80% of the rural population do not get these services. Multidisciplinary approach for the treatment of mentally ill is confined to only few institutions. Importance is attached to treat the mentally ill patients and not much thought is given to prevent mental illness and promote mental health.

DEVELOPMENT OF PSYCHIATRIC NURSING IN INDIA

In the nursing curriculum in India there was no component of psychiatric nursing. The Health Survey's Committee's Report in 1949 recommended preparation of nursing personnel in psychiatric nursing also.

- The Committee also recommended that the existing institutions like the Bangalore Mental Hospital and Ranchi Mental Hospital should start with the training of nursing personnel.
- In 1956, one year – Post certificate course in psychiatric nursing was started as NIMHANS.
- In 1964, Mudaliar Committee made recommended that there is need to prepare a large number of psychiatric nurses.
- ICN that nursing curriculum should have a component of psychiatric nursing.
- In 1965, ICN included psychiatric nursing as a compulsory course in the BSc Nursing program.
- In 1965 – 66 psychiatric nursing component was added in the GNM.
- By 1975, psychiatric nursing was offered as elective subject in MSc Nursing at the Rajkumari Amrit Kaur College of Nursing, New Delhi (RAK).
- In 1990, 4 colleges started MSc. Psychiatric Nursing Bombay, Chandigarh, Ludhiana and Vellore.
- In recent revision GNM syllabus the content of psychiatric nursing has been dealt with in more depth, PhD (Nursing) also started in 1996.

Future in Psychiatric Nursing

1. **PUGH:** Psychiatric Units in General Hospital already formulated but not success. So, it should be developed, to all General Hospital itself to provide care for the psychiatric patients.

2. **Community Health Centre**: To promote mental health and prevent mental illness through community health center. It already implemented in few states in India, but not fulfilled completely.
3. **Deinstitutionalization:** Avoid hospital admission all the cases. Treatment should be provided by the community itself.
4. **Tele-medicine:** Through the computer can translate the innovative treatment for the psychiatric condition from one country to another.

Advanced and Systematic Care: Like psychotherapy, behavioral therapy, physical therapy should have all the mental institution.

BIBLIOGRAPHY

1. Bhattacharya RN and Chatterjee SB: "Problems of Committed Mental Patient". Indian Journal of Psychiatry 1978;20(3):267-73.
2. Carstairs GM and RL Kapur. The Great Universe Of Kota: Stress change and mental disorders in an Indian Village, 1976.
3. Chakrabarty A. Psychotherapy revisited. Indian Journal of Social Psychiatry 1995;2:4-9.
4. Isac MK (Ed). A Decade of Rural Mental Health Centre Sakalwara, A Report (1978), Bangalore: National Institute of Mental Health And Neuro Sciences.
5. Khanna BC, NN Wing, VK Sharma. General Hospital Psychiatric Clinic-an Epidemiological Study. Indian Journal of Psychiatry 1974;16(3):211-29.
6. Neki JS. "A reappraisal of Guru-Chela Relationship as a Therapeutic Paradigm". Int Ment Health Res, Newsletter 1974;16:2-5.
7. Neki JS. "Psychotherapy in India traditions and trends": In Psychiatry in India: (ed) Dr. Alan De Souza and Dr. Mas D.A. De Souse, Bhalani Book Depot, 1984;339-42,344.
8. Sethi BB, Trivedi JK. Drug Abuse in a rural population. Indian Journal of Psychiatry 1979;21, 211.
9. Wig NN, S Akhtar. "Twenty five years of psychiatric research in India", Indian Journal of Psychiatry 1974;16(1):48-64.
10. Wig NN. "Indian concepts of mental health and their impact on the care of the mentally ill", International Journal of Mental Health 1990;18(3):71-80.

4 Classification in Psychiatry

INTRODUCTION

Classification is the process by which the complexity of phenomena is reduced by arranging them into categories according to some established criteria for one or more purposes.

A classification of mental disorders consists of a list of categories of specific mental disorders grouped into various classes on the basis of some shared characteristics.

Major classifications of mental disorders are:

1. International classification of diseases (ICD – X).
2. Diagnostic statistical manual classification of mental disorders (DSM – IV).

Purposes of Classification of Mental Classification

The purposes of classification of mental classification of mental disorders always involve in the broadcast sense, communication, control and comprehension.

Communication

A classification enables users to communicate with each other about the disorders with which they deal. This involves using names of categories as standard shorthand ways of summarizing certain agreed on important features of categories that would otherwise require use of a larger number of terms.

Control

Ideally involves the ability either to prevent their occurrence or modify their courses with treatment. For that reason, control is the most important purpose of a classification of mental disorders.

Comprehension

Comprehension implies understanding the causes of mental disorders and the processes involved in their development and maintenance. Frequently, a mental disorder can be treated effectively without understanding either its cause or its pathological process, comprehension is not an end in itself but is desired because it usually leads to better control of the disorder.

History of Official Classification

1840 : The I official system for tabulation mental disorder in US with one category – idiotic and insane together.

1880 : 7 categories (Mania, Malancholia, Monomania, Paresis, Dementia, Dipsomania, Epilepsy).

1889 : A system adopted by American Psychiatric Association called as Standard classified nomenclature of diseases.

1935 : Classification was only for chronic patients proved inadequate for use with World War II Psychiatric causatives, acute disturbances, psychosomatic, personality disorders.

1948 : WHO Revised

International list of causes of Death (1900) it was revised every 1/20 year 6th revision renamed as manual of the International Classification of Diseases, injuries, causes of death, which contained for the first time a classification of mental disorder entitled "mental, psychoneurotic and personality disorder" with 10 categories psychosis, 9 categories of psycho neurosis, 7 categories of disorder of character, behavior of intelligence.

ICD – 10 – 1992 → International statistical classifications of diseases and related health problems — earlier called as International classification of diseases – injuries and causes of death – 10th Revision, 1992.

- WHO's classification for all diseases and related health problems.
- Chapter 'F' – Classifies psychiatric disorders as mental and behavioral disorders.
- Codes them on an alphanumeric system from F00 to F99.
- ICD 10 – is now available in several versions, some important versions are – 1. Clinical descriptions and Diagnostic Guidance (CDDG), 2. Diagnostic criteria for research (DCR), 3. Multi–axial classification version, 4. Primary care version.
- It is based on classification to causes – Mental and behavioral disorders based on ICD
  - F00 – F09 – Organic mental disorders.
  - F10 – F19 – Mental and behavioral disorders due to psychiatric substance use.
  - F20 –F29 – Schizophrenia, Schizotypal and Delusional disorders
  - F30 – F39 – Mood disorders.
  - F40 – F48 – Neurotic, stress–related and somatoform disorders.
  - F50 – F58 – Behavioral syndromes – associated with physiological disturbance.
  - F60 – F69 – Disorders of adult personality and behavior.
  - F70 – F79 – Mental retardation.
  - F80 – F89 – Disorders of psychological development.
  - F90 – F98 – Behavioral and emotional disorders with onset usually occurring in childhood and adolescence.
  - F99 – Unspecified mental disorders.

I. DSM – IV (Diagnostic and statistical manual of mental disorders – IV Edition, 1994).

- APA's Classification of mental disorders.
- It have mainly 5 Axes.
  - Axis I : Clinical psychiatric Axis
  - Axis II: Personality disorders and mental retardation.

- Axis III: General medical conditions.
- Axis IV: Psychological and environmental problems.
- Axis V: Global assessment of functioning – Past one year

- It based on Antic view.

DSM I: In 1951, US with representation of American Psychiatric Association developed an alternative to mental disorder section of ICD – 6 which was published in 1952.

It replaced the outdated mental disorders section of ANA and first time provided a glossary of definition of categories.

DSM II: In 1965, by American Psychiatric Association it encouraged multiple diagnosis by clinician unlike DSM – I and the word "Reaction" was eliminated.

DSM – III: In 1974 – 1980 was published using poly diagnostic criteria and multi axial system, i.e.

Axis I	-	Mental disorder and additional codes.
Axis II	-	Personality disorder and specific development of disorder.
Axis III	-	Physical disorder
Axis IV	-	Severity of psychosocial stressors (7 point rating scale).
Axis V	-	Highest level of adaptive functioning past year.

Features of DSM – IV: The fourth edition of DSM of mental disorder published in 1994, is latest and most up to date classification of mental disorder. It correlated with 10th edition of WHO's ICD.

Basic Features of DSM – IV: DSM IV attempts the describe what manifestation of mental disorder are:

- Specific diagnostic criteria are provided for each mental disorder.
- Describes each disorders in terms of associated features, specific age, culture and gender and prevalence.
- Provides explicit rule when information is insufficient by category NOIS.

DSM – IV TR (Diagnostic and Statistical Manual of Mental Disorders – IV Edition/Text Revision, 2000).

5 Conceptual Models

INTRODUCTION

Mental health professionals practice within the framework of a conceptual model of psychiatric treatment. A model is a way of organizing a complex body of knowledge, such as concepts related to human behavior.

Models help clinicians by suggesting:

- Reasons for observed behavior
- Therapeutic treatment strategies
- Appropriate roles for patient and therapist

Models also provide for the organization of data and it allows the clinician to measure the effectiveness of the treatment process and facilitate research into human behavior.

Conceptual model provides philosophical, pragmatic orientations to the service and scientific knowledge of rendering better service, responsibilities and accountability. Models are symbolic representation of phenomena. Models depict a theory or conceptual scheme through the use of symbols and diagrams.

THEORETICAL APPROACH TO MENTAL ILLNESS

The treatment of the mentally ill and their management depend mainly on the philosophy related to mental health and mental illness. The various models or theoretical approaches influencing current practice are:

1. Psychoanalytical model
2. Interpersonal model
3. Social model

4. Existential model
5. Communication model
6. Behavioral model
7. Medical model
8. Nursing model.

1. PSYCHOANALYTICAL MODEL/PSYCHODYNAMIC MODEL

Psychoanalytical model derived from the work of Sigmund Freud, a Viennese physician (1856-1939). It is based on the concept of intrapsychic conflict with in the individual. In 1890, Sigmund Freud explained the theories of the mind. The subsequent work from by Freudian followers has greatly added and changed many of the Freudian initial concepts.

Psychoanalysis system was presented both theoretical and practical side.

Theoretical side it presented a theory to understand and explain the human cycle.

Practical side its studies human behavior and also as a therapy treat mentally ill.

BASIC CONCEPTS

- **Psychic Energy/Psychic Determinism:** All mental activities, consciousness and unconsciousness, meaningful and purposeful activities with previous life experiences. The human organism is a complicated energy system deriving from all the instincts or desires or need fulfillment. The form of energy, which operates the three system of personality, is called as 'psychic energy'. It performs psychological work, i.e. thinking, perceiving, recalling, reasoning and analyzing, etc.
- **Instincts or Drives:** The motivating force that determines the behavior of an individual, they originate form biosomatic processes and are experienced as urges, wishes. An instinct is the mental representative of a bodily made. Freud used the word instinct in his theories as an energy of all the life instinct, i.e. libido. It is some of psychic energy, which imparts direction to psychological process.

The aim of the instinct is the removal of a bodily need. When the instinct is fulfilled, the individual will get psychological and physiological satisfaction and the source of the instinct is eliminated, e.g. hunger drive.

- **Cathexis:** Utilization of energy in the image of an object or in discharge action upon an object that will satisfy an instinct is called as, 'cathexis'. The total energy of the id is utilized in object —cathaxis.
- **Anticathexis:** The urging forces are to satisfy instinct; cathexis and the checking force are anticathexis. The ego and superego possesses anticathexis. Ego and superego check the action of id with their own forces.

The psychoanalytical approaches based on the following theoretical explanation. They are:

- Topographic theory of mind
- Structure theory of mind
- Psychosexual developmental theory.

TOPOGRAPHIC THEORY OF MIND

According to this theory the mind structure of the human psyche was divided into 3 layers they are conscious mind, subconscious mind, and unconscious mind.

Conscious Mind

Upper portion of the mind occupies only one tenth of our total psyche or mental life. All mental activities are meaningful and purposeful. The conscious mental process of thinking is based on reality principle. It is a special sense organ of attention concerned with registration of stimuli from both within (internal) and outside (environmental influence). Here, the person aware of time, place and persons/individuals. The ideas, perceptions, feelings, and images that we are aware of at any movement of our mental life are said to lie with in the conscious part of the psyche.

Subconscious Mind or Preconscious Mind

Just beneath the conscious layer lies the subconscious mind. It stores all type of information just beneath the surface of awareness. It can be clearly brought to the level of conscious at a moment's notice whenever required. Thus, all experiences or knowledge that have been gained or learned by an individual through various types of experiences or training. It is a liaison between the unconscious mind and conscious mind with access to both. The unconscious mental content can reach the conscious mind only through the preconscious mind.

The preconscious mental content can easily become conscious with the focusing of attention. It is not present at the birth, but develops in childhood paralleling the ego development. Censor lies here that maintains the repressive behavior.

Unconscious Mind

The conscious mind was denoted from its status as the largest and most important region of the mind to the lesser status of being, a quality of mental phenomena. It is the underneath layer of brain, much of the mental activities lies outside the sphere of conscious, but this unconscious mental activity is influential in determining the conscious thought and behavior, even if it is not available to the voluntary recall.

The unconscious mind contains ideas and affects the repressed material (repression mechanism, i.e. wishes, desires, feelings, derives, motives, etc) can only reach the conscious through preconscious, when the censor is relaxed, e.g. dreams or abreaction or overpowered, e.g. slips of tongue and free association. The unconscious mind is based on pleasure principle (Id).

- It is characterized by primary process of thinking found in young children, mentally retarded children, severe psychotic clients and in dreams.
- It includes thoughts, wishes, urges, feelings, fantasies that would be considered an unacceptable or danger, if they become conscious or if the individual acted upon them. They usually strive and agitate to come up to subconscious or conscious

layers, in disguised forms (dreams or reveries). This hidden treasure of mental life belonging to the conscious is responsible for most of our behaviors.

- It differs from normal thinking.
- It strives for immediate discharge of drive/energy.
- It lacks contacts with reality, full of contradictions.
- Freud asserts what we do and how we behave is always determined by the forces residing in our unconscious and not by the choices of conscious mind.
- It lacks organization and logical connection.
- Sometimes exhibits automatic behavior, deriving from work without thinking about it.

STRUCTURE THEORY OF MIND

Sigmund Freud (1923) divided the mental apparatus into three dynamic components:

- Id
- Ego
- Superego.

Id: Legislator of the Personality

At birth, the personality is all id. The sole function of the id is to serve the instincts by seeking objects that will satisfy them. It is the psychic representation of derives or wishes and the source of mental energy and of the individual.

It is totally unconscious, containing the basic drives and instincts concerned with survival, sexual drive, eating, fulfillment of all other bodily needs (Eros/life instinct) and aggression, murder, fistfights, arson (Thonatos/death instinct –destructive force).

Qualities – it has the qualities like, it must get what it wants and when it wants, in this way id is quite selfish and unethical. It is characterized by primary process of thinking and is based on pleasure principle, no reality and no rules. It considers only satisfaction of its own needs and drives. The only urge of this drive is immediate gratification. The energy of the id is used for institutional gratification by means of reflex action and wish fulfillment.

The aim of both processes is to utilize the instinctual energy that will eliminate the need and bring response to the individual. When id is blocked by superego or ego processes it tries to break through resistances of ego and superego and discharge itself in fantasy or action. Id cannot satisfy the vital needs of life through reflex action or wish fulfillment alone, consequently the person just has to learn the difference between images and reality, if he is going to survive, i.e. ego.

Ego: Executive of the Personality

According to Freud (1933), the ego emerges when psychic energy is diverted from the id to energize important cognitive process such as perception, learning, logical reasoning. Ego is primarily determined and guided by the reality principle. It is intermediately determined and guided by the reality principle. It is intermediately between 3 sets of forces, i.e. the instinctive, irrational demands of the id, moral demands of the superego. It is extended to all the 3 layers of the mind for exercising its balancing role (to control id in terms of reality and to appease the superego).

Ego is predominantly conscious, though some parts are unconscious, so ego maintains balance between id and superego on the one hand and the reality on the other. Ego is the seat of conscious, intellectual, self-preservative and defense functions of mental apparatus. Individual is trying to get harmony between internal environment (mind) and to external world.

The ego also invests some of psychic energy to block the ids irrational impulses. Freud stressed that the ego is both servant and master to the id. The ego's mastery is reflected by its ability to delay gratification until reality is served. The ego continues to serve the id as an executive serves subordinates, pondering several alternative course of action and selecting a plan that will best satisfy the id's basic needs.

Ego's functions are manifested as:

1. Maturational functions, motor activity, sensory function, language, cognition, memory, etc.

2. Developmental functions, e.g. defenses, signal anxiety, reality testing, object relationships, sexual development, identity and overall integration of personality. It encompasses conscience and ego ideal. Conscience- judgmental and self criticism are effectively regulated (the individual have sense of what he should do or he should not do, feel or think). Ego ideal – the aspirations and values. Both conscience and ego ideal will develop through the transfer of prohibitions, permissions, expectations and values from external authority figures (usually parents) to an internal agency.

Superego: Judicial Branch of Personality

It is predominantly unconscious subdivision of mental apparatus from the ego and strives for protection rather than for pleasure or reality. It is the direct anticathesis of id and represents the ethical and moral aspect of the psyche. It consists of punitive conscience and non-punitive conscience; both derive from the effect of parental influence on the ego. The parental influences not only include the effect of actual parents but also of the important people in the surrounding environment.

Fear of punishment and a desire for approval cause the child to identify him with the moral percepts of parents. The open criticisms, prohibitions, guilt arousing statements and punishments are introjected as conscience. Superego develops in the 5 yrs age of the child, it is idealistic in nature. On the other hand, the approvals and reward become introjected as the ego ideal. Superego is also punished with the power to reward or to punish. The power is done by ego-ideal; punishment is done by the conscience.

Examples

If an individual happens to see a good saree on the shop window, the id might say 'I like it', 'I want it' but ego will control that wish with a warning "no, you cannot have it just like that unless you go in and pay money and bye it, or else you will get in trouble if you just have it and you do not have the money to bye it", whereas superego might say "no, you cannot just take it like that because it belongs to the shop keeper and it is wrong to take that for you yourself without paying". It is a balance of these three forces that results in acceptable behavior.

PSYCHOSEXUAL STAGES

Freud viewed the sex instinct as the most important of the life instincts because he often found that the mental disturbances of his patients revolved around childhood sexual conflicts that they had repressed. Freud has described psychosexual development of the individual from the birth to adulthood. These stages are gradual, sequential, emergence of sexual instincts starts from infancy to adulthood (genital sexuality). These stages reflect the interaction between physical and nervous system maturation and individual experience (development). The sexual energy is referred to as libido. As the sex instinct matures, its energy (libido) gradually shifts from one part of the body to another and the child enters a new stage of psychosexual development. Freud called these stages distinct imprints on the developing psyche (i.e. the mind or personality).

The psychosexual stages/phases are:

Oral Phase (0-1 ½ yr)

Infant will have drive and gratifications through the oral region. Mouth is the 1st sex organ and gives pleasure to the child. Feeding was thought to be a particularly rich source of oral gratification. It consist of 2 phases:

(i) oral erotic phase (sucking, chewing and feeding)

(ii) Oral sadistic phase (biting).

Fixation at and regression to this stage leads to dependent personality traits, schizophrenia, severe mood disorder, alcohol dependence syndrome and drug dependence behavior Ego development begins toward end of this stage until then id dominates the infant.

Anal Phase (11/2 -3 yr)

Child gets gratification through the anal and perianal area. During this stage anal sphincter control is achieved and the primary focus shifts to the anal zone and the behaviors are associated with retention and expulsion. Major achievement in this stage, i.e. anal sphincter control is achieved through toilet training. It consist of 2 phases

(i) Anal erotic phase (excretion)

(ii) Anal sadistic phase (holding and letting go at his will).

Fixation at anal sadistic phase leads to obsessive compulsive personality traits and obsessive-compulsive disorder.

Phallic Phase/Oedipal Phase (3-5 yr)

Major site of gratification is the genital area. Genitals become the primary source of interest, discharge and organization of urges leads to wishes and fantasies. All children at this age develop a strong incestuous desire for the parent of the other sex. He called this period the phallic stage because he believed that the phallus (penis) assumes a critically important role in the psychosexual development of both boys and girls.

The Oedipus complex is both the central theme of phallic stage and a core concept of early psychoanalytic theory. The Oedipus complex (boys) and Electra complex (girls) include the wish of the child for an exclusive and quasiadult libidinal relationship with the parent of the opposite sex. This wish includes a desire to exclude and replace the same sex parent, who is perceived as a rival and love for the parent of the opposite sex.

Conflict results from the fear of parental displeasure and retaliation and from attachment to the same sex parent. Boys experience this fear of retaliation as castration anxiety, whereas girls fear the loss of mothers love and approval. Fixation at this stage leads to sexual deviations, sexual dysfunction and neurotic disorder.

Latency Phase (5-12 yr)

This is a stage of relative sexual quiescence. Superego is at formulated at this stage. Sexual drive is channelized into socially appropriate goals like development of social interpersonal relationships, acquisition of knowledge and new skills, engage in academic and socialization activities. Children prepare their own sex and neglect opposite sex. This latency period continues until puberty, when the child suddenly experiences a number of biological changes that make the beginning of Freud final psychosexual stage. Fixation at this stage leads to neurotic disorders.

Genital Phase (12-18 yr)

With the onset of puberty comes maturation of the reproductive system, a flooding of the body with sex hormones and according to Freud, a reactivation of the genital zone as an area of sexual pleasure. The underlying goal of the sex instinct now becomes biological reproduction through sexual intercourse. It is associated with explicit neuroendocrine and biosomatic maturational components. An adult sexuality develops child will develop the capacity for intimacy and respect for others.

Gradual release from parental control with more influence of peer group is seen. However, adolescents face conflicts in learning how to manage these new sexual urges in socially acceptable ways. Throughout adolescent and young adulthood, libido is invested in such activities as forming friendships, preparing for a career, courting, masturbation, fall in love with own self by taking interest in beautifying and adoring their bodies and getting married — activities that prepare the individual to eventually satisfy the mature sex instinct by having children. Here, Freud believed that people remain for the rest of their lives. Fixation at genital phase leads to neurotic disorders.

BASIC ASSUMPTIONS

- All human behavior is caused and thus is capable of explanation. Human behavior, however insignificant or obscure, does not occur randomly or by chance. Rather, all behavior is determined by prior life events.
- All human behavior from birth to old age is driven by an energy called the libido. The goal of the libido is the reduction of tension

through the attainment of pleasure. The libido is closely associated with physiological or instinctual drives (e.g. hunger, thirst, elimination and sex). Release of these drives results in the reduction of tension and experience of pleasure. Hence the pleasure principle is operative when pleasure seeking behaviors are used.

- Maturity is associated with the ability to invent and use substitutive or distinguished forms of gratification. The ability to delay pleasure in favor of more acceptable behavior is based on reality principle.
- Thought processes deriving from the id are characterized by their illogic, confused from and preverbal content. Such thought processes are called as primary process thinking and are often reflected in verbalization of mentally ill people (schizophrenia and psychotic individuals).
- The superego is the personality structure containing the values, legal and moral regulations and social expectations that thwart free expression of pleasure seeking behavior. Society and the family determine the content of the superego and sets limitations over the individual.
- Ego represents reality and is capable of postponing pleasure until an appropriate time, place or object is available. Ego acts in mature and adaptive behavior. It uses mental mechanisms to maintain inner harmony and balance.
- The human personality functions on 3 levels of awareness – conscious, preconscious, and unconscious.
- Human development unfolds through 5 innate psychosexual stages — oral, anal, phallic, latent and genital. These stages extend throughout the lifespan; the 1st 6 yr of life determine the individual's long-term personality characteristics.

PSYCHOANALYTICAL PROCESS

Psychoanalysis, described by Freud, make use of free association 7 dream analysis to affect reconstruction of personality. Free association – refers to the verbalization of thoughts as they occur, without any conscious screening. Analysis of the patient's dreams helps to gain additional insight into his problem and the resistances. Thus dreams symbolically communicate areas of intrapsychic conflict. The therapist then attempts to assist the patient to recognize his intrapsychic conflicts through the use of interpretation.

The patient is an active participant, feely revealing all thoughts exactly as they occur and describing all dreams. By termination of therapy, the patient is able to conduct his life according to an accurate assessment of external reality and is also able to relate to others uninhibited by neurotic conflicts.

ADVANTAGES OF PSYCHOANALYSIS

- Good method to study the human behavior.
- Child centered education was imported by identifying needs, instincts and wishes of children.
- By identification of earlier childhood experiences, childhood education was modified by giving a maximum freedom to the children for expression of their biological urges and minimum interference in the course of their natural growth and development.
- Identification of behavioral deviations became easier, thereby precautionary measures for preventing the problems related to maladjusted personalities.
- It promotes presentation of mental health and timely identification and treatment of the behavioral problems of individuals.
- It highlighted the importance of catharsis for relearing pent up emotions, repressed desires and wishes and also the importance of planning co-curricular activities, hobbies and freedom of expression for children in education and training.
- It also contributed to highlight the role of sex in one's life in terms of shaping the personality and determining the behavior.
- Sex education has been developed stages of psychosexual development, need for spontaneous expression of the sex instinct, changing the attitude of individuals towards sex as natural, essential, biological function.

ROLE OF THE PATIENT AND THE PSYCHOANALYST

The patient is to be an active participant, freely revealing all thoughts exactly as they occur and describing all dreams. The psychoanalyst is a shadow person; while patient is expected to reveal all his thoughts, feelings, the analyst reveals nothing personal.

APPLICATION TO NURSING

This theoretical perspective has helped mental health professionals to understand psychopathology and stress related behaviors. More importantly, this theory illustrates the importance of not taking human behavior at face value. That is, it helps the psychiatrist-mental health nurse to discern and explore the meaning behind human behavior.

ERIC ERIKSON'S PSYCHOSOCIAL THEORY

Trust vs Mistrust (Birth-18 months)

Major developmental task – to develop a basic trust in the mothering figure and be able to generalize it to others

Achievement – self confidence, optimism, faith in the gratification of needs 7 desires and hope for the future.

Nonachievement – emotional dissatisfaction with the self and others, suspiciousness, and difficulty with IPR.

Autonomy vs Shame/Doubt (18 months- 3 yr)

Major developmental task- to gain some self control and independence with in the environment

Achievement – sense of self-control and ability to delay gratification, a feeling of self-confidence in one's ability to perform.

Nonachievement – lack of self-confidence, a lack of pride in the ability to perform, a sense of controlled by other, and a range against the self.

Initiative vs Guilt (3-6 yr)

Major developmental task – to develop sense of purpose and the ability to initiate and direct one's own activities

Achievement – ability to exercise restraint and self-control of inappropriate social behaviors. Assertiveness and dependability increase, and the child enjoys learning and personal achievement. The conscience develops, thereby controlling the impulsive behavior of the id. Initiative is achieved when creativity is encouraged and performance is recognized and positively reinforced.

Nonachievement – feeling of inadequacy and a sense of defeat. Guilt is experienced to an excessive degree, even to the point of accepting liability in situations for which one is not responsible.

Industry vs Inferiority (6-12 yr)

Major developmental task – to achieve a sense of self confidence by learning, competing, performing successfully and receiving from significant others, peers and acquaintances.

Achievement – sense of satisfaction and pleasure in the interaction and involvement with others. The individual masters reliable work habits and develops attitudes of trustworthiness. Industry is achieved when encouragement is given to activities and responsibilities in school and community.

Nonachievement – difficulty in IPR owing to feeling of personal inadequacy. The individual can neither co-operates and compromises with others in group activities or problems solves or complete tasks successfully. Individual may manipulate or violate the rights of others to satisfy his or her own needs or desires.

Identity vs Role Confusion (12-20 yr)

Major developmental task – goal is to integrate the task mastered in the previous stages into a secure sense of self.

Achievement – sense of confidence, emotional stability and a view of the self as a unique individual. Commitments are made to a value system, to the choice for a career. Identity is achieved when adolescents are allowed to experience by making decisions that influences their lives.

Nonachievement – sense of self- consciousness, doubt and confusion about one's role in life.

Intimacy vs isolation (20-30 yr)

Major developmental task – to form an intense lasting relationship or commitment to another person, a cause, an institution and create effort

Achievement – capacity for mutual love and respect between 2 people and ability of an individual to pledge a total commitment to another. The intimacy goes for beyond the sexual contact between 2 people. It describes a commitment in which personal sacrifice are made for another, whether it be another person or if one chooses, a career or another type of cause or endeavor to which an individual elects to devote his or her life. Intimacy is achieved when an individual has developed the capacity for giving of oneself to another.

Nonachievement – withdrawal, social isolation and aloneness. The individual is unable to form lasting, intimate relationships often seeing intimacy through numerous superficial sexual contacts. No career established; he or she may have a history of occupational changes. The task remains unresolved when love in home has been deprived or distorted through the younger years.

Generativity vs Stagnation or Self Absorption (30-65 yr)

Major developmental task – to achieve the life goals established for oneself while also considering welfare of future generations.

Achievement – sense of gratification from personal and professional achievement and from meaningful contributions to others. The individuals is active in service it and to society.

Nonachievement – lack of concern for the welfare of others and total preoccupation with the self. He/she becomes withdrawn isolated and highly self indulgent, with no capacity for giving of the self to others. The task remains unresolved when earlier development tasks are not fulfilled.

Ego Integrity vs Despair (65 – death)

Major developmental task – during this stage, the goal is to review one's life and drive meaning from both positive and negative events, while achieving a positive sense of self at this stage in life.

Achievement – sense of self-worth and self acceptance as one reviews life goals, accepting the same were achieved and some were not. The individual drives a sense of dignity from his/her life experiences and does not fear death, rather viewing it as another stage of development.

Nonachievement – sense of self contempt and disgust with how life has progressed. The individual would like to start over and have a second chance at life. He/she feels worthless and helpless to change. Anger, depression and loneliness are evident. The focus may be on past failures or perceived failures.

2. INTERPERSONAL MODEL

1953, Harry Stack Sullivan is the originator of interpersonal relations theory. He argued that a personality can never be isolated from the complex of interpersonal relations in which the person lives. In his view, people's responses to interpersonal experiences cause them to develop personifications (mental representation of themselves and others)

Images of self fall into 3 categories:

(i) Good me personification
(ii) Bad me personification
(iii) Not me personification— contains aspects of self and maintains them in the unconscious.

He believed that, the personality continues to develop even after childhood. He identified seven stages of personality development.

1. Infancy
2. Childhood
3. Juvenile era
4. Preadolescence

5. Early adolescence
6. Late adolescence
7. Adulthood

Basic Assumptions

- Human beings are essentially social being.
- Hyman personality is determined in the context of social interactions with other human beings.
- Anxiety plays a central role in the formation of human personality by serving as a primary motivator of human behavior. Especially anxiety is important in building self-esteem and enabling a person to learn from their life experiences.
- Self esteem is an important facet of human personality that forms in reaction to the experience of anxiety. Interaction with significant others conveying disapproval or other such negative meanings contribute to self system formation.
- Security mechanisms are used to reduce or avoid the experience of anxiety. These security mechanisms include sublimation. Selective inattention and dissociation.
- Early life experiences with parents, especially the mother, influence an individual's experiences development throughout life.
- Human development proceeds through 7 stages of development— Infancy childhood, juvenile era, preadolescence, early adolescence, late adolescence, adulthood.

Basic Principles of Interpersonal Theory

a. Development proceeds through various stages, in each stage there is involvement of different patterns of relationship, e.g. in infancy- need for contact was fulfilled by the parents.
    - In child- active participation in activities and interaction with adults will be observed.
    - In preadolescent and adolescent- detachment from parents and attachment with peer group increases.
    - In early adulthood – intimate relationship with heterosexual groups resulting into marriage and family formation.

- If any failure to make progress satisfactory through various stages may result into maladaptive behavior.

b. Anxiety has direct relationship in the personality formation, e.g. for fulfillment of basic needs of an infant will depend on caregiver, lack of any of these needs will lead to develop mistrust or anxious or insecure and may prone for maladjustment.

c. Early life experiences (attachment with care takers to the infant especially mother) will influence individual's development throughout his life. This lasting effect produced by personifications, feelings, attitudes, ideas and forms as the result of experiences with anxiety and needs satisfaction with the mothering one.

d. Social exchange – social relationship is established to meet the mutual needs. Each person needs mutual help, recognition from others for self identification.

e. Social roles – every individual has to perform specific social role set by the society, e.g. teacher, mother, priest, etc.

f. Interpersonal accommodation – 2/more persons interact with each other and establish certain goals to build a satisfying relationship. It enables the nurse to understand clients' background, relationship with significant people, etc.

Interpersonal Therapeutic Process

The interpersonal therapist, like the psychoanalyst, explores the patient's life history. Components of self-esteem are to defined, including the security operations that are used to defend the self.

The process of therapy is essentially a process of re-education as the therapist helps the patient identify interpersonal problems and then encourages the patient to try out more successful styles of relating. Therapy is terminated when the patient has developed the ability to establish human relationships therapy meeting his basic needs.

Role of the Patient and the Interpersonal Therapist

Sullivan describes the therapist as a participant observer, who should not remain detached from the therapeutic situation. The

Effects of Interpersonal Therapeutic Approach

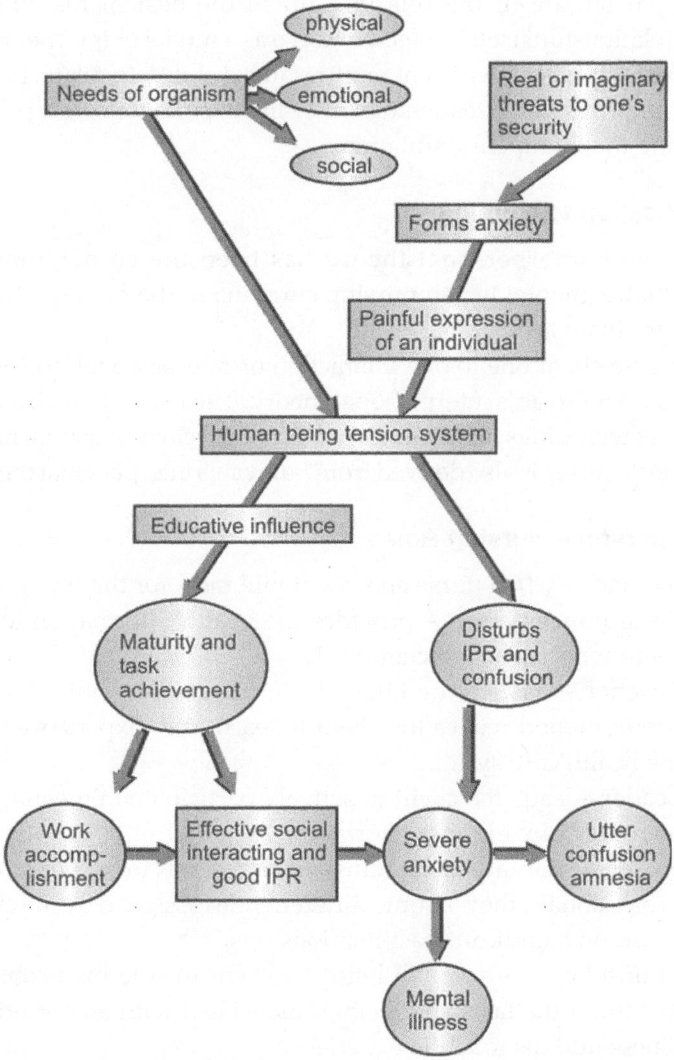

therapist's role is to actively engage the patient to establish trust and to empathize. He will create an atmosphere of uncritical acceptance to encourage the patient to speak openly.

The patient's role is to share his concerns with the therapist and participate in the relationship to the best of his ability. The relationship itself is meant to serve as a model of interpersonal relationships. As the patient matures in his ability to relate, he can then improve and broaden his other life experiences with people outside the therapeutic situation.

Application to Nursing

Sullivan's interpersonal theory has been the cornerstone of psychiatric mental health nursing curricula in the undergraduate and graduate levels.

Nurse-client one to one interaction or interpersonal process is based on Sullivan's interpersonal theory. The use of interpersonal process recordings in the clinical aspect of psychiatric mental heath nursing courses is also derived from Sullivan's interpersonal theory.

Interpersonal Nursing Roles

- Stranger – when nurse and client will meet for the first time.
- Reassurance person – provides the health information to the client who plays conscience role.
- Teacher – assists the client in learning about his disease condition and makes the client to learn from experience with the health care system.
- Leader – leads the client to actively participate in meeting his own needs by his own efforts.
- Surrogate parent – client transfers his feelings to the health care professionals; they assume different roles assigned by the client based on significant past relationships.
- Counselor – nurses will help the client to sole his problems integrates the facts and feelings associated with an episode of illness into his total life experience.
- The therapist – will assist the client to meet their needs and gains satisfaction and attained personal growth. Therapist will effectively perform their roles; self awareness is essential for practicing effectively in interpersonal model.

3. SOCIAL MODEL

Introduction

The social environment has influenced on the individual and his life experiences. Thomas Szasz (1961, 1993, and 2002) and Gerald Caplan (1964) believed that culture will have strong effect over the mental illness and prescribing therapy. Community movement in psychiatric nursing has been based on social factors and its significance. It is a response of the philosophy of the social theories.

Social View of Behavioral Deviation

- Social factors are responsible for deviant behavior.
- Deviance is culturally defined.

For example, a particular aspect of behavior which is normal to one society may be eccentric to other cultural setting or psychotic in another.

Thomas szasz (1961) in his "myth of mental illness" state that, people are responsible for their own behavior. He has the control over whether to confirm to the societal norm and social expectation. He apposed to describe, deviant behavior as 'illness', he believed that illness can occur in the body, which affects the behavior. He distinguished the biological condition, i.e. centered to illness and the social role i.e. focuses of deviancy. No physiological disruption can be demonstrated to cause most deviancies.

General Caplan (1964) has also studied deviant behavior from a social perspective. He has extended 'public health model' to the 'mental health field'. He focused specially on 'primary prevention', i.e. avoidance of the occurrence of specific diseases. Caplan believed that certain social situations.

For example, poverty, illiteracy, inadequate education, family instability, crises in life, social derivation, etc. will predisposes the individuals to expose for mental illness. Deprivation in any stage of the life cycle results in limited ability to cope with stress. The person who has inadequate or few environmental supports may predispose to maladaptive coping responses and exhibits pathological behavior.

If adequate strategies will be utilized by an individual with adequate situational social support crisis may be the root cause or an opportunity for growth.

Social Therapeutic Process

Thomas Szasz advocates, freedom has to be given to the psychiatric clients to select their own therapeutic modality and the therapist. The clients have to receive the knowledge on 'effective modes of psychotherapy'. Szasz disapproves the community mental health movement to place mental health care with in the reach of every citizen.

Gerald Caplan supports 'community psychiatry' and 'community mental health movement'. Health professionals have to act as 'consultants' to educate community on 'primary preventive measures'. These consultations have to help the general population (counselee centered case consultation approach). It improves interpersonal relationships. Consultation has to be focused on work situation. Its aim is to combat the societal problems. Positive social change will have effect on prevention of mental illness.

Role of Social Therapist

Thomas Szasz: he believe that,

- Therapist has to help the client, only if the patient requests help.
- Therapist has to promote positive change among the clients; it should not have any influence of coercion, e.g. The threat of hospitalization, if the client, not following therapist recommendation.
- Protect the client from social demands, which were against his will related to coercive treatment.
- Therapist has moral and ethical obligation towards the client.

Gerald Caplan: He insisted on,

- Moral approach to therapeutic services. Society has a moral obligation to provide a wide range of therapeutic services covering 3 levels on prevention.
- Professionals and nonprofessionals will have consultant skills (e.g. clergy, police, bar attenders, beauticians, etc.). This can be

trained to refer people who need professional help for appropriate resources.

- Therapist will be involved in community activities (like domiciliary visits conducting health education sessions to focus groups) to promote community involvement and understanding of individuals within community.

Role of the Client

Thomas Szasz view:

- Patient has to define the problem (which has to be solved)
- Client will have liberty to involve activity in the therapeutic process.
- He has to have satisfaction with the change, which he has to chose and give value in his life style.

Gerald Caplan's view:

- Client plays 'consumer role' and select the appropriate level of help from a wide assay of service (3 levels of preventive services); client can select and implement appropriate preventive measure, which will help him not to become a patient.

  For example, short-term psychotherapy and appropriate environment support in time of crisis situations.

4. EXISTENTIAL MODEL

Satre, Heikegaard are the philosophers of existential model. The theory focuses on person's present experience provide less attention to the person's past.

Existential View of Behavioral Deviation

Behavioral deviation will occur:

- If the individual is out of touch with him or his environment or when he poses self-imposed restrictions or inhibitors.
- When individual is not free to choose from among alternative behavior.
- When the individuals avoids socially acceptable and responsible behavior.

Manifestations of Behavioral Deviation

- Helplessness
- Sadness
- Lonely/aloof
- Self-criticism
- Lack of awareness
- Prevent participating in authentic and rewarding relationships with others (self approbation).
- Surrenders to the demand of others
- Psychiatric clients lost the values which gives meaning for the existence; the world is absurd, gives invalid demands.
- Lack of commitment
- Hazy identity
- Sense of unreality
- Will not accept the painful realities of life
- Altered sense of time, self absorption.

Existential Therapeutic Process

The therapeutic process assumes that the patient must be able to choose freely from what life has to offer. The therapeutic goal is to return the patient to an authentic awareness of his being. The existential therapeutic process focuses on the encounter. The client is helped to accept and understand his past, to live present and to look forward to the future.

Role of Existential Therapist

- Therapist acts as a guide, director and role model
- Provide warmth and caring, give values to the clients
- Helps the client to find his way from the alienation of madness to the areas where the client has to consider change
- Treats the client as an adult; inculcates hope and trust.

Role of Client

- Client is active in therapy
- Client must be open and honest; ready for change.
- Works toward the challenges kept by the therapist.

Therapies Based on Existential Model

- **Reality therapy:** William Glasser invoked this therapy; client is helped to identify the life goals and guide the ways to accomplish his goals. Certain needs are inculcated in client like feeling of loved, worth while, sense of responsible, capacity for about topics related to behavior. Therapist will help the client to orient towards present.
- **Psychosynthesis:** Reberto Assagioli explained 'self' is considered as 'inner center of awareness and peace'. Guided imaginary and meditation techniques will be used to achieve self awareness and control over the course of his life. Develop mental stages like pre-personal (do I exist), personal (if I exist, who am I), transpersonal (what is the meaning for my life) were explained.
- **Rational emotional therapy:**
  Cognitive oriented therapy: Albert Ellis identified this therapy. Confrontation forces the client to assume responsibility for his behavior. Client is encouraged to accept as he is to make risks and challenges, try out new behaviors or action oriented for both therapist and client.
- **Gestalt therapy:** Frederick S Paris emphasized it. Therapist will encourage the client to identify the feelings which will enhance self awareness, self acceptance. It makes the client to be sensitive for the other aspects of existence.
- **Logo therapy:** Future oriented therapy – Viktor E Frank explained the therapy, client is oriented towards spiritual meaning of his life (logos) - primary life force. Helps the client to become aware of his responsibleness; the client is guided to take control of his own life 7 determines meaning for him.
- **Encounter group therapy:** Williams C Schultz and Carl Rogers explained the establishment of intimate interactions in a group situation. The client is expected to assume responsibility to his behavior, feelings in stress. Group exercises are practices. Group members are encouraged to exchange their thoughts and feelings.

5. COMMUNICATION MODEL

Introduction

The theorists Eric Eerne, Paul Walzlawick and his associates emphasized the importance of communication; they studied the pragmatics of human communication. Communication system is one of the characteristics that distinguish human beings from lower orders of animal life.

The word communication comes from the Latin word '*communicare*' which means ' to share, to impart and to partake'.

Definition

A two-way process by which information is exchanged between individuals through a common system of symbols, sins or behavior

— Webster's New Collegiate Dictionary.

Meaning

Communication refers to the reciprocal exchange of information, i.e. the transmission and sharing of ideas, opinions, beliefs, facts and attitudes between persons or groups and families.

It is goal directed process in which people use verbal or nonverbal means, i.e. system of symbols, gestures, and signs to convey a message.

Communication Process

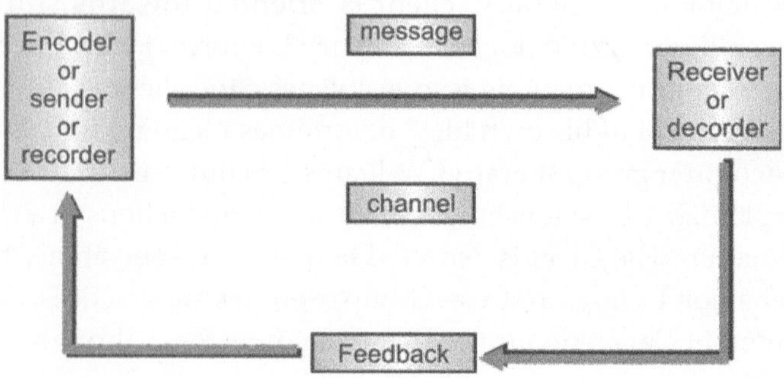

Basic Assumptions

- The understanding of the meaning of behavior is based on the clearity of communication between the sender and receiver.
- Breakdown in successful transmission of information causes anxiety and frustration.
- All behavior is communication, whether verbal or non-verbal.
- Disruptions in behavior may then be viewed as a disturbance in the communication process, and as an attempt to communicate.

Communication View of Behavioral Deviations

Deviant behavior may be viewed as an attempt to communicate, the message may be masked or distorted the route may be indirect, but the end result of behavior is still the transmission of a message to others who are able to perceive it.

Eric Berne (the Founder of Transactional Analysis)

People communicate in any one of the 3 ego states — parent, adult, and child. These terms do not refer to the actual status in life, but to the concept that the person acts like parent, adult or child.

A communication unit refers to as a 'transaction'. Complementary transactions occur when the message sent from one ego state to another is responded to as expected, the ego state, e.g. 'bring me a cup of coffee, please'— parent; 'get it yourself, I am busy' – child.

Types of transaction results in communication block — the 4 most common crossed communications are the following;

- Adult to adult – child to parent (transaction)
- Adult to adult – parent to child (counter transference)
- Child to parent – adult to adult (exasperating)
- Parent to child – adult to adult (impudent).

Watzlawick and Other Communication Pragmatists

They explained deviant behavior is based on disrupted communication patterns;

(i) The 1st is an effort not to communicate which in self defeating because it is impossible.

(ii) The 2nd disrupted communication pattern is a lack of cognitive levels of communication, when a person makes a statement about himself, the other may confirm, reject or discomfort it. Human relationships are the symmetrical (equality) or complimentary (difference).

Communication Therapeutic Process

The therapist will locate the disruption in behavior with in the communication process; interventions are made in patterns of communication. The communication pattern may take place in individuals, groups or families. The communication pattern is 1st assessed and the disruption diagnosed. The patient is then helped to recognize his own disrupted communication.

Therapies/Techniques Based on Communication Model

- **Transactional analysis:** It helps the client to recognize their ego states in them and others and to identify the crossed transactions. The emphasis is on authenticity and responsibility for the self. The client will work to discover his script, once identified; the script can be modified to meet the person's adult needs and to facilitate healthy relationship.
- **Neurolinguistic programming:** It focuses on the sensory channel (visual, auditory and kinesthetic) through which people receive information. Each person develops a preference for their own communication. For example, I can see, that you are depressed (visual); can you tell what is upsetting you, 'I would like to listen' (auditory); 'you feel upset right now' (kinesthetic). It plays an important attention to both words and nonverbal communication.

Mirroring techniques – helps the client to increase the other person's comfort level, e.g. body gestures, respiratory rate, speech pattern, etc.

Milter Erickson, hypnotherapist believed that people will have the resources, they need to manage their lives, but for various reasons do not have access to their internal resources. Hypothesis helps the people to identify and make use of their strengths. Activities carried out that would help them to learn new behavior pattern. The therapist along with neurolinguistic programming uses additional techniques such as the usage of metaphor, story telling and hypothesis.

- **Therapeutic double blind technique:** This technique was developed by Paul Walzawick. According to this theory, there are 2 ways to induce change in therapy.

i. To tell the person to change, which he probably would have done, if he was able to do so.

ii. Tell him not to change.

It enhances his awareness of his behavior, increases tension and may stimulate him to change. Any behavior is expected to result in a change.

Role of Communication Therapist

- Communication therapist induces change in the client by intervening the communication process.
- Feedback is given to the client on his success in communicating.
- Effective communication will be reinforced.
- For ineffective communication the alternatives can be discussed.
- Therapist also demonstrates how to relate to others clearly.
- Non verbal communication also emphasized in harmony with verbal behavior.
- Therapist will teach the principles, types and importance of effective communication.

Role of the Patient

- The willingness of the client is essential for the analysis of his style of communicating and to accept the change.
- Significant others support, i.e. situational support is also need to bring change in communication pattern of the client.
- Client has to participate actively in identifying the ego states, games and sports.

- Change in communication system of one individual will have influence over the other. It acts as a stimulant; change in over lasting, if it takes place at the system level.

Application to Nursing

This theory helps mental health nurses to understand the communication process and to correct communication disturbances.

6. BEHAVIORAL MODEL

Introduction

It is derived from 'learning theories' focused on client's actions, not on thoughts and feelings. Behavioral approach is used frequently to control the undesirable behavior. Prominent therapists of behavioral theory/model/therapy include HJ Eysenck Joseph Wolpe, BF Skinner, Ivan Pavlov and John Watson.

Basic Assumptions

- Behavior is a response to a stimulus from the environment.
- Either adaptive or maladaptive behavior is learnt.
- Change in behavior leads to change in the cognitive and affective spheres.
- Therapists will emphases on qualitative aspect of observable behavior.
- Deviations from the norm are habitual responses that can be modified through application of learning theory.
- Positive responses are reinforced. The response is strengthened by repetition of the learning sequence. Reinforcement is essential to get the response. Positive response is reward for selected behavior.
- Human beings are passive organisms that can be shaped or conditioned to do anything, if correct responses are rewarded or reinforced.
- Maladaptive behavior can be unlearnt and replaced with adaptive behavior, if the person receives an appropriate stimulus to eliminate the maladaptive learning.

Techniques of Behavioral Theory

- Systemic desensitization
- Operant conditioning procedures for increasing adaptive behavior:
  a. Positive reinforcement
  b. Token economy
- Operant conditioning procedures to teach new behavior:
  a. Modeling
  b. Shaping
  c. Chaining
  d. prompting
- Operant conditioning procedures for decreasing maladaptive behavior:
  a. Time out
  b. Response cost
  c. Punishment
  d. Ignoring/extinction
  e. Restitution
- Assertiveness training and social skills training
- Aversion therapy
- Flooding
- Reciprocal inhibition

Role of Patient and the Behavioral Therapist

The approach is that of a teacher and a learner. Therapy considered to be complete when the symptoms subside.

Therapist

- The therapist is an expert in behavior therapy who helps the patient unlearn his symptoms and replace them with more satisfying behavior.
- The therapist uses the patient's anxiety as a motivational force towards learning.
- The therapist teaches the patient about behavioral approaches and helps him develop behavioral hierarchy.
- The therapist reinforces desired behaviors.

Patient

- As a learner the patient is an active participant in the therapy process.
- Patient practices behavioral techniques.
- Does homework and reinforcement exercises.

Application to Nursing

Nurses commonly use behavioral techniques in a wide variety of mental health settings. Additionally, nurses who work with clients having physical disability, chronic pain, chemical dependency and rehabilitation centers also apply these techniques.

Role of the Nurse

- Nurses have to keep in mind, the principles of learning while administering behavioral therapy for the clients.
- Use behavioral approaches like positive reinforcement, relaxation techniques.
- Involves the client and significant people in provision of care.
- Positive responses will be reinforced.

7. MEDICAL MODEL

Introduction

Medical model dominates much of modern psychiatric care. Physicians are viewed as the leaders of the team when this model is in effect. It focuses on the diagnosis of a mental illness 7 further treatment is based on confirmed diagnosis. The interpersonal aspect of the medical model varies widely from intensive insight oriented intervention to brief, superficial medication supervision session.

Other health care professionals may be involved in family assessment, referral system, therapeutic and rehabilitative modalities. Somatic treatments, pharmacotherapy, electroconvulsive therapy and psychosurgery are major components of therapeutic process.

In medical model, cautious exploration of situation based on scientific process will be used to identify the causes of mental illness.

Elements of other models of care may be used in conjunction with the medical model.

Meaning

Medical model refers to modern psychiatric care which is based on traditional physician – patient relationship.

Basic Assumptions

- Medical model believes that deviant behavior is a manifestation of a disorder of the central nervous system.
- It suspects that psychiatric disorders involve an abnormality in the transmission of neural impulses, difficulty at the synaptic level and neurochemicals such as dopamine, serotonin and norepinephrine.
- It focuses on the diagnosis of a mental illness and subsequent treatment based on this diagnosis.
- Environmental and social factors are also considered in the Medical model. They may be either predisposing or precipitating factors in an episode of illness.
- Another branch of research focuses on stressors and the human have a physiological stress threshold that may be genetically determined.

Medical Therapeutic Process

- To explore the causes of mental illness, the physician collects the total history of the client either from the client (if he is able to give) or significant others and through the review of medical records (secondary sources).
- Physical examination, mental status examination, diagnosis studies and observation of the behavior of the client will be carried out to formulate preliminary diagnosis.

Treatment is initiated once diagnosis is made. Somatic treatments including pharmacotherapy, pharmacotherapy, electroconvulsive therapy and occasionally psycho surgery are major components of therapeutic process.

- Physician establishes therapeutic nurse – client relationship to foster trust and compliance with treatment plan.
- Therapist will take the help of other health care professionals for implementing therapeutic plan.
- Therapist will encourage the client to utilize coping mechanisms to overcome stress.
- Response to treatment can be evaluated on the basis of objective observations of systematic behavior and the subjective assessment.
- When the client will achieve satisfactory functional level therapy will be terminated.

Role of the Therapist

- The therapist will acts as leader of health care team, he will be viewed as healer, identifies the cause for mental illness by significant scientific methods.
- Physician initiates therapeutic plan, guides the team members in implementing therapeutic activities.
- Encourages and councils the client in best utilization of client's defense mechanism to overcome stress

Role of the Client

- Client will accept his illness and come forward to obtain the treatment.
- Clients are not encouraged to question the therapists' decision; he will try to follow the therapist instructions to fight against mental illness.
- When observable satisfactory improvement occurs in client's condition therapy will be terminated.

Application to Nursing

- Psychiatric mental health nurse uses medical model for assessment, diagnosis, planning, implementing and evaluating nursing care to the patient.

- This model helps psychiatric mental health nurse to understand the physiological changes occurring due to psychiatric disorders.

8. NURSING MODEL

Introduction

In nursing model, human behavior is viewed in holistic perspective. Nursing care focuses in the meeting the total needs of individual in response to actual or potential health problems. Nursing model concentrates its attention to meet the biological, psychological and sociocultural needs of clients. Nurses establish a therapeutic nurse-client relationship and they will represent the client's needs to health team members and significant others.

The prominent nursing theorists who have developed models for nursing care delivery includes Hildegard Peplau (1952), sister Callista Roy (1979), Martha Rogers (1970), Ida Jean Orlando, Nightingale (1860), Henderson (1955), Abdellah (1960), Dorothea Elizebeth Orem (1971), king (1971), Newman (1972), Leininger (1978), Watson (1979), Brenner and Wrubel (1989).

Nursing View of Behavioral Deviations

- Behavior is viewed on a continuum from healthy adaptive responses to maladaptive responses that indicate illness.
- Each individual is predisposed to respond to life events in unique ways. These predispositions are biological, psychological, sociocultural, and the sum of the person's heritage and post-experiences.
- Behavior is the result of combining the predisposing factors with precipitating stressors. Stressors are life events that the individual perceives as challenging, threatening or demanding. The nature of the Behavioral response depends on the person's primary appraisal of the stressor and his secondary appraisal of the coping resources available to him.

- A stressor that has primary impact on physiological functioning also affects the person's psychological and sociocultural behavior. For instance, a man who had a myocardial infarction may also become severely depressed, because he fears he will lose his ability to work.
- On the other hand, the patient who enters the psychiatric inpatient unit with major depression nay be suffering from malnutrition and dehydration because of his refusal to eat or drink.

The holistic nature of nursing encompasses all of these facets of behavior and incorporates them into patient care planning.

Hildegard Peplau's Nursing Theory

Peplau's, 'mother of psychiatric nursing' formulated 'interpersonal theory' in 1999, which is applicable for nursing practice in general and psychiatric mental health nursing. It focuses primarily on the nurse-client relationship. Peplau theory describes explains, predicts 7 to some extent, permits central of the sequence of events occurring in the nurse-client relationship.

Process of Peplau's Theory

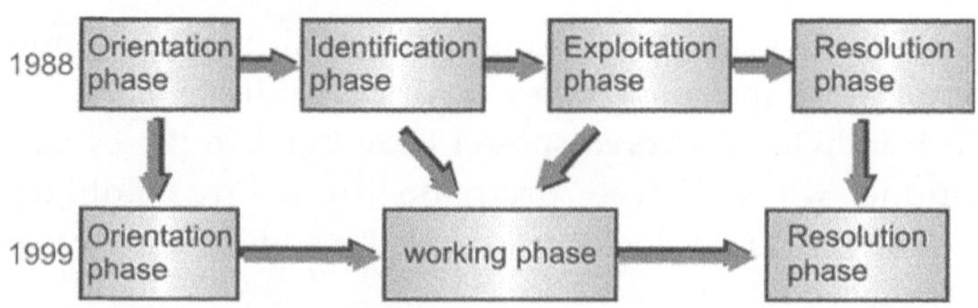

It consists of 4 phases:

i. Orientation phase
ii. Identification phase
iii. Exploitation phase
iv. Resolution or termination phase.

i. **Orientation phase:** The nurse and the client will meet as strangers and they assume the role stranger as they do not know each other. Nurse and the client will exchange social amenities and then proceed to clarity each other's roles.

ii. **Identification phase:** Nurse will encourages the client to express their feelings and tries to correct misconceptions of client, nurse will formulate nursing diagnosis based on previous life and health care experience. They learn each others as unique persons, as a result client experiences acceptance and develops high degree of trust in nurse and other health care professionals.

iii. **Exploitation phase:** The nurse will try to understand the importance of nurse–client relationship and begins to test alternative ways of coping methods when health problems arises and formulates goals for the future; client learns the problem solving techniques.

The nurse assumes the role of resource expert and teacher as they provide guidance and teach the client alternative ways of coping techniques in meeting client's need and assist the clients in utilization of problem solving techniques.

In 1977, Peplau combined identification phases and exploitation phase formulated 'working phase', where the client starts to respond to those selectively who can meet the felt needs, gains self control takes measures to become independent. Nurse will maintain therapeutic nurse-client relationship in a no-judgemental manner.

iv. **Resolution or termination phase:** The nurse assumes the role of leader and surrogate parent to ensure the client's needs addressed and guide the client in problem solving techniques. Nurses will act as counselor. The client will regress during illness and having dependency needs associated with earlier developmental stags; nurses will act as parents and counsels.

Termination phase starts from the orientation phase itself. in this phase, the relationship terminates and client experiences this phase as a freeing process in which the client's felt needs are met and attains personal maturity and nurse experiences professional fulfillment.

Role of Nurse

- Resource person
- Technical expert
- Teacher
- Leader
- Surrogate parent
- Counselor

Peplau's theory continues to apply to today's nursing scene, especially with respect to long-term psychiatric care in outpatient and home health settings.

Orems Theory

Dorothea Elizebeth Orem is a pioneer in developing her nursing theory in 1950. self care deficit theory is based on capacities of the client and required nursing care behavior or the activities. This theory is considered as an 'inductive theory' and also classified as 'behavioral model nursing theory'.

Orem's theory is a three part theory of self care, the three theories that make up the general theory are:

- Self care
- Self care deficit
- Nursing systems.

Self care theory – states that adults deliberately learn and perform actions to direct their survival, quality of the life and wellbeing.

Self care deficit theory – nursing is required because of inability to perform self care as the result of limitations.

Nursing system theory – is the product of nursing in nursing systems by which nurses use the nursing process to help the individual to meet their self care requisites and build their self care or dependent care capacities.

The three theories form the overall self care deficit theory.

Types of Self Care

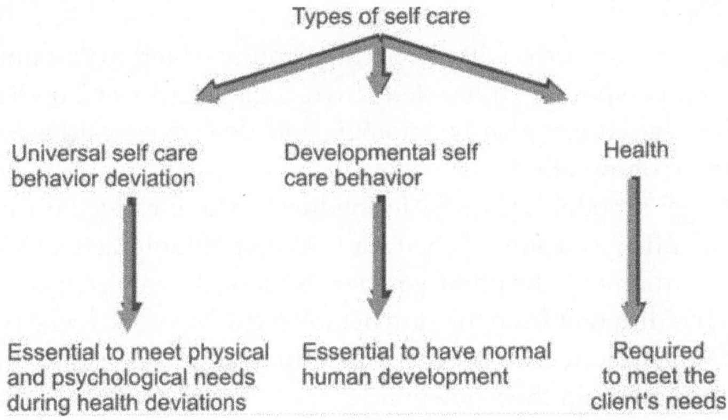

Components of Nursing Process

a. **Assessment** – focuses on the client's self care demand, self care agency, and self care deficit.
b. **Nursing diagnosis** – derived from analysis of assessment information.
c. **Plan** – based on the information obtained in the assessment.
d. **Nursing implementation** – implementation done by using nursing approach. Nursing approach is needed to meet the client's needs can be categorized as:
   i. Wholly compensatory — in which the client does not participate behaviorally in self care.
   ii. Partially compensatory — in which the client and nurse participate behaviorally in meeting the clients' self care needs.
   iii. Educative- developmental — in which the client meets self-care needs with minimal nursing assistance.

To implement the required nursing approach, the nurse uses one of 5 behaviors

i. acting or doing for the client
ii. guiding
iii. supporting
iv. providing
v. Teaching.

SYSTEM ORIENTED THEORY (MARTHA ROGER)

Introduction

This theory concerns with the nature of human kind from a unique nursing perspective. It has deductive, logical forms of 2 bodies of knowledge. It can also be anologic and detective as it based on minimal observation.

Roger's model focuses the individual as a 'unified whole' cannot be identified as a sum of their parts in consent interaction within the environment, the unitary person is viewed as an 'energy field' which is different from the sum of biological, physical, social parts. Nursing practice helps the individual to achieve maximum wellbeing within their potential.

Premises of Roger's Theory

- Human being is characterized by openness and having continuous mutual interaction with the environment.
- Human organism is having energy field which is having constant mutual interaction with the energy fields of the environment are in a constant exchange of energy and matter and with other human organisms. This dynamic mutual interaction can be perceived as 'wave patterns or auras'.
- Energy fields are characterized by organized patterns or designs.
- Human existence is the human beings capacity to transcend conventional concepts of time space interaction.

Principles

- Human life proceeds in one direction along a spiral like course. Human organisms are open systems with energy fields having mutual interaction with the energy fields of environment along a unidirectional spiral through time and space known as, 'complimentarity' which permits occurrence of 'paranormal phenomena'.
- To reduce interference and restore order and complimentarity, the person has the capacity to transcend time and space.

- Humans are capable of imagery, thought, abstraction, language, sensation and emotions.

Goals of Nursing

- To maintain and promote the maximal health potential of clients.
- To prevent disease.
- To formulate nursing diagnosis.
- To provide rehabilitative nursing care.

Strengths of Roger's Theory

- The theory is holistic and considers the entire field of phenomena associated with nursing practice. It addresses the total environmental aspects like psychological, social, physiological and physical realms of human existence and related them to nursing.
- The theory addresses the spirituality of human existence by explaining universe and the occurrence of paranormal experiences.
- Focused on the nature of human evolution.
- The theory has the potential to contribute the psychiatric mental health nursing's understanding of family, group and community systems.
- Broadens the mind and imagination of nurses in the field of nursing by developing field of nursing research.

Weaknesses

Its terminology is overly complex. The absence or weakness of logical bridges or transitions between the conceptual components confuses the theory's content.

ADAPTATION MODEL/ROY'S THEORY

Introduction

Callista Roy used Harry Helson's theory of learning and adaptation to organize nursing concepts in a logical pattern. Roy's work can be typed as, 'analogic theory' as it is widely used in all nursing fields like nursing research, nursing clinical practice 7 nursing education 7 professional trends which are interconnected.

It is also classified as 'behavioral theory'. Roy presents her work as a model rather than a theory as it describes the practice and generates testable hypothesis. It resents comprehensive view of the overall nursing processes. It is least useful in psychiatric nursing.

Goals of Nursing

To promote the clients adaptation in health and illness nurses will keep constant efforts to change, manipulate or block the stress producing stimuli which will affect the client. Nurse will assist the client to cope more effectively by reducing stressful stimuli.

Assumptions

- Adaptation is an ongoing process occurring within the living systems. The purpose of adaptation process is for 'survival, growth and reproduction' and mastery and gaining higher levels of adaptation.
- Roy's theory assumes that all human beings are adaptive systems can respond to changing stimuli.
- If the change is positive, which promotes the person's integrity brings adaptive changes.
- If the change does not promote the person's integrity and hinders to fulfill goals, then it is considered as maladaptive.
- Two coping mechanisms for adaptation are used:
  - Regulator mechanism pertains to physiologic needs and processes, e.g. chemical, neural and endocrine responses
  - Cognitive mechanism — are related to higher brain functioning such as social, perceptual, information processing, judgment, emotions functions.

Nursing Process

It involves two levels of assessment of behavior,

1. Observation of behaviors related to four adaptive modes which will be used by the client to adapt

   i. Physiological mode, e.g. oxygenation, nutrition, elimination, rest and activity, fluid electrolyte and acid balance; sensory perception, neurological and endocrine function.
   ii. Self concept mode, e.g. spiritual and psychological aspects of the person
   iii. Role function mode, behavior expected of a person in interaction with another.
   iv. Interdependence mode, e.g. interpersonal relationships with both individual and in groups; love and belonging and affection need.
2. Identification of stimuli:-
   i. Focal stimuli – the immediate dominant stimuli affecting the client, e.g. injury, specific illness, stressors.
   ii. Contextual stimuli – includes environment, e.g. the client's family and other background factors related to focal stimuli.
   iii. Residual stimuli – e.g. client's previous background, beliefs, attitudes, and tracts related to focal and contextual stimuli.
3. Formulation of nursing diagnosis and goal setting:
   - Stating the diagnosis by listing the observed behavior along with influencing stimuli.
   - The adaptive responses or the behaviors that are being sought.
   - Goal setting- based on promoting adaptive responses.
4. Nursing intervention
5. Evaluation

Strengths

- Clear language
- Uses standard form of the nursing process
- Focuses concretely on observable behaviors exhibited by the client indicating need for nursing intervention.
- Nursing behavior is described in precise and a concrete-term focuses on observable behavior increases the potential for individualized client.

Weakness

- Four adaptive modes are overlapping in meaning and function; hence these modes need to be operationally defined to reduce overlap and redundancy.
- Subjective evaluation to determine whether it is adaptive or maladaptive.
- Adaptation conveys a variety of meanings.

System Model (Newman, 1995)

The Newman systems model is a unique system based perspective that provides a unifying focus for approaching a wide range of nursing concerns. It is a comprehensive guide for nursing practice, nursing research, nursing education and nursing administration. This model is based on concepts related to stress and reaction to stress within environment, hence this theory is applicable to psychiatric setting. The stressors from within or outside the system seek to disrupt system balance or stability. System reactions may be positive or negative.

Concepts Related to System

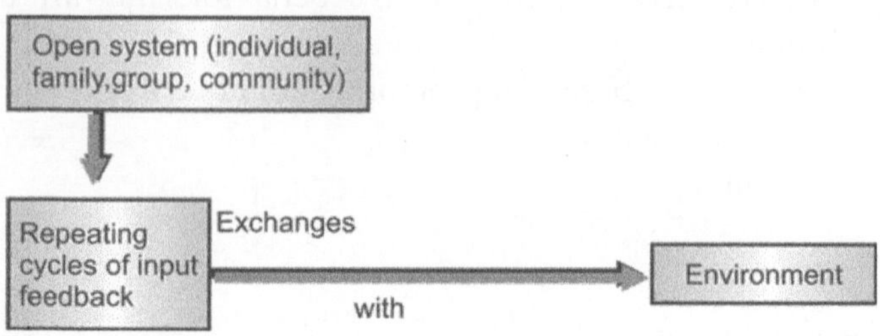

Types of Variables

Newman explained five types of variables

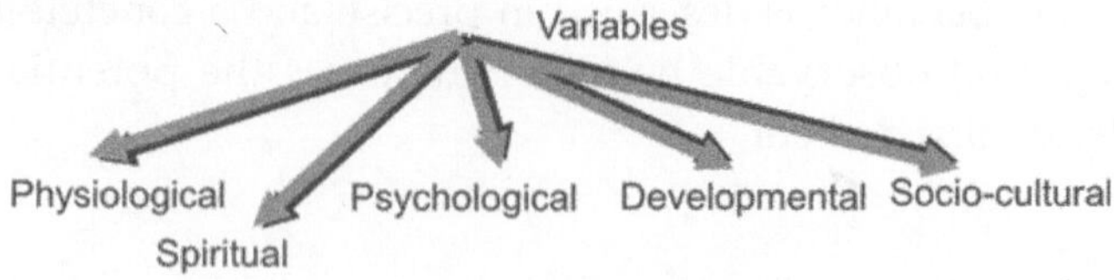

Physiological variables – deals with the body, its structure and its functions.

Psychological variables – mental relationships and process.

Developmental variables – developmental process which need for the system matures.

Socio-cultural variables – function of the system which involves social and cultural interactions and expectations.

Spiritual variables – system's spiritual beliefs and their influence.

Production of System

The core system represents basic survival factors. The system core is surrounded by lines of resistance to protect the system functions. The line of resistance activated when the stressors involve the normal line of defense. Resistance will protect the system and allow for reconstruction or return to system stability.

The next layer of protection is the normal line of defense. It represents the system's usual level of wellness or dynamic stability. When stressors invade the defense system reacts in the form of illness.

The outer boundary of protection if the flexible line of defense; stressor encounter initial line of protection; flexible line protects normal line of defense, the greater the protection available to the system.

Stressors

Stressors are stimuli places demand on a system creates tension and instability at any time. System may be affected with one or other stressor.

- Intrapersonal – with in the system boundary
- Interpersonal – from outside the system boundary but proximal to the system
- Extrapersonal – greater distance outside the system boundary

Environment

Newman explained three types of environment:

i. Internal environment – forces and factors influences that occur inside the system.
ii. External environment – pressurizes outside the system.
iii. Created environment - symbolizes system wholeness exemplifies the exchange between the internal and external represents the unconscious mobilization of all system variables (sociocultural and psychological).

Preventive Measures

Newman described the interventions to maintain the stability of system through preventive measures.

- Primary preventive measures — preventive measures results before stressors invade the normal line of defense. By strengthening the flexible line of defense through preventing or reducing the risk factors.
- Secondary preventive measures — occurs after the system reacted to the invasion of a stressor; these preventive measures will strengthen the internal lines of resistance to protect the system care, energy and basic energy.

6 Therapeutic Communication and Therapeutic Relationship

INTRODUCTION

Nurse patient relationship is significant in psychiatric nursing too.

The objective of psychiatric nursing is – the promotion for mental health, prevention of mental illness and care and rehabilitation of the patient with mental illness.

TYPES OF RELATIONSHIP

The types of relationship can be social and therapeutic or professional.

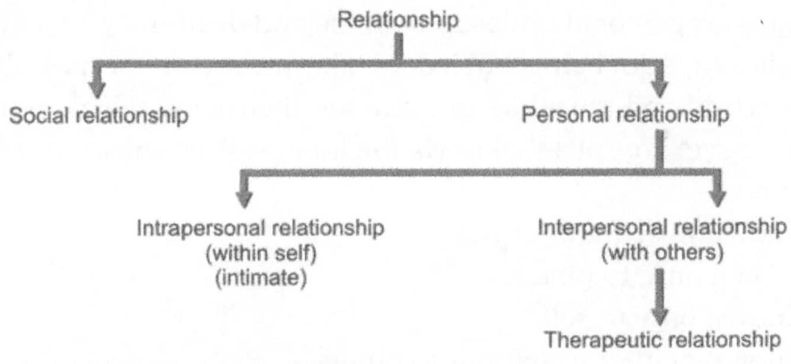

PERSONAL QUALITIES OF THE NURSE

The key therapeutic tool the psychiatric nurse uses is oneself. Thus self analysis is the first building block in providing quality nursing care.

Awareness of the self: Effective helpers must be able to answer the question, who am I? Self awareness is a key part of the psychiatric nursing experiences. The nurse's goal is to achieve authentic, open and personal communication. The nurse must be able to examine the personal feelings, actions and reactions. This also has been described as emotional competence. A good understanding and acceptance of the self allow the nurse to acknowledge a patients differences and uniqueness.

Campbell has identified a holistic model of self awareness that consists of **four** interconnected components: psychological, physical, environmental and philosophical.

The psychological components include knowledge of emotions, motivations, self concept and personality. Being psychologically self aware means being sensitive to the feelings and outside events that affect those feelings.

The physical component is the knowledge of personal and general physiology, as well as of the bodily sensations, body image and physical potential.

The environment component consists of the sociocultural environment, relationships with others and the knowledge of the relationship between humans and nature.

The philosophical component is the sense of life having meaning. A personal philosophy of life and death may or may not include a superior being, but it does take into account responsibility to the world and the ethics of behavior. Increasing self awareness: - no one ever completely knows the inner self, as shown in **Johari window**.

1. Known to self and others
2. known only to others
3. Known only to self
4. Known neither to self nor to others.

Johari window

Known self Known others	Unknown self Known others
known self unknown others	Unknown self Unknown others

Quadrant 1 is the open quadrant: it includes the behaviors, feelings and thought known to the individual and others. Quadrant 2 is called as the blind quadrant because it includes all things that others know but the individual does not know. Quadrant 3 is the hidden quadrant; it includes the things about the self that only the individual knows. Quadrant 4 is the unknown quadrant, containing aspects of the self that are known to the individual and others. Taken together, these quadrants represent the total self.

The goal of self awareness is to increase the area of quadrant 1 while reducing the size of the other three quadrants. To increase self knowledge, it is necessary to listen to the self. This means the individual allows the genuine emotions to be experienced; identifies and accepts personal needs and move the body in free, joyful and spontaneous ways. It includes exploring personal thoughts, feelings, memories and impulses. The next step in the process is to reduce the size of the quadrant 2 by listening to and learning from others. The final step involves reducing the size of the quadrant 3 by self disclosing or relieving to others important aspect of the self.

Compare A and B. A represents a person with little self awareness whose behaviors and feelings are limited. B, however, shows an individual with great openness to the world. B represents an individual who has an increased capacity for experiences of all kinds: joy, hate, work and love. This person also has few defenses and can interact with people spontaneously and honesty with others.

Clarification of Values

Awareness helps the nurse to be honest and avoid the unethical use of patients to meet the personal needs.

Value systems: - Values are concepts that are formed as result of life experience with family, friends, culture, education, work and relaxation. Value systems provide the framework for many daily decisions and actions. By being aware of value systems, nurses can identify situations in which value systems are in conflict. Many therapeutic relationships test the nurse's values, e.g. a patient may describe a sexual behavior that the nurse finds unacceptable; a patient may talk about the divorce where as the nurse may strongly believe that marriage contracts should not be broken; or a patient may be a born again Christian but the nurse may not believe in God or religion.

Value clarification Process: It allows the individual to discover their values by assessing, exploring and determining what those values are and what priority they hold in decision making process. Seven criteria are used to determine the value. These criteria should be considered in relation to a person's strongest value and tested against the persons own definition of a value.

The three criteria of choosing relay on the person's cognitive abilities, the two criteria of prizing emphasize the emotional or affective level, and the two criteria of acting have a behavioral focus.

The Mature Valuing Process

It is complex. There is no guarantee that the choice made will prove to be self-actualizing. The valuing process in the mature person has the following characteristics:

- It is fluid and flexible
- the valuing experience is tied to a particular time and experience.
- Personal experience provides the value information.

Exploration of feelings: The nurses should be open to, aware of and in control of their feelings so that they can be used to help the patient. The feelings that the nurse have serve an important purpose. In helping others, nurses have many feelings; elation at seeing a patient improves: disappointment when a patient regresses, distress when a patient refuses the help, anger when a patient is demanding or manipulative and power when a patient express strong dependence on the nurse.

Serving as a role model: A nurse has an obligation to model maladaptive and growth producing behavior. If a nurse has a chaotic personal life, it will show in the nurse's work with patients, decreasing the effectiveness of care. The effective nurse has a fulfilling and satisfying personal life that is not dominated by conflict, distress, or denial and that the nurses approach to life conveys a sense of growing, hopefulness, and adapting.

Altruism: Altruism is concern for the welfare of others. It does not mean that an altruistic person should not expect adequate compensation and recognition or must practice denial or self sacrifice. A sense of altruism also can apply to changing social conditions to meet human welfare needs. One goal of all helping professional should be to create a people –serving and growth facilitating society. So the necessary goal of nurse is to work to change the larger structure and process of society in ways that will promote the individuals health and well-being.

Ethics and responsibility: Nurse's sense of ethics is the need to assume responsibility for behavior. This involves knowing limitations and strengths and being accountable for them. As a member of health team nurse has ready access to the knowledge and expertise of other people; these resources should be used appropriately.

Details about Social and Therapeutic Relationship

	Therapeutic Relationship	*Social Relationship*
Technique	It is a planned therapeutic relationship	It just happens with mutual interests
Objective	Helping the patient	Having fun together satisfying needs of each other
Interaction time	Interactions are planned for specific time and place	It may be planned, unplanned and by chance 2 people met.
Duration	The length of relationship will depend on the goals. Time is limited	This varies and may last for years
Accountability	The nurse focus on goals during her relationship	It is shared, both are responsible
Acceptance	The nurse accepts the patient as "here and now" without any prejudgement	Acceptance of relationship based on shared values and beliefs

Termination	It is planned and discussed with the patient	Relationship may exist life long/may terminate gradually

THERAPEUTIC COMMUNICATION

Introduction

Communication refers to the reciprocal exchange of information, ideas, belief, feelings and attitudes between persons. Communication is very significant in nursing.

Definition

1. Communication is a process by which information is exchanged between individuals through a common system of symbols, signs or behaviour.

— Webster's New Collegiate Dictionary.

"The nurse directs the communication towards the patient to identify his current health problems, plans, implements and evaluates the action taken".

— Bimla Kapoor, 2002.

"Promotes mutual understanding, establishes constructive relationship between the nurse and the client'.

— Kozier, 2004.

"It is a process, in which the nurse utilizes a planned approach to learn about the client".

— Potter A, 1997.

Therapeutic communication is an interpersonal interaction between the nurse and client during which the nurse focuses on the client's specific needs to promote an effective exchange of information.

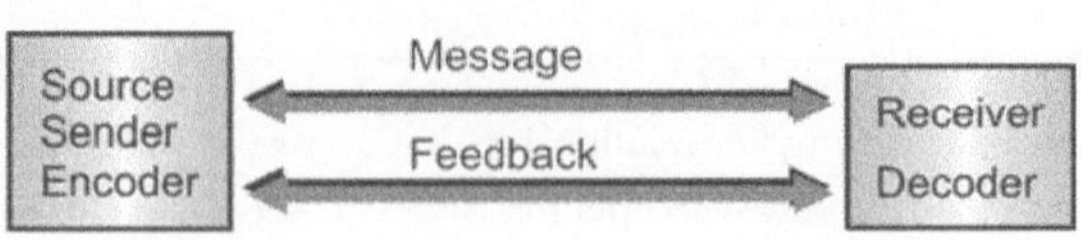

Purposes/Goals/Functions

- To achieve self realization, self acceptance, self respect, personal identity, personal integration.
- To formulate good interpersonal therapeutic relationship.
- To satisfy needs and to achieve realistic personal goals.
- Permits the client to express their thoughts truly, openly.
- Aids in clarification of internal conflicts and frustrations of the client.
- Improves client ego strengths.
- Encourages socialization and family interaction process.
- Treats communication problems.
- Modifies maladaptive behavior into adaptive behavior.
- motivates the client to utilize new coping strategies
- helps the nurses to identify and intervene appropriate nursing approaches
- Assess the client to develop self control and utilizes problem solving skills in attacking the problems.
- Implement nursing process effectively.

Importance of Thereapuetic Communication

The importance of therapeutic communication is that it allows the patient to express thoughts, concerns and emotions in a safe non-threatening environment.

Modes/Types of Communication

People communicate in various ways. Written communication is a means to document and convey information to the others. The writer selects and organizes words in way that is eligible and comprehensible to the reader. This is an important component in nursing practice because documentation in client's records informs treatment and care.

Verbal Communication

It involves the spoken word. It is an exchange using the elements of language. Taken alone verbal communication can convey the factual information accurately and efficiently. It is less effective means of communicating feelings or nuances of meaning, and it represents only a small part of total human communication. Another limitation of verbal communication is that the words can change meaning with different cultural groups or subgroups because words have both denotative (actual) and connotative (suggested) meaning. The effective psychiatric nurse uses verbal communication sensitively to promote mutual respect based on understanding and acceptance of cultural differences. The nurse also may communicate respect for the patient's dialect by adapting to the patient's linguistic style by using fewer words, more gestures or more expressive facial behaviors.

Nonverbal Communication

Nonverbal communication includes everything that doesn't involve the spoken or written words, including all of the five senses, it is often unconsciously motivated and may more accurately indicates the person's meaning than the words being spoken.

Types of Nonverbal Behaviors

Following are the brief description of five categories of nonverbal communication.

Vocal Cues or Paralinguistic Cues

Include all nonverbal qualities of speech, e.g. pitch, tone of voice, loudness or intensity, rate and rhythm of talking, and unrelated nonverbal sounds such as laughing, groaning, nervous coughing and sounds of hesitation.

Action Cues

Action cues are body movements, sometime referred as kinetics. They include automatic reflexes, posture, facial expression, gestures, mannerisms and actions of any kind.

Object Cues

Object cues are the speaker's intentional and nonintentional use of all objects. Dress, furnishings, and possessions all communicates something to the observer about the speaker's sense of self.

Space

Provides another nature to the clue to the nature of relationship between two people. The zone of space includes

1. Intimate space: up to 18 inches. This allows maximum interpersonal sensory stimulation.
2. Personal space: 18 inches to 4 feets used for closed relationship.
3. Social consultative space: 9-12 feets. Less personal and less interpersonal.
4. Public space: 12 feet and more. Used in speech giving and other public occasions.

Touch

Involves both personal space and action. Touch can express a desire to connect with the person as a way of meeting them or relating to them. It can be a conveying something to the person as a way of meeting them or relating to them. It can be a way of expressing or conveying something to another, such as concern, empathy or caring.

Methods of Nonverbal Communication

Rapport: The harmonious feeling experienced by two people who hold one another in mutual respect, acceptance, and understanding.

Empathy

- Empathy is that degree of understanding, which allows one person to experience how, another feels in a particular situation.
- Empathy is neither sympathy (feeling sorry for another person) nor compassion (that quality of love or tenderness that causes one person to suffer along with another).

Body Language: Remember that actions speak louder than words. A person will generally pay more attention to what you do than what you say. Think about the following nonverbal messages and what they might reveal.

- Facial expressions (smile, frown, blank look, grimace).
- Gestures/mannerisms (fidgeting, toe tapping, clenched fists).
- Eye behaviors (avoiding eye contact, staring, wide eyes).
- Use (and avoidance) of touch or physical contact.
- Posture (erect, slouching, leaning toward/away from someone).
- Walk.

Silence: Silence can be an extremely effective communication tool. It can be used to express a wide range of feelings.

- Silence can be used to communicate the deepest kind of love and devotion, when words are not needed.
- Silence can be a cold and rejecting sort of punishment, the "silent treatment" received for coming home late or forgetting an anniversary.
- Silence can be used in an interview or conversation to encourage the other person to "open up." Conversely, it can be used to intentionally create anxiety and discomfort in the other person.

Listening: As a patient speaks, think about what he must be feeling. Sometimes, as a listener, you must cut through layers of words to get to the real message. You must read between the lines. Pick up the underlying meaning of the message (intent); don't rely entirely upon the obvious or superficial meaning (content)

Meta Communication

Which is the communication about the communication or lack thereof it. It is an implicit but integral part of the message and is an interpersonal bridge between verbal and nonverbal components communication

It refers to how the message should understand by the receiver, e.g. the message "you look fresh and lovely today" is conveyed with wrinkles of the fore head. So, the receiver must interpret the sincerity of the sender in giving the compliments.

COMPONENTS OF THERAPEUTIC COMMUNICATION

Crucial components of therapeutic communication are.

- Confidentiality
- Privacy
- Respect for boundaries
- Self-disclosure
- Use of touch
- Active listening
- Observation skills

Use of touch

As intimacy increases, the need for distance decreases. Touch is a powerful communication tool. It can elicit both positive and negative reactions, depending on the people involved and the circumstances of the interaction. Touch is a very basic and primitive form of communication, and the appropriateness of its use is culturally determined.

Types of Touch

Touch can be categorized according to the message communicated (Knapp, 1980)

1. **Functional -professional**: This type of touch is impersonal and business like. It is used to accomplish a task, for examples, a tailor who is measuring a customer for a suit or a physician examining a patient
2. **Social -polite:** This type of touch is still rather impersonal, but it conveys an affirmation or acceptance of the other person, for example, a handshake
3. **Friendship-warmth:** Touch at this level indicates strong linking for the other person, a feeling that he or she is a friend, for example, laying one's hand upon the shoulder of another.
4. **Love-intimacy:** This type of touch conveys an emotional attachment or attraction for another person, for example, to engage in a strong, mutual embrace
5. **Sexual arousal:** Touch at this level is an expression of physical attraction only, for example, touching another in the genital region.

Some cultures encourage more touching of various type than others. The nurse should understand the cultural meaning of touch before using this method of communication in specific situations.

Therapeutic Use of Touch in Mental Health

Touching a client can be comforting and supportive when it is welcome and permitted. The nurse should observe the client of cues that show if touch is desired or indicated. For example, holding the hand of a sobbing mother whose child is ill is appropriate and therapeutic. If the mother pulls her hand away, however, she signals to the nurse that she feels uncomfortable being touched. The nurse also can ask the client about touching (e.g. would it help you to squeeze my hand ?)

Although touch can be comforting and therapeutic, it is an invention of intimated personal space. Some clients with mental illness have difficulty understanding the concept of personal boundaries or knowing when touch is or not appropriate. Consequently most psychiatric inpatient, outpatient, and ambulatory care units abroad have policies against clients touching one another or staff. Unless they need to get close to a client to perform some nursing care, staff members should serve as role models and refrain from invading clients personal and intimate space. When a staff member is going to touch a client while performing nursing care, he or she must verbally prepare the client before starting the procedure. A client with paranoia may interpret being touched as a threat and may attempt to protect himself or herself by striking the staff person.

Trust is a critical element which you may have to establish or just maintain. In some cases you will automatically be accorded trust because of your role and setting.

Empathy is the ability to put oneself in the other's place and see things from his/her perspective. You do this by really listening to what he/she is expressing, and then acknowledging it. For example, if the other person has been talking about struggling with illness and family responsibilities, you might say, "It must be very hard for you now, feeling awful but trying to keep up your family responsibilities". If the person has been talking about something in a very angry tone, you might say, "That must make you mad as h—." Saying, "I know how you feel" does not convey empathy, instead it is usually at least "off putting" if not infuriating to the other person. Even if you've had a very similar experience and the person to whom you're speaking is well aware of your similar experience, "I know how you feel." is probably not an effective response—we all experience things differently, and you never really know how someone else feels unless s/he tells you.

Respect is conveyed verbally and non-verbally. It includes both respecting the other for who he/she is and what he/she is expressing. It's important to note here that there are cultural differences in how respect and lack of respect are conveyed.

Congruence involves genuineness or authenticity. You aren't trying to be someone you're not or convey something you don't mean. It includes congruence of your verbal and non-verbal communication, as well as congruence of your message and its expression. In other words, you come across as being sincere, and meaning what you say.

Self awareness is being aware of how your thoughts, feelings, and behavior can help to convey other elements like congruence, respect, and empathy. The person with self awareness can comfortably move the focus away from self and onto the other.

Listening is a key element in therapeutic communication, and is discussed in further detail in the following slides.

ELEMENTS OF COMMUNICATION

Communication which is the basic to human interaction is a complex process. It has 5 main components:

1. Sender— the Sender (Communicator)

It is the originator of the message .To be an effective communicator, he must know –his objectives clearly defined, his audience (its interest and needs), his message, channels of communication, his professional ability and ties and limitations. The sender's purpose must be translated into a code. This is done with language or nonverbal signals, such as gestures, facial expressions, or body cues. The process of getting the purpose translated into the code is called encoding. Encoding results in a message.

2. Receiver

The receiver is the target of the communication and must be able to understand or decode the message. This can be a single person or a group. The audience may be of 2 types— the controlled and the uncontrolled. A controlled audience is one which is held together by a common interest. It is a homogenous group. An uncontrolled or free audience is one which has gathered together from motives of curiosity. This type of audience poses a challenge to the ability of the educator.

3. Message

A message is the information which the communicator transmits to the receiver, to receive, understand, accept and act upon. It may be in the form of words, pictures or signs. A good message must be: in line with the objective, meaningful, based on felt needs, clear and understandable, specific and accurate, timely and adequate, fitting the audience, interesting, culturally and socially appropriate.

4. Channels of Communication

By channel is implied the "physical bridges" or the media of communication between the sender and receiver.

Media systems — the total communication effort is based on 3 media systems.

a. Interpersonal communication — the most common channel of communication is the interpersonal or face to face communication. It is particularly important in influencing the decisions of the undecided persons. Also it has a motivational effect over mass media.
b. Mass media — mass media have the advantage of reaching a relative larger population in a shorter time than is possible with other means. Being one-way channels of communication, mass

media carry messages only from the centre to the periphery; feedback mechanisms are poorly organized, e.g. of mass media include TV, radio, printed media, etc.

c. Folk media — every community has its own network of traditional or folk media such as folk dances, singing, dramas, etc. These are important channels of communication close to the cultural values of the rural population.

5. Feedback

Feedback means that the sender and receiver use one another's reaction to produce further messages. It is the flow of information from the audience to the sender. If the message is not clear or otherwise not acceptable the audience may reject it outright. The feedback thus provides an opportunity to the sender to modify his message and render it acceptable.

Understanding the elements of communication process is useful because sometime specific difficulties in communication can be traced to one or more of these elements. A basic example is a client who speaks a different language from the nurse. In this case the nurse needs to attend to the communication channel. An interpreter may be needed to help carry the messages or help the client to decode nurse's message.

Problems in encoding process also may occur, for example, in clients with thought disorders or certain forms of brain damage. The brain has intent to communicate but impairment in encoding results in a garbled message.

FACTORS OR VARIABLES THAT INFLUENCE COMMUNICATION

- Perceptions and stereotypes
- Environmental factors — personal space
- Values
- Emotions
- Sociocultural issues
- Knowledge
- Clarity, timing and relevance

- Perception
- Values, attitudes, beliefs
- Culture
- Social status
- Gender
- Age/developmental level
- Environment
- Verbal and nonverbal communication.

THESORIES OF COMMUNICATION

1. Therapeutic Communication

According to Berlo, under 4 headings as the SMCR model, where 'S' is source, 'M' stands for message, 'C' is channel used for communicate and 'R' is receiver.

In therapeutic communication the nurse directs the communication toward the patient to identify his current health problems, plan, implement and evaluate the action taken.

- It is a 2 way process.
- Both sender and receiver need to have commonness for effective communication.

2. Ruesch's theory

Theory of communication that considers communication as the social matrix (framework) for health care was developed by J. Ruesch in the late 1950s. He believed that communication included a broad range of activities that were designed to affect another person. Communications were viewed as a circular process, whereby messages traveled from within one person to another person and back again.

Events within the sender prompt the sending of a message. The message is then transmitted to one who receives it, processes it internally and responds. Successful communications occur when agreement about the meaning of the message has been reached. Communications are unsuccessful when there is a lack of agreement or understanding of the message. Ruesch (1961) coined the term disturbed communications to describe unsuccessful interactions that he believed resulted from interference in the sending or receiving of the messages, inadequate mastery of the language being used, insufficient information, or little or no opportunity for feedback.

Therapeutic communications are distinguished from ordinary communications by the intent of one of the participants to bring about a positive change. According to Ruesch's view therapist is one who direct exchanges to bring about more satisfying social relations. They try too understanding the nature of client's distresses and developing an understanding of their problems.

3. Transactional Analysis Model

Transactional analysis (TA) is the study of the communication or transactions that take place between people; it uncovers the sometimes unconscious and destructive ways ("games") in which people relate to each other. This approach to personality was developed by Berne (1964). a psychiatrist who made transactional analysis a popular theory through his classic book, Games People Play: The Psychology of Human Relationships. It is a method of therapy as well as a model of communication.

The cornerstone of this theory that each person's personality is made up of three distinct components called ego states. An ego state is a consistent pattern of feeling, experiencing, and behaving. The three ego states that make up personality are the parent ego state adult ego state, and child; ego state. It is as though three people reside in each person; the "parent" incorporates all the attitudes and behaviors the individual was taught (directly or indirectly) by parents; the "child" contains all the feelings the individual had as a child; and the "adult" deals with reality in a logical, rational, computer like manner.

The parent and child ego states are made up of the feelings, attitudes, and behaviors that are remnants of the past but can be re-experienced under certain conditions. The parent .ego state consists of all the nurturing, critical and prejudicial attitudes, behaviors, and experiences learned from other people, especially parents and teachers. The adult ego state is the reality-oriented part of the personality. It gathers and processes information about the world and is objective, emotionless, and intelligent in its approach to problem solving. The child ego state is the feeling part of the personality. In it resides feeling of happiness, joy, sadness, depression, and anxiety.

Berne's model of communication makes it possible to diagram transactions using these ego states. A transaction or communication between two people can be complementary, crossed, or ulterior. In a complementary transaction the arrows in the ego state diagram are parallel, and the communication flows smoothly.

Complementary Transaction

Crossed Transaction

It takes place on two levels; the social or overt, level and the psychological, or covert, level. These transactions tend to be destructive because the communicators conceal their true motivations. One of the best known examples of this is the "Why don't you.... Yes But" game. This game involves one person asking for a solution to a problem: however every suggested solution is negated, until the helper is silenced. On the surface, the interaction is two adults problem solving. In reality, one person is using the child ego state to show what a bad parent the other person is.

Ulterior Transaction

Neurolinguistic Programming

The basis for neurolinguistic programming lies in the work of Milton H. Erickson who until his death in 1980 was considered the greatest medical hypnotist of his time. Richard Sandler and John Grinder spent several years doing careful and systematic analyses of Erickson's work and extensive writings. Using their observations as a framework, they developed a method for analyzing and an individual's system of communication based on the theory that any effective communication is a state of hypnosis. Effective communication alters a person's state of consciousness. By learning the patterns of an individual's communications, one is able to achieve more effective and fulfilling interactions. Patterns include eye accessing clues (ways in which people move their eyes while thinking), different language patterns and the pace and rhythm of speech.

Nurses, therapist and other professionals are finding the principles of neurolinguistic programming a valuable asset for communications. Because neurolinguistic programming is a powerful tool for communicating, specialized training is recommended.

CHARACTERISTICS OF THERAPEUTIC COMMUNICATION

The nurse has to process certain characteristics to develop and maintain therapeutic relationship. It is broadly divided into:

- Response dimension
  - Genuineness
  - Respect
  - Empathetic understanding
  - Concreteness
- Action dimension
  - Confrontation
  - Immediacy
  - Nurse self disclosure
  - Patient self disclosure
  - Catharsis
  - Role play.

RESPONSIVE DIMENSIONS

The nurse must possess certain skills and qualities to establish and maintain a therapeutic relationship. Specific core conditions for facilitative interpersonal relationship can be divided into responsive dimension and action dimensions. The responsive dimensions include geniuses, respect, empathetic understanding and concreteness. The responsive dimensions are crucial in a therapeutic relationship establish trust and open communication. The nurse's goal is to understand the patient and to help the patient gain self understanding and insight.

Genuineness

Genuineness means that the nurse is an open, honest, sincere person who is actively involved in the relationship. Genuineness means that the nurse's response is sincere, that the nurse is not thinking and feeling one thing and saying something different. Whatever the nurse shows must be real and not merely a professional response that has been learned and repeated.

Respect

Respect also called as no possessive warmth or unconditional positive regard does not depend on the patient's behavior. Caring, liking and valuing are other terms for respect. Respect can be communicated in different ways: by sitting silently with a patient who is crying, by genuine laughter with the patent over a particular event, by accepting the patients request not to share a certain experience, by apologizing for the hurt unintentionally caused by a particular phase, or by being open enough to communicate anger or hurt caused by the patient.

Empathetic Understanding

Empathy is the ability to enter into the life of another person and to accurately perceive his or her current feelings and their meanings. Rogers (1975) described it as "to sense the clients private world as if it were on your own, but without losing the as if quality. There are two types of empathy. The first is basic empathy. It involves the natural, universal human capacity to feel for others. The second type is trained empathy, which is taught and learned in relation to helping others. It is also called as clinical empathy or professional empathy.

Development of Empathy

Empathic understanding consists of a number of stages. If patients allow nurses to enter into their private world and attempt to communicate their perception of feelings, nurses must be receptive to this feeling; nurses must be receptive to this communication.

Next nurse must understand the patient's communication by putting themselves in the place of patient. Nurses must then step back into their own role and communicate understanding to the patient.

Empathic Responses

First the nurse needs to provide genuineness and unconditional positive regard for the patient. Then the understanding conveyed to the patient through empathy gives him or her personhood or identity. The patient incorporates these aspects into a new changing self concept. Once self concept changes, behavior also changes, thus producing the positive clinical outcome of therapy.

Empathetic Functioning Scale

Kalisch (1973) devised the nurse –patient empathetic functioning scale, which describes 5 categories of empathy.

Category 0 and 1: The nurse ignores the patient's feelings, goes off on a tangent or misinterprets what the patient's feelings. The nurse at this level may be uninterested in the patient or concentrating on the fact of what the patient says rather than on current feelings and experiences. The nurse is doing something other than listening, such as evaluating the patient, giving advice or thinking about personal problems or needs.

Category 2: A middle level of empathy shows that the nurse is making an effort to understand the patient's feelings. They are required initially to build an atmosphere of trust and openness.

Categories 3 and 4: High levels of empathy communicate "I am with you"; the nurses responses fit perfectly with the patient's current feelings and experiences. The nurse responses also serve to expand the patient's awareness of hidden feelings through the use of clarification and reflection. Such empathy is communicated by the language used, voice qualities and nonverbal behavior, all of which reflect the nurses seriousness and depth of feeling.

Concreteness

It involves using specific terminology rather than abstractions when discussing the patient's feelings, experiences and behavior. It avoids vagueness and ambiguity. It has three functions: to keep the nurses responses close to the patient's feelings and experiences, to foster accuracy of understanding by the nurse, and to encourage the patient to attend to specific problem areas. In the orientation phase, concreteness should be high. It is essential for the formulation of specific goals and plans. In the working phase, it should be at a low level to facilitate a thorough self-exploration. High levels are again desirable a t the end of the working phase, when patients are engaging in action and during the termination phase.

ACTION DIMENSIONS

The action oriented conditions for facilitative interpersonal relationship are confrontation, immediacy, therapist self disclosure .catharsis and role play.

Confrontation

It is an expression by the nurse of perceived discrepancies in the patient's behavior. The three categories of confrontation are listed in the following (Carkhoff, 1969):

- Discrepancies between the patients expression of what she or he is and what he or she wants to be
- Discrepancies' between the patient's verbal self expression and nonverbal behavior
- Discrepancies between the patient's verbal expressed experience of himself or herself and the nurses experience of him or her.

Confrontation is an attempt to by the nurse to make the patient aware of incongruence in his or her feelings, attitudes, beliefs and behaviors. It also may lead to the discovery of ambivalent feelings in the patient. It is not limited to negative aspects of the patient. It includes pointing out discrepancies involving resources and strengths that are unrecognized and unused. It requires that the nurse collect sufficient data about the patient's history and accumulate sufficient perception and observations of verbal and nonverbal communication so that validation of reality is possible. The nurse must have developed an understanding of the patient to perceive discrepancies, inconsistencies in the word and deed, distortions and defenses. The nurse must be willing and able to work through the crisis after confronting the patient. Without this commitment confrontation lacks therapeutic potential and can be damaging to both patient and nurse.

Timing in relationship: Before confrontation nurse should assess the following factors:

- The trust level in the relationship
- The timing
- The patients stress level
- The strength of the patient's defense mechanisms
- The patients perceived need for personal space or closeness
- The patients level of rage and tolerance for hearing another perception.

Patients have the capacity to deny or accept nurse's observation and their response to the confrontation can serve as a measure of its success or failure. Acceptance indicates appropriate timing and patient readiness. Denial by the patient provides nurses with additional information that the patients are resisting change and are unwilling to enlarge their view of reality at this time. In the orientation phase, the nurse should use the confrontation infrequently. In the working phase of the relationship, more direct confrontation may focus on specific patient discrepancies. The nurse may confront the patient with areas of weakness or shortcomings or may focus on the discrepancies between the nurses perception of the patient and the patients self perception. This expands the patient's awareness and helps the patient move to higher levels of functioning. Confrontation is especially important in pointing out when the patient has developed insight but has not changed the behavior. Inexperienced nurses often avoid confrontation.

Immediacy

Immediacy involves focusing on the current interaction of the nurse and the patient in the relationship. It involves sensitivity to the patient's feelings and a willingness to deal with these feelings rather than ignore them. It is not possible or appropriate for the nurse to focus continually on the immediacy of the relationship. It is most appropriate to do so when the relationship is not progressing. It is also helpful to look at the immediacy when the relationship is progressing particularly well.

Nurses Self Disclosure

Self-disclosures are subjectively true, personal statements about the self, intentionally revealed to another person. The nurse may share experiences or feelings that are similar to those of the patient and may emphasize both similarities and differences. It is an expression of genuineness and honesty by the nurse and is an aspect of empathy. Criteria for self disclosure include the following:

- To model and educate
- To foster the therapeutic alliance
- To validate reality
- To encourage the patients autonomy

The nurse should disclose in response to statements made by the patient. If the nurse's disclosure is away from what the patient is experiencing, it can distract the patient from the problem or cause feelings of alienation. A patient who is experiencing severe anxiety may feel threatened by the nurses self disclosure, e.g.

Patient: When he told me he didn't want to see me again, I felt like slapping him and hugging at the same time. But then I knew the problem was really me and no one could ever love me.

Nurse: When I broke off with a man I had been seeing. I felt the anger, hurt and bitterness you just described. I remember thinking I would never date another man.

In this example, nurse self disclosed to emphasize that the

patient's feelings were natural. She also reinforced the external causes for the separation (boyfriend's decision to leave versus the patient's inadequacy) and implied that, with time, the patient will be able to resolve the loss.

Emotional Catharsis

Emotional catharsis occurs when patient is encouraged to talk about things that are most bothersome. It brings fears, feelings and experiences out into the open so that they can be examined and discussed with the nurse. Forcing emotional catharsis on the patient could precipitate a panic episode because the patient's defenses are attacked without sufficient alternative coping mechanisms available.

If the patient has difficulty in expressing feelings, nurses may help suggesting how they or others might feel in the patients' specific situation. Some patients respond directly to the question "How did that make you feel?"

Role Playing

It involves acting out a particular situation. It increases the patient's insight into human relations and can deepen the ability to see the situation from another person's point of view. Role playing consists of the following steps:

- Define the problem
- Creating a readiness for role playing
- Establishing the situation
- Casting the characters
- Briefing and warming up
- Acting
- Stopping
- Analyzing and discussing
- Evaluating

One of the specific way in which role playing can be used to resolve conflicts and increase self awareness is through a dialogue that requires the patient to take the pat of each person or each part of a problem. If the conflict is internal, the dialogue occurs in the present tense between the patients conflicting selves until one part of the conflict overweighs the other. If the conflict involves a second person, the patient is instructed to imagine that the other person is sitting in the chair across from you. The patient is told to begin the dialogue wants and resentments about the other person. Then the patient changes the chairs, assumes the role of another person and responds to what was just said. It not only helps the patient in expressing feelings and opinions but also gives a reality for the probable response from the other party involved in the conflict.

THERAPEUTIC COMMUNICATION TECHNIQUES

1. **Listening**: Listening is an active process of receiving information and examining reaction to the messages received. It is not simply hearing. It is essential to reach any understanding of the patient. It is the first rule of therapeutic-nurse relationship. The patient should be talking more than the nurse during the interaction. Listening is sign of respect and is powerful reinforcer. Active listening involves all the nurse's senses, e.g. maintaining eye contact and receptive nonverbal communication which helps to convey the nurse's interest and acceptance
2. **Broad openings:** Here the nurse is encouraging the patient to select topics for discussion. Patient should be welcomed to the communication with warmth and respect. Patient should feel that nurse is ready to listen. Open-ended questions result in fuller, more revealing answers, e.g.
   What are you thinking about?
   Can you tell me more about that?
   What shall we discuss today?
   Domination of the interaction by the nurse or rejecting the responses by the nurse results in poor therapeutic relationship.
3. **Questioning:** The nurse skillfully asks open-ended questions during the initial admission. Interviewing skills are necessary to avoid asking too many personal questions in one session. Questions should be to achieve relevance and depth.

How come you stopped taking your medication?
Tell me how you feel now?

4. **Restating:** Nurse is repeating of the main thought the patient has expressed. It also indicates that the nurse is listening, validating, reinforcing or calling attention to what has been said. Usually a part of patient's statement is repeated. When restating patient should not feel the nurse is reassuring, judgmental or defending, e.g.
"Your mother left you when you were 5-year-old?
5. **Clarification:** Here, the nurse makes specific questions to help clear up a specific point patient makes by attempting to put in to words vague ideas or unclear ideas of the patient. Patient's verbalizations may not be clear when overwhelmed with emotions. Nothing should be allowed to pass to the patient that nurse does not hear or understand, e.g.
"I am not sure what you mean. Could do tell me about it again?"
Failure to probe and assumed understanding result in poor communication.
6. **Reflection:** By reflection nurse is directing back the patient's ideas, feeling, questions or content. Reflection lets the patient know that the nurse has heard what was said and understand the content. Reflection of the feelings let the patient know that the nurse is aware of what the patient is feeling. It signifies understanding, empathy, interest and respect for the patient. Other techniques may not represent empathetic understanding.
"You are looking sad and tense. Is it related to what you have explained?"
Reflecting techniques can be used incorrectly, when stereotyping patient's response, inappropriate timing of reflections and inappropriate cultural experience and educational level of the patient.
7. **Focusing:** Focusing helps the patient expand o a topic of importance and also helps in analyzing in detail. It helps the patient talk about life experiences or problem areas and accepts the responsibility for improving them. If the goal is to change thoughts, feelings or beliefs, the patient must first identify and

down them. It allows the patient discuss central issues and keeps the communication goal-directed.
"I think you should talk more about your relationship with your husband?"

8. **Sharing perceptions:** It involves asking the patient to verify the nurse's understanding of what the patient is thinking or feeling. For example, nurse is interviewing an alcoholic patient.
   Patient: My wife and children are so good. They love me. But I do not know what happened to me. I can't care tem. I can't stop drinking.
   Nurse: You seem to be very disappointed with your drinking. Am right about that?
   If used inappropriately sharing perceptions can make the patient feel challenging, reassuring, and testing
9. **Theme identification:** Themes are underlying issues or problems experienced by the patient that emerge repeatedly during the course of the nurse-patient relationship, like anxiety, depression.
   "It sounds like that is very important to you. You have mentioned it a very few times."
10. **Silence:** Here, the nurse use lack of verbal communication for a therapeutic reason. It allows the patient to think and gain insights. Silence on the part of nurse has varying effects, depending on how the patient perceives it. To a vocal patient silence on the part of nurse may be welcome, but with a depressed or withdrawn patient, the nurse's silence may convey support, understanding, and acceptance.
11. **Humor:** Humor is basic part of our personality and has a place in therapeutic nurse-patient relationship. It is the discharge of energy through the comic enjoyment of imperfect. It may be helpful with a patient experiencing mild to moderate anxiety. Humor should be consistent with social and cultural values.
12. **Informing:** Informing or giving information is nurse shares simple facts with the patient. This skill is use in patient education like when to take medication, necessary precautions and side effects.

"I think you need to know more about your medication works" Informing should not fall in to giving advice.

13. **Suggesting:** Suggesting is the presentation of alternate ideas. As a therapeutic technique, it is useful intervention in the working phase of the relationship. Suggesting or giving advice can be non-therapeutic. Patient may take nurse's advice and still have an unsuccessful outcome, the patient returns to blame nurse.
14. **Confrontation:** Confrontation involves anger and aggression. The therapeutic dimension is assertiveness rather than aggression. Confrontation is an attempt by the nurse to make the patient aware of incongruence in is or her feelings, attitudes, beliefs, and behaviors. It may also help in discovery of ambivalent feelings in the patient. The nurse must be ready to work with the patient through the crisis after confronting the patient. With out this commitment the confrontation lack therapeutic potential and may damage nurse-patient relationship.
15. **Role playing:** Role playing involves acting out a particular situation. It increases patient's insight in to human relations can deepen the ability to see the situation from another person's point of view. Role playing can be used for attitude change and to promote self-awareness.

One of the specific ways in which role playing can be used to resolve conflicts and increase self-awareness is through a dialogue that requires the patient to take the part of each person or each side of the problem. If the conflict is internal, the dialogue occurs in the present tense between the conflicting selves until one part of the conflict outweighs the other. If second person is involved, the patient is told to begin the dialogue by expressing wants and resentments about the other person. Then, the patient changes chairs assume the role other person, and responds to what was said. This way patient can express feelings and opinions and gives reality base for the probable response from the other party involved in the conflict.

Therapeutic communication techniques	*Examples*
1. Using silence	The client says: "We drink and smoke a lot here." The student thinks…how can that be…drinking alcohol in a state hospital? But says nothing…using silence…the client then says: "yes we drink a lot of cokes and smoke a lot."
2. Accepting	"Yes" or "I follow what you said"
3. Giving recognition	"I notice you combed your hair."
4. Offering self	"I'll sit with you awhile."
5. Using broad openings	"What would you like to talk about?" "Tell me what's bothering you."
6. Using general leads (using neutral expressions to encourage continued talking by the client)	"Go on. "Ummm..I am listening" "Tell me about it"
7. Placing the event in time or sequence	"Was this before or after…?" "What seemed to lead up to…?"
8. Making observations	"You appear tense" "I notice you are biting your lips."
9. Encouraging description of perceptions	"What do you think is happening to you right now…?"
10. Restating	Client: "I can't sleep. I stay awake all night." Nurse:"You have difficulty sleeping"
11. Reflecting	Patient: "Do you think I should tell the doctor?" Nurse: "Do you think you should tell the doctor?"
12. Focusing	"This point seems worth looking at more closely." "You said something earlier that I want you to go back to."
13. Exploring	"Would you describe that more fully."
14. Giving Information	"My name is…I am a student nurse.."
15. Seeking clarification	"What would you say is the main point of what you said?"
16. Presenting reality	"Your mother is not here…I am a nurse." Patient: "Did you bring my car today?" Nurse: "No, you do not have a car. I drove my car here today."
17. Voicing doubt	"That's hard to believe." "Really?"

Contd...

Contd...

Therapeutic communication techniques	*Examples*
18. Seeking consensual validation	
19. Verbalizing the Implied	
20. Encouraging evaluation (asking for the client's view of the meaning or importance of something)	"How important is it for you to change this behavior?"
21. Attempting to translate into feelings	"From what you say, I suspect you are feeling relieved."
22. Suggested collaboration	"Let's see if we can figure this out.."
23. Summarizing	"Let's see, so far you have said..."
24. Encouraging formulation of a plan of action	"What will it take to reach your goal of not hitting anyone?"
25. Identifying themes ..asking client to identify recurrent patterns in thoughts, feelings, and behaviors	"So what do you do each time you drink too much and it's time to go home?" What is the major feeling you have about all men?"

NONTHERAPEUTIC COMMUNICATION TECHNIQUES

- Be defensive or challenging the client
- Ask the client "why"
- Change the subjects
- Give advice or approval or disapproval
- Make value judgment
- Make stereotypical comments
- Place the client's feeling on hold
- Provide false reassurance

BARRIERS TO THERAPEUTIC COMMUNICATION

- Not listening properly (actually in therapeutic nurse patient relationship, nurse is active listener).
- Maintaining dominance in therapeutic interaction will not benefit both (either to nurse or to the client).
- Giving reassurance, false hopes will not contribute the therapeutic relationship.
- Too much probing into personal matters in the beginning usually goes wrong.

- Making stereotyped comments shows that you are not interested towards the client.
- Without listening to the client's feelings and problems, if the nurse goes on changing the topic or bringing unrelated topics, the patient will be discouraged from discussing his problem.
- If nurse offer challenges to the client, it will not work out.
- Too much advising the client is not good in TNPR.
- Belittling the patient will reinforce withdrawal features of client. for example, if the depressed patient expresses, 'I have nothing to live, I am worthless', then the nurse also expresses, 'I also felt the same way' like that will make the client to further goes into withdrawal behavior.
- Utilizing denial process in therapeutic nurse patient relationship.

STEPS IN THERAPEUTIC COMMUNICATION

1. Assessment, how to gather information
2. Diagnose
3. Planning and setting goals
4. Implementation
5. Evaluation

THERAPEUTIC COMMUNICATION SKILLS REQUIRED FOR THE PSYCHIATRIC NURSE

Skills are the ability or efficiency of the nurse to utilize their knowledge systematically and effectively in proficiency manner.

- General ability, e.g. ability to listen, interprets, speak and express through writing.
- Special abilities, e.g. observation and its interpretation
  - Process the therapeutic interaction to attain goals.
  - Ability to ascertain
  - Ability to differentiate and follow when to be silent, speak, smile, interact.
  - Ability to wait, proceed, speed

Participate actively and maintains therapeutic nurse patient relationship.

THERAPEUTIC NURSE-PATIENT RELATIONSHIP

Introduction

A relationship is defined as a state of being related or a state of affinity between two individuals one to one relationship is the end result of a series of planned purposeful interaction between human being, a nurse and patient.

Characteristics of the Relationship

The goals of a relationship are:

1. Achieving the patient's optimal growth.
2. Self-realization, self-acceptance and an increased genuine self-respect.
3. Sense of personal identity.
4. An ability to form intimate, interdependent, interpersonal relationships.
5. Improved functioning and increased ability to satisfy needs.
6. Achieve realistic personal goals.

Types of Relationship

The types of relationship can be social, intimate and therapeutic relationship.

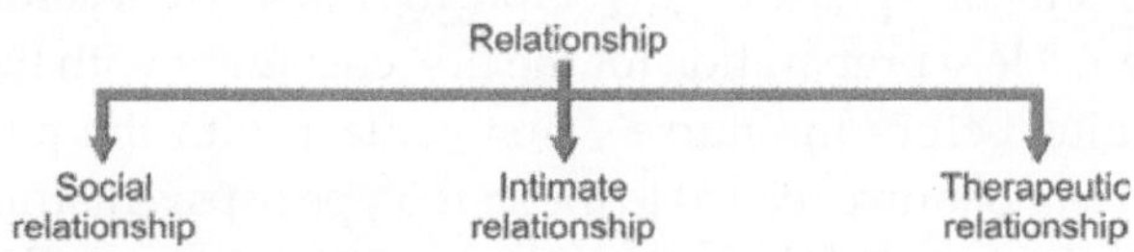

Social Relationship

It is just happens with mutual interests for satisfying needs of each other. (e.g.) work colleagues.

Intimate Relationship

It is a relationship between two individuals committed to one another, caring for and respecting each other (e.g.) partner type.

Therapeutic Relationship

Nurse – client (or) Therapist – client work together toward the goal.

Definition of Therapeutic Relationship

"One to one relationship is the end result of a series of planned purpose interaction between two human being, a nurse and a patient".

— Travelbee Joyce (1971)

Phases of Therapeutic Relationship

A vital characteristic of nurse patient relationship is the sharing of behaviours, thoughts and feelings. Peplau (1962) identified tasks of the relationships. The therapeutic interpersonal relationship is the means by which the nursing process is implemented.

Tasks of the relationship have been categorized into 4 phases:

i. The preinteraction phase
ii. The orientation (introduction) phase
iii. The working phase
iv. The termination phase

The Preinteraction Phase

The preinteraction phase begins before the nurse's first contact with the patient. Here preparation for the first encounter with the client.

It begins before the nurse's first contact with the patient. A common fear of nurse related to the stereotype of psychiatric patient as violent. Because this is the picture portrayed by the media, many nurses are afraid of being physically hurt by the patient's outburst of aggressive behavior. Other fear is related to nurses questioning their own mental health status. Nurses may fear mental illness and worry that exposure to psychiatric patients might cause them to lose their own needs. Other tasks of this phase include gathering data about the patient if information is available and planning for the first interaction with the patient.

Task

1. Obtaining available information from case sheet, chart, significant others, and other health team members.
2. Initial assessment is begun.
3. Prepare self for working activity.

The Orientation Phase

The introductory contract between client and nurse first meet.

It is the introductory phase that the nurse and patient first meet. One of the nurses concerns is to find out why the patient sought help and whether it was voluntary.

Formulating Contracts

The tasks in this phase of relationship are to establish a climate of trust, understanding, acceptance and open communication and formulate a contract with the patient.

The elements of a nurse-patient contract:

- Name of the individual
- Roles of nurse and patient
- Responsibilities of nurse and patient
- Expectations of nurse and patient
- Purpose of the relationship
- Meeting location and time
- Conditions for termination
- Confidentiality

Exploring Feelings

Both the nurse and patient may experience some degree of discomfort and nervousness in the introductory phase.

Reasons patient have difficulty seeking help:

- It may be difficult to see or admit one's difficulties, first to oneself and then to another.
- It is not easy to trust or be open with strangers
- Sharing personal problems with another person can threaten one's sense of independence, autonomy and self-esteem.

- Solving problems involves thinking about something that may be unpleasant, viewing life realistically, deciding on a plan of action, and then carrying out whatever it takes to bring about a change.

Other tasks of the nurse in the orientation phase of the relationship include the following:

- To explore the patient's perceptions, thoughts, feelings and actions.
- To identify the pertinent patient problem
- to define mutual, specific goals with the patient

Task

1. Introduction of nurse and client.
2. Creating an environment for the establishment of trust and rapport.
3. Establishing a contract for interventions.
4. To explore the patient's perceptions, thoughts, feelings and actions.
5. To identify pertinent patient problems.
6. To identify the client's strengths and limitations.
7. Formulating nursing diagnosis.
8. Setting goals.
9. Developing a plan of action.

The Working Phase

Most of the therapeutic work is carried out during the working phase. Most of the therapeutic work is carried out during the working phase. The nurse helps the patient to master anxieties, increase independence and self-responsibility and develops constructive coping mechanisms. Actual behavior change is the focus of this phase. Patient often display resistance during this phase. As the relationship develops the patient begins to feel close to the nurse.

Task

1. Maintaining the trust and rapport.
2. Promoting the client's insight and perception of reality.

3. Develop realistic self concepts and promote self confidence.
4. Develop a plan of action, implement the plan and evaluate the results of the plan.
5. Help client to change her/him dysfunctional behaviour.

Barriers

1. *Transference:* When the client unconsciously displaces or transfers to the nurse family formed toward a person from his/her past.
   Transference can interfere with the therapeutic interaction when the feeling being expressed include anger and hostility. The patient perceives the nurse as his daughter and starts behaving with her like a father.
2. *Counter transference:* It refers to the nurse's behavioural and emotional response to the client.
   When the nurse perceives a male patient like her father and gives him the same care that she would have given to her father. It is called Counter Transference.

Termination Phase

During this phase, learning is maximized for both the patient and the nurse. Reasons for termination are, the client may be discharged from the hospital, in the case of a student nurse, it ma be the end of a clinical rotation.

Termination is one of the most difficult but most important phases of the therapeutic nurse-patient relationship. It is the time to exchange feelings and memories and to evaluate mutually the patient's progress and goal attainment.

Criteria for determining patient readiness for termination:

- The patient experiences relief from the presenting problem
- The patients functioning has improved
- The patient has increased self-esteem and a stronger sense of identity
- The patient uses more adaptive coping responses
- The patient has achieved the planned treatment outcomes

Together the nurse and patient review the progress made in

treatment and the attainment of specified goals. Feelings of rejection, sadness, loss and anger are expressed and explored. It may be helpful to prepare the patient for termination by decreasing the number of visits, incorporating others into the meetings or changing the location of the meetings. The reasons behind a change should be clarified so that the patient does not interpret it as rejection by the nurse.

Task

1. Bringing a therapeutic conclusion to the relationship.
2. Focus on the future.
3. Provide necessary referral to others on the health team.
4. A plan for continuing care.
5. Feeling's about termination of relationship are recognized and explored.

BIBLIOGRAPHY

1. Bimla K. Text Book of Psychiatric Nursing. New Delhi: Kumar Publishing House, 2006(2)
2. Mary TC. Psyhiatric Mental Health Nursing– Concept of Care (3rd ed.) Philadelphia: FA Davis Publishers, 2002.
3. Stuart GW, Laria MT. Principles and Practices of Psychiatric Nursing (1st ed.) Philadelphia: Mosby Publishers, 2001.

7 Therapeutic Impasses

The commonest four impasses are:
- Resistance
- Transference
- Countertransference
- Boundary violations

RESISTANCE

Resistance is the patent's reluctance or avoidance of verbalizing or experiencing troubling aspects of oneself. The term was first coined by Freud. Resistance is often caused by patient's unwillingness to change when the need for change is recognized. Patient usually displays resistance during the working phase of nurse-patient relationship, because greater part of problem-solving occurs during this phase.

Resistance may be due to:
- Nurse who has moved too quickly or too deeply into the patient's feelings in to the patient's feelings
- Intentional or unintentional communication of lack of respect
- Nurse who is an inappropriate role model for therapeutic behavior
- Secondary gain — Favorable environmental, interpersonal, and situational changes occur and material advantages as a result of the illness (secondary gain can become a powerful force in perpetuating an illness because it makes environment more comfortable).

TRANSFERENCE

Transference is an unconscious response in which the patient experiences feelings and attitudes toward the nurse that were originally associated with other significant figures I his or her life.

- They may be triggered by superficial similarity, such as facial features or speech, or by personality style or trait.
- These reactions are the patient's attempt to reduce anxiety.
- The nurse may be viewed as an authority figure from the past such as parent figure, or lost loved object, such as former spouse
- Transference reactions are harmful to the therapeutic relationship only if they are ignored and unexplained.

Types of transference are particularly problematic in nurse-patient relationship:

Hostile transference

Dependent reaction transference

1. Hostile Transference

Patient may express hostility by uncooperativeness, negativism and hostile silence. If the hostility and anger are internalized, this resistance is expressed as depression and discouragement. Patient may terminate the relationship on the grounds that there is no chance of getting well. If hostility is externalized the, the patient may become critical, defiant, and irritable and may express doubts about nurse's training, experience or competence. Patient may attempt to compete with the nurse by reading books on psychology and debating intellectual issues rather than working on real life problems.

2. Dependent Reaction Transference

This resistance is characterized by patient who are submissive, subordinate, and irritating and who regard nurse as godlike figure. Patient continues to demand more of the nurse.

Management of Transference and Resistance

Resistance and transference can be difficult problems for the nurse. The psychiatric nurse must be ready to be exposed to such powerful positive and negative emotional responses from the patient.

- Resistance may be due to the nurse and patient have not arrived a mutually acceptable goals or plans of action. The appropriate action here is to return to the goals, purposes and roles of the nurse and patient relationship.
- The analysis of the resistance or transference should be directed toward the patient gaining awareness of these motivations and learning about being completely responsible for all actions or behavior.
- The first thing nurse must listen to the patient.
- When transference or resistance is recognized clarification and reflection of feelings can be used. Clarification gives the nurse a more focused idea of what is happening. Reflection of the content may help patients become aware of what has been going on their own mind, e.g.

  Nurse may say "I sense you are struggling with yourself. Part of you want to explore the issue of your of your marriage and another part says 'No-I'm not ready yet".

COUNTERTRANSFERENCE

It is a therapeutic impasse created by the nurse's specific emotional response to the qualities of the patient. This is inappropriate to the content and context of therapeutic nurse-patient relationship. It is transference applied to the nurse. It is natural that nurse feels warmth toward or liking for some patients more than others. The nurse also will be genuinely angry about the actions of some patient. But in countertransfernce, the nurse's responses are not justified by reality. Here nurse identify the patient with individuals from their past, and personal needs interfere with their therapeutic relationship.

Types

1. Reactions of intense love or caring
2. Reactions of intense disgust or hostility
3. Reactions of intense anxiety often in response to resistance by the patient

Examples:

- Difficulty in empathizing with the patient in certain problem areas
- Feeling of depression during or after a session
- Feeling or anger or impatience because of the patient's unwillingness to change
- Argument with the patient or a tendency to push before the patient is ready
- Personal or social involvement with the patient
- Dreams about or preoccupation with the patient
- Sexual or aggressive fantasies about the patient

  Other forms include staff involve in countertransference
- When they over-react the patient's aggressive behavior, ignore available patient data that would promote understanding
- Ignoring patient's behavior that does not fit the staff's diagnosis, minimizing a patent's behavior, joking about or criticizing a patient or becoming in caught up in intimidation.

The nurse must be constant look out for countertransference, become aware when it occurs and work with it to promote therapeutic goals. The nurse must use self-examination throughout the relationship. Following questions are helpful:

How do I feel about the patient?

Do I feel sorry or sympathetic for the patient?

Am I afraid of the patient?

Do I get extreme pressure out of seeing the patient?

Do I want to protect, reject, or punish the patient?

Countertransference can be harmful to the relationship; it should be dealt as soon as possible. The nurse should discover the source of the problem. When it is recognized the nurse can exercise control over it. If required help, the nurse can seek individual or group supervision.

'Problem patients' may elicit strong negative feelings such as anger, fear and helplessness in the mind of nurse. Such patients should be dealt with patience and action should be directed to making patient responsible for his own behavior. Nurse should review patient's needs and problems and use responsive dimensions of genuineness, respect, empathetic understanding, and concreteness.

BOUNDARY VIOLATIONS

Here the nurse goes beyond the boundaries of therapeutic relationship and establishes a social, economic, or personal relationship with a patient. Boundary violation is involved whenever a nurse is doing or thinking of doing something special, different or unusual for a patient. Situations where possible boundary violations can happen:

1. The patient takes the nurse to a lunch or dinner.
2. The nurse regularly reveals personal information to the patient.
3. The nurse accepts free gifts from the patient.
4. The nurse agrees to meet the patient for treatment outside the usual therapeutic setting without therapeutic justification.

Types

1. **Role boundaries**-Problems with role boundaries require the insight of the nurse and the setting of firm therapeutic limits with the patient.
2. **Time boundaries**-Odd and unusual hours that have no therapeutic necessity.
3. **Place and space boundaries**-Usually in an office or a hospital unit, outside that requires strong therapeutic rationale.
4. **Money boundaries**-regarding fee.
5. **Gift and service boundaries**-Gift acceptance may place undue obligations to the patient.
6. **Clothing boundaries**-Dress appropriately in a therapeutic manner.

7. **Language boundaries**-Addressing the patient and nurse's choice of words in implementing care. Too familiar, sexual, off-colour or leading language are boundary violations.
8. **Self-disclosure boundaries**—Inappropriately timed self-disclosure and that lacking therapeutic value.
9. **Post-discharge social boundaries**—Post-discharge social contact raise the question of boundary violation.
10. **Physical contact boundaries**— Sexual contact.

8 Physical Methods of Therapy

1. ELECTROCONVULSIVE THERAPY (ECT)

Introduction

In 1900 – 1930 specific treatments for mentally illness patients were not known much. One of the reasons could be the causes of psychiatric illness were not clearly identified. However, the technological changes and constant research various treatment modalities have been adopted.

These are: somatic therapy which includes psychopharmacology, electroconvulsive therapy, insulin coma therapy and psychosocial therapy.

History

A much safer from of convulsive therapy was used by Certetti and Bini in 1938. They called it EST or Electroshock therapy. Later, this method of treatment came to be known as ECT or electro convulsive therapy.

Definition

Electroconvulsive therapy is a physical/somatic therapy in which with the help of two electrodes, current is passed through the temporal region in between the two hemispheres on the brain, to produce a grand mal type of seizures.

ECT is a treatment in which a grand mal seizure is artificially induced in an anesthetized patient by passing an electrical current through electrodes applied to the patient's head.

[The induction of a grand mal seizures through the application of electrical current to the brain].

Indications

According to APA's Task Force on ECT, in 1976, gave its report which provided clear guidelines for the use of ECT and declared it to be a safe and effective method of treatment".

Indications are:

1. Major severe depression:
   - With suicidal risk
   - With stupor
   - With poor intake of foods
   - With psychotic features
   - With unsatisfactory response to drugs.
   - Where drugs are contraindicated.
2. Severe catatonic:
   - With stupor
   - With poor intake of food and
   - With unsatisfactory response to drug
3. Severe psychosis:
   - With risk of suicide, homicide
   - With unsatisfaction response to drug
   - Where drugs or contraindications
4. Mania
5. Schizophrenia
6. Schizo-affective
7. Postpartum psychosis
8. Organic mental disorders — organic mood syndrome, organic hallucinosis
9. Medical disorders: Organic catatonia , NMs, EPS

Contraindications

A. Absolute

Presence of raised intra cranial tension, is only absolute contra indication.

B. Relative:

1. Severe HT
2. Recent MI
3. CVA
4. Severe pulmonary disease
5. Retinal detachment.

Method

Two types:

1. Direct ECT:
   ECT is given in the absence of muscular relaxation and general anesthesia. All other steps are same.
2. Modified ECT: (Indirect)
   ECT is modified by drug-induced muscular relaxation and general anesthesia.

Procedure

- ECT is usually administered in the morning after an overnight fast. If given at any other time during the day, the patient should be empty stomach for atleast 4 hrs. No oral medication should be given in the morning.
- The bladder and bowel should be emptied just before the treatment.
- Dentures, if present should be removed and loose teeth should be ruled out.
- Tight clothing and metallic, sharp objects should be removed from the person's body.
- Hand Bath – to remove extra oil from the head.
- Pre medications should start 0.6mg of atropine through IV slowly. It decrease oral secretions and prevent vagal stimulation during ECT.
- Anesthetic agent like thiopentone (150-250 mg) and muscle relaxant like Succinyl choline (0.5-1.5 mg/kg)
- 100% O_2 administered before giving ECT.
- Now a mouth gag is inserted between the teeth, to prevent tongue bite during the convulsion.

- Electrodes are moistened with saline (or) gelly and are applied on head.
- The places of electrode placement is also cleaned with normal saline is applied.
- One attendant places are hand each of both things near the knee joint, while another attendant holds the shoulders.
- The usual dose of obtaining an adequate seizure response to 70 – 110 rots for 0.1 – 1 seconds.
- After the seizure has occurred, mouth gag is removed, secretions are sucked from oral cavity and oxygen mask is applied.
- The patient is made to rest, for about 30 minutes to 1 hour on bed after the treatment is over.

Technique/Application: Two types

1. **Bilateral ECT:** This is the standard form of ECT most commonly used. Each electrode is placed 2.5 – 4 cm above the midpoint, on a line joining the tagus of ear and lateral canthus of eye.
2. **Unilateral ECT:** Electrodes are placed only on onside of head, usually non-dominant side. Another one electrodes can place anywhere the head.
   Bilateral: More effective/Side effects also
   Unilateral: Safer, less effective

Pretreatment Evaluation

1. Informed consent for the patient and patient relatives.
2. Detailed medical and psychiatric exam.
3. Physical examinations.
4. Lab investigation – Hb, Tc, DC, ESR, Urine – routine, X-ray, EEG, etc.
5. Eye test — fundus test

Mechanism of Action

The exact mechanism by which ECT affects a therapeutic response is unknown. Several theories exist, but the one to which the most credibility has been given is the biochemical theory. A number of researchers have demonstrated that electric stimulation results in significant increases in the circulating levels of several neurotransmitters. These neurotransmitters include serotinin, norepinephrine and dopamine, the same biogenic amines that are affected by antidepressant drugs.

- One point is clear that the efficacy ECT is linked with production of generalized tonic – clonic seizures lasting atleast 25 – 30 sec.
- ECT exact mechanism is unclear.
- Hypothesis:
  ECT – affects the catecholamine pathway between diencephalons and limbic system.
- It regulates of B1 reception in cortex and hippo campus.

Duration of Therapy

Usually 6 – 10 treatment are sufficient. Some, needed 15 treatment times.

The treatment should be spaced, so that no more than 3 ECTs given/week. (i.e.) alternative days only can give ECT.

Side Effects

1. Deaths – 1:1000 to 1:10,000.
2. Memory disturbances (anterograde and rectrograde) very common.
3. Confusion
4. Headache, prolonged apnea, prolonged seizure, muscle ache, apprehension.

[ECT does not cause brain damage]

2. PSYCHOSURGERY

Psychosurgery is the surgical intervention to sever fibers connecting one part of the brain with another (or) to remove, destroy, or stimulate brain tissue with the intent of modifying or altering disturbances of behaviour, thought content or mood for which no organic pathological cause can be demonstrated by established tested techniques.

Definition

It is a surgical intervention to severe fibres connecting one part of brain with another, or to remove, destroy or stimulate brain or tissue, with the intent of modifying, behaviour, thought or mood disturbances, for which there is no underlying organic pathology.

— APA's Task Force

History

From technical, therapeutic and theoretical view points, it is now evident that psycho surgery covers two distinct time periods, the first upto the 1950s, the second the years since then.

During the first period, frontal lobes were the only site of operation: in the second, the operations have been limited to the limbic system.

Prefrontal lobotomy: Initiated in 1936 by **Egas Moniz**, a Portuguese psychiatrist, the first attempt to alleviate assaultive behaviour who reported a small series of cases about 50 years ago.

Freeman, a neuro psychiatrist and **Watts,** a neurosurgeon, introduced prefrontal lobotomy in the US in 1937. Therefore it is called Standard Lobotomy. In 1949, **Moniz** was awareded the Nobel prize for medicine.

Anatomy

It is believed that limbic system for closely linked with normal and abnormal emotional reactions. Limbic system is closely connected with frontal and temporal lobes, midbrain and other parts of brain by many connecting fibres.

One major part of limbic system believed to be important in emotional experience, is Papez circuit. This is an important circuit, which lies within limbic system connects lingulate bundle, hippocampus, anterior thalamus, fornix and septum.

Indications

Because the effects of psychosurgery are permanent its continued use is limited to special cases such as,

1. Severe in capacitating OCD, depression and phobia.
2. Intractable severe pain.
3. A very small number of schizophrenia, uncontrollable with other methods of treatment.
4. Intractable seizures (rarely).
5. Proposed for a variety of other psychiatric disorders such as chronic alcoholism, drug addicting, personality disorders and sexual psychopathy.

Techniques

- Before any procedure, an informed consent must be obtained.
- Currently all techniques use stereostatic methods, so, it is precise and side effects produced are few.

Available Procedures

- Bimedical leucotomy, orbital under cutting.
- Rostral leucotomy, prefrontal leucotomy.
- Stereotactic tractotomy.

Types of Psychosurgery

1. Modified leucotomy
2. Biomedical orbital undercutting.

Other Operations

1. Cingulonotomy – OCD
2. Amygdolotomy and thalamotomy (in aggressive, violent)
3. Temporal Lobectomy (in aggressive and intractable)
4. Temporal lobe epilepsy

Method

- Electrocoagulation
- Freezing
- Thermocoagulation
- Yttrium – 90 seeds
- Laser

Side Effects

1. Mortality rates varying from 0.5 to 5%.
2. Deaths were often due to hemorrhages from several, often aberrant, vessels.
3. 15% of patients, epilepsy occurred.
4. Apathy, lack of drive.
5. Emotional flatners or slight euphoria.
6. Loss of judgement/Uninhibited behaviour.
7. Some patients become incontinent and vegetable like.

3. PSYCHOPHARMACOLOGY

Psychopharmacological agents treat specific symptoms of neurobiological illnesses with significant effectiveness, although side effects and adverse reactions of drug therapy require expertise and sound clinical judgement on the part of the nurse.

Definition

Medication that affects psychic function, behaviour or experience.

Classification of Psychotropic Drugs

These psychotropic drugs can be classified as follows:
1. Antipsychotic agents
2. Antidepressants agents
3. Mood-stabilizing agents
4. Antianxiety agents
5. Antiparkinsonians
6. Antiepileptics
7. Miscellaneous drugs

Antipsychotic Drugs

The original drugs from the 1950's used to treat psychosis are called "typical" or "conversional" antipsychotic drugs. The newer or second generation antipsychotic drugs from the 1990s are called "atypical" or "novel" anti psychotic drugs. Thus their development again revolutionized the treatment of psychosis.

Indications

Used in the treatment of acute and chronic psychosis, antiemetics, intractable hiccoughs, Taurette's disorder.

The major uses for anti psychotic drugs are in the treatment of schizophrenia, schizoeffective disorder, organic brain syndrome with psychosis, and delusional disorder.

Their short-term use may be indicated in severe depression with psychotic features and in substance-induced psychosis, aggressiveness and behavioral problems seen in patients with pervasive developmental disorders and in elderly patients with dementia and delirium with agitation and psychosis.

Action

The exact mechanism of action is not known. These drugs are thought to work by blocking post synaptic dopamine receptors in the basal ganglia, hypothalamus, limbic system, brainstem and medulla. Newer medications may exert antipsychotic properties by blocking action on receptors specific to dopamine, serotonin, and other neurotransmitters.

Contraindications

These drugs are contraindicated in clients with known hypersensitivity. They should not be used when CNS depression is evident, when blood dyscrasias exist, in clients with Parkinson's disease or in clients with liver, renal or cardiac insufficiency. Diabetic clients, respiratory insufficiency, prostatic hypertrophy or intestinal obstruction.

Classification

Chemical Class	*Trade Name*	*Dose Range (mg/day)*
I. PHENOTHIAZINES		
A. Aliphatics		
1. Chlorpromazine (CPZ)	Megatil	300 – 1500
	Thorazine	75 – 400
2. Triflupromazine	Siquil	100 – 400

Contd..

Contd..

Chemical Class	*Trade Name*	*Dose Range (mg/day)*
B. Piperidines		
1. Thioridazine	Thioril	300 – 800
	Mellaril	150 – 800
C. Piperazines		
1. Triflourperazine	Espazine	15 – 60
	Stelazine	4 – 40
2. Prochlorperazine	Stemetil	45 – 150
	Compazine	15 – 150
3. Fluphenazine hydrochloride	Anatensol	5 – 30
4. Thiopreperazine	Majeptil	15 – 45
II. THIOANTHENES		
A. Aliphatics		
1. Chlorprothixene	Tractan	75 – 600
B. Piperazines		
1. Thioxthixene	Navane	6 – 60
2. Flupenthixol	Fluanxol	3 – 40
3. Flupenthioxl decanoate	Fluanxol Depot	-
III. HUTYROPHENONE'S		
1. Haloperidol	Haldol	1 – 100
2. Trifluperidol	Triperidol	0.5 – 8.0
3. Haloperidol Decanoate	Senorm – LA	-
IV. DIBENZOXAZEPINE		
Loxapine	Loxitane	20 – 250
V. DIPHENYL BUTYL PIPERIDINES		
1. Pimozide	Orap	4 – 20
2. Penfluridol	Flumap	20 – 60/week
VI. ATYPICAL ANTIPSYCHOTICS		
A. Dibenzodiazepines		
Clozapine	Clozaril	300 – 900
	Sizopin	50 – 450
B. Dibenzothiazepine		
Qiatiapine	Seroquel	300 – 750
C. Thienobenzodiazepine		
Olanzepine	Zyprexa	5 – 20
D. Arylpiperidylindole		
Sertindole	Serdolect	12 – 14
VII. OTHERS		
A. Rauwoffia alkaloids	Resperpine	Serpasil 0.5 – 50

Side Effects

1. Anticholinergic effects
   a. Dry mouth
   b. Blurred vision
   c. Constipation
   d. Urinary retention
2. Nausea; GI upset
3. Skin rash
4. Sedation
5. Orthostatic hypotension
6. Photosensitivity
7. Decreased libido; retrograde ejaculation, gynecomastia, amenorrhea, and weight gain.
8. Extrapyramidal symptoms (EPS)
   i. Pseudoparkinsonism (tremor, shuffling gait, drooling, rigidity)
   ii. Akinesia (Muscular weakness).
   iii. Akathisia (Continuous restlessness and fidgeting)
   iv. Dystonia (involuntary muscular movements of face, (spasms), arms, legs and neck).
   v. Oculogyric crisis (uncontrolled rolling back of the eyes).
   vi. Tardive dyskinesia (bizarre facial and tongue movements, stiff neck, and difficulty swallowing).
   vii. Neuroleptic malignant syndrome (NMS).

This is a rare, but potentially fatal, complication of treatment with neuroleptic drugs.

Onset can occur within hours or even years after drug initiation and progression is rapid over the following 24 to 72 hours.

Symptoms include severe parkinsonian muscle rigidity, hyperpyrexia upto 107°F, tachycardia, tachypnea, fluctuations in blood pressure, diaphoresis, and rapid deterioration of mental status to stupor and coma.

Discontinue neuroleptic medication immediately, monitor vital signs, degree of muscle rigidity, intake and output, level of consciousness.

The physician may order bromocriptine (Parlodel) or dantrolene (Dantrium) to counteract the effects of NMS.

ANTIDEPRESSANT DRUGS

Antidepressants are used for the treatment of depressive illness. These are also called as mood elevators and thymoleptics. Research has been proposed that serotonin, norepinephrine and other neurochemicals are dysregulated in mood disorders.

Indications

Antidepressant medications are used in the treatment of

- Dysthymic disorder
- Major depression with melancholia or psychotic symptoms
- Depression associated with organic disease
- Alcoholism
- Schizophrenia
- Mental retardation
- Depressive phase of bipolar disorder
- Depression accompanied by anxiety
- Child psychiatric disorders (enuresis, ADD with hyperactivity, school phobia and somnambulism)
- Post-traumatic stress disorder.

Action

These drugs ultimately work to increase the concentration of norepinephrine, serotionin, or dopamine in the body. This in accomplished in the brain by blocking the reuptake of these neurtransmitters by the neurons (tricyclics, selective serotonin reuptake inhibitors and others).

It also occurs when an enzyme, monoamine oxidase (MAO), that is known to inactivate norepinephrine, serotonin and dopamine, is inhibited at various sites in the nervous system (MAOIs).

Contraindications

- Individuals with hypersensitivity
- Individuals with angle-closure glaucoma
- Individuals with hepatic, renal or cardiac insufficiency
- Benign prostatic hypertrophy

Classifications

Chemical Class	*Trade Name*	*Dose Range (mg/day)*
A. Tricyclics		
1. Imipramine	Antidep	75 – 300
2. Amitriptyline	Tryptomer	75 – 300
3. Doxepine	Doxetar	75 – 300
4. Tri-imipramine	Surmontil	75 – 300
5. Clomipramine	Anafranil	75 – 300
6. Dotheipin	Prothaiden	75 – 300
B. Tetracyclics		
1. Mianserin	Depnon	30 – 120
2. Maprotiline	Ludiomil	75 – 225
3. Amoxapine	Demolox	150 – 400
C. Bicyclics		
1. Zimeldine	-	50 – 300
2. Viloxazine	-	100 – 300
E. Selective serotonin reuptake inhibitors:		
1. Fluxetine	Fludac	10 – 80
2. Fluvoxamine	Faverin	50 – 300
3. Paroxetine	Paxil	10 – 50
4. Sertraline	Serenata	50 – 200
5. Citalopram		
F. Monoamine oxidase inhibitors:		
1. Isocarboxacid	Marplan	10 – 30
2. Phenelzine	Nardil	15 – 90
3. Tranylcypromine	Parnate	30 – 60

Side Effects

1. **For all classification:** Dry mouth, sedation, nausea, discontinuation syndrome.

2. **For tricyclics:** Blurred vision, constipation, urinary retention, orthostatic hypotension, reduction of seizure threshold, tachycardia, arthythmias, photosensitivity and weight gain.
3. **For SSRIs:** Insomnia, agitation, headache, weight loss, sexual dysfunction, serotonin syndrome.
4. **For MAOIs:** Hypertensive crisis, occipital headache, palpitations, nausea/vomiting, nuchal rigidity, fever, sweating, marked increase in blood pressure, chest pain and coma.
5. **Miscellaneous side effects:** Prolonged or inappropriate penile erection, hepatic failure, skin rashes, EKG changes, hyper-pyrexia, direct myocardial depression, tachycardia and seizures.
6. **Serotonin syndrome (SS):** SS is a life-threatening emergency resulting from excess central nervous system. 5 – HT caused by combining 5 – HT enhancing drugs or administering SSRIs too close to the discontinuation of MAOIs.

   SS – symptoms are confusion, disorientaiotn, mania, restlessness/agitation, myoclonus, hyper reflexia, diaphoresis, shivering, tremor, diarrhoea, ataxia, headache.

   Discontinue all serotonergic drugs immediately anti convulsants for seizures, serotonin antagonist drugs may help.

Clonazepam for myoclonus, lorazepam for restlessness/ agitation, other symptomatic care as indicated; do not reintroduce serotonin drugs.

MOOD STABILIZING DRUGS

Bipolar disorder is a common, recurrent and often severe psychiatric illness associated with high rates of morbidity and mortality if left untreated.

Mood-stabilizing Drugs

1. Antimania:	**Usual dose (mg/day)**
Lithium	600 – 2400
Lithium citrate	600 – 2400
2. Anticonvulsants:	
Valproic acid	15 – 60 mg/kg/day
Valproate	

Lamotrigine		300 – 500
Carbamazepine – Tegretol		200 – 1600
Topiramate – Topamax		200 – 400
Tiagabine – Gabatril		4 – 32

3. **Thyroxin and T_3:** -
4. **Calcium channel blockers**

Verapamil	Calan	240
Nifedipine	Adalat, Procardia	240
Nimodipine	Nimotop	60 – 120

Antimanic Drugs

Antimanic agents are called "mood stabilizers". Lithium is medication of choice to treat mania and bipolar disorders. Approximately 80% of clients treated with lithium respond, when lithium is in effective, carbamazepine may be used.

Indication

The major use of an antimanic agent is for treatment of mania and recurrent manic episodes.

Antimanic Drugs

Lithium and Carbamazepine

LITHIUM

It is a medication that is like no other in psychiatry. It is natural salt, found in nature in the form of lithium carbonate and used in exactly the same form medicinally. It courses through most natural bodies of water and can be found in heavy concentration in rock formation around the world. There is a common misconnection that people take lithium medicinally to correct a lithium deficiency. This is not so. Lithium is not an element that is necessary for our bodies to function, so there is no such thing as a lithium deficiency.

Mode of Action

The specific biochemical mechanism of action of antimanic agents is unclear.

Lithium abolishes the excitement, euphoria and insomnia and mania without causing sedation. It produces many neuro chemical changes in the CNS, which may be related to its interaction with distribution of sodium and potassium across the cell membrane. It alters neurotraumatic activities in the brain.

Inhibits the release of thyroid hormone and testosterone rebalances disturbed circadian rhythms; changes cell membrane function.

One of these effects may be responsible for its mood stabilizer properties, but as yet no one knows which.

Nor epinephrine and serotonin in the part of CNS involved in emotion. It may decrease the activity of nerve impulse, resulting in depression (or) increase in the nerve impulse causing mania.

Lithium also helps in maintaining the sodium concentration in the brain, thereby regulating the mood swings as well as impulse along the nerve cells.

Indications of Lithium

It is used primarily in the treatment of bipolar disorder.

- Both acute manic and depressive episodes.
- Bipolar disorder
- Cyclic mood disorders
- Borderline personality
- Schizoaffective disorder
- Alcoholism

Contraindications

1. Renal Impairment: 80% of lithium dose is reabsorbed in the proximal renal tubules and excreted by the kidneys (acute and chronic renal failure).
2. Cardiovascular problems
3. Cerebreller disorder
4. Diabetic mellitus
5. Electrolyte imbalance
6. Hypertension
7. Hypothyroidism

8. Sodium depletion/receiving diuretics
9. During pregnancy and lactation: When it is taken by a women during the first trimester of pregnancy, it causes a slight increase in cardiac abnormalities in the fetus.

Absorption and Distribution

Lithium is readily absorbed from the entire gastrointestinal tract. Serum levels peak in 1.5 to 2 hours with lithium carbonate or they peak in 4 to 4.5 hours with a slow release preparation. Lithium does not bind to plasma proteins and is distributed non uniformly throughout body water. It reaches equilibrium after about 5 to 7 days of regular intake.

Lithium has an elimination half life of almost 24 hours. Although non significant losses occur through the skin or in the feces, about one-fifth on the lithium ion is eliminated through renal excretion during each circulations cycle of the kidneys. This process is dependent on Glomerular Filtration Rate (GFR) and Sodium balance and it varies considerably as a function of fluctuations in these parameters. Lithium is reabsorbed primarily in the proximal tubules together with Sodium, although the loop of Henle and Distal nephron may play some role. A decrease in plasma sodium levels, resulting from diuretics, excessive sweating and reduced sodium intake, initiates a compensating increase in sodium reabsorption accompanied by lithium reabsorption.

Distribution

Therapeutically effective plasma levels of lithium lie between 0.6 - 1.2 mEq/L of plasma but can be a low as 0.2 mEq/L in elderly. Serious toxicity can result from plasma levels above 2m Eq/L.

Medication Interactions

Avoid concurrent use of lithium and iodine. Cautions clients to avoid preparation containing iodides.

Iodomethacin and Phenylbutazone elevate serum lithium levels. It is important to observe for changes in serum lithium levels which these or other non steroidal anti-inflammatory medications are given with lithium.

Dosage

Lithium dosage is guided to plasma levels. Generally requires 600 to 1800 mg of lithium carbonate per day. Maintenance dosage is usually lowered to 900 to 1200 mg/day. Obtain plasma levels of 0.5 to 1.3 mEq/L 8 to 12 hr after last dose.

Side Effects

Side effects can be summarized under various systems as well as according to the serum lithium levels in the blood.

A. According to Various Systems

- Central nervous and autonomic nervous system
- Tremors, muscle irritability, tinnitus (Ringing or tinkling sound in the ears that is purely subjective) confusion, slurred speech, convulsion and blurred vision.
- Cardiovascular system: Arrhythmia, hypotension, bradycardia, generalized oedema.
- Gastrointestinal: Euthyroid goiter, myxedema.
- Urinary: Albuminuria, oliguria, Polyuria
- Allergic: Drying and thinning of hair, alopecia, itching.

B. According to Serum Lithium Level

Serum Lithium level	Symptoms
1.2 – 2 mEq/L	Drowsiness, vomiting, abdominal pain, lethargy, dizziness, confusion, ataxia.
2 – 2.5 mEq/L	Anorexia, persistent nausea and vomiting, blurred vision, seizure, acute circulating failure, stupor, coma.
Above 2.5 mEq/L	Generalized convulsion oliguria, death.

Guidelines for Use

Lithium is available in several forms; tables and capsules that are regular or slow – release and in liquid form. Lithium is not available in injectable forms. The solid form is lithium carbonate and liquid form is lithium citrate. The liquid form is used for people who are unable to swallow the solid form and occasionally in beginning of treatment to ensure compliance in clients who "cheek" or "tongue" their medications, (i.e.,)hide the tablets or capsules under their tongue or their cheek only to spit them out after they are out of the nurse's sight.

Before Lithium Therapy

Both thyroid and kidney functions are measured. In most setting triodothyronine T3 and thyroxine T4 (or) TSH. Blood levels are drawn as thyroid function measures, serum creatinine is used as a rough measures of kidney function. These tests are usually repeated periodically (every 6 months to a year) throughout the course of lithium treatment to measure any changes in the thyroid and kidney that result from prolonged lithium administration.

Check in blood – Hemoglobin, WBC (DC), serum electrolyte, serum calcium and phosphate, BUN, Thyroid function.

Urine – Complete urine analysis.

Others – ECG, Weight, Blood pressure, pregnancy (doubt).

During Therapy

Weigh clients before therapy. Excessive weight gain or edematous swelling of wrists and ankles can occur. Teach the client to keep a weekly weight record.

Monitor blood pressure regularly. If weight gain is excessive or trouble some to the client, it is not due to fluid retention, teach the client about a calorie – restricted diet and encourage daily exercise.

Lithium is not contraindicated in diabetic clients, but it may increase the serum insulin level. The drug may also cause polydipsia and polyuria. Monitor the blood glucose levels and serum electrolyte levels to help avoid additional problems. Monitor intake and output as needed.

Lithium may reach toxic levels in the kidney in the presence of dehydration or electrolyte depletion. Medical attention for prolonged diarrhoea or vomiting and to avoid activities that cause excessive sweating. Stress the importance of an adequate fluid intake.

Assess for signs of altered kidney function; fluid retention, unexplained weight gain, new signs of lithium of lithium toxicity, polyuria or nocturia.

Some clients find persistent hand tremors embarrassingly suggest that the client decrease caffeine consumption or on physician's approval, take most of the daily lithium dose at bedtime or reduce the dose slightly.

Metallic taste may be nuisance but is not serious. Taking lithium with meals may lessen nausea.

Hypothyroidism: Usually orders thyroid hormone replacement such as levethyroxine or desiccated thyroid.

Edema: A moderate salt restriction.

Nausea: Abdominal discomfort, recommend that the client take lithium with meals, a glass of milk or a snack.

Tremor: Recommend that the client reduce or eliminate caffeine – containing beverages.

Alternative to Lithium

Lithium is effective in about 70%. People who take it, for 30% who do not respond, there are several alternative that can be used either alone or in combination with lithium. First three alternative are: Anti seizure medication

- Carbamazepine (regretol)
- Sodium Valproate/Valporic acid
- Clonazepam

Carbamazepine

Blood level of carbamazepine is between 4 to 12 mg/ml.

Side Effects

Nausea, vomiting, sedation, dizziness, light headedness, clumsiness, ataxia, rash, blurred vision, dry mouth, urinary retention and bone marrow suppression.

Bone marrow suppression is dangerous and is guarded against by teaching clients the warning signs and drawing a period CBC every 2 to 4 weeks.

Warning signs of bone marrow suppression are anemia such as weakness, pallor, fatigue, signs of platelet suppression such as easy bruising or bleeding; bleeding gums, petechiae and signs of WBC suppression such as high fever and sore throat.

Recently some clients who fail on all these mood stabilizer agents have benefited from the calcium channel blocker verapamil.

Nurse's Role

- Give medicine during or after meat to decrease gastric irritability. It will also reduce the metallic taste in the mouth.
- Make observation of the side effects. Record and report immediately.
- Make note of serum lithium level, and observe the side effects and plan the nursing intervention.
- Weight should be recorded before lithium therapy. Excessive weight gain/swelling of ankles or wrists should be noted. Weekly weight record should be maintained.
- Intake/output chart is to be maintained to note the kidney functioning.
- Fluid intake is to be balanced because retention of fluid will increase weight.
- Any change in the diet should be reported immediately. Less intake of diet will affect the lithium level in blood.
- Salt should not be restricted in the diet unless instructed by physician.
- Advise the patient not to increase or decrease medicine unless advised.

ANTIANXIETY AGENTS

Anxiety is a normal emotion under circumstances of threat and is part of the fight-or-flight instinct necessary for survival.

This section divides anti anxiety and sedative–hypnotic drugs into 2 categories.

The benzodiazepines and several nonbenzodiazepine antianxiety drugs. The benzodiazepines are the most widely prescribed drugs in the world.

Indications

It also called anxiolytics and minor tranquilizers.

1. Anxiety disorders, anxiety symptoms
2. Acute alcohol withdrawal
3. Skeletal muscle spasms
4. Convulsive disorders
5. Status epileptics
6. Preoperative sedation.

Action

Anti anxiety drugs depress subcortical levels of the central nervous system (CNS), particularly the limbic system and reticular formation. They may potentiate the effects of the powerful inhibitory neuro transmitter gamma – aminobutyric acid (GABA) in the brain, thereby producing a calming effect. All levels of CNS depression can be affected, from mild sedation to hypnosis to coma.

Contraindications

1. Individuals with hypersensitivity
2. Pregnancy and lactation
3. Narrow – angle glaucoma
4. Shock
5. Coma
6. Hepatic or renal dysfunction

Classifications

I. Benzodiasepines

The Benzodiapines are thought to reduce anxiety because they are powerful potentiators of the inhibitory neurotransmitter GABA.

Mode of Action

The exact mechanism of action of benzodiazepines is not clear. Actions based benzodiazepine receptors.

1. BDZ Receptor I, which is linked with GABA receptor and involve din medication of sleep.
2. BDZ Receptor II, it is involved in cognition, and motor control.

Examples:

1. Very short acting
   Triazolam
   Midazolam
2. Short acting
   Oxazepam
   Lorazepam
   Alprazolam
   Estazolam
3. Long acting
   Chlordiazepoxide
   Diazepam
   Flurazepam
   Prazepam
   Clonazepam

II. Non benzodiazepine

Buspirone, a non benzodiazepine anxiolytic drugs, is a potent antianxiety agent with no addictive potential and for the treatment of generalized anxiety disorder.

Examples:

1. Carbamates:
   Meprobamate, tybamate and carisoprodol

2. Piperidinediones:
   Glutethimide
3. Antihistaminics:
   Diphenydramine, hydroxyzine and pro-methazine
4. Beta – (β) blockers:
   Propanolol

III. Barbiturates

Barbiturates can be divided into 4 main types.

1. Long acting:
   Action is more than 8 hours. Ex: Phenobarbital
2. Intermediate acting:
   Action is 5 – 8 hours. Ex: Amobarbital
3. Short acting:
   Action is 1 – 5 hours. Ex: Secobarbital
4. Ultra short acting:
   Action is less than 1 hour. Ex: thiopentone, methohexital

Side Effects

1. Drowsiness, sedation
2. Ataxia, dizziness
3. Feelings of detachment
4. Increased irritability or hostility
5. Anterograde amnesia
6. Nausea, headache, confusion, depression and urinary incontinence.

Alcoholic Drugs

1. Disulfiram (tetraethyl thiuram disulfide)

It is a drug that can be administered to individuals who abuse alcohol as a deterrent to drinking. This drug interrupts the metabolism of alcohol, causing a build up of a toxic substance in the body if the person uses alcohol in any form.

Disulfiram works by inhibiting the enzyme aldehyde dehydrogenase, thereby blocking the oxidation of alcohol at the stage when acetaldehyde is converted to acetate. This results in an accumulation of acetaldehyde in the blood, which is thought to produce the symptoms associated with the disulfiram alcohol reaction. The physiological response may include a severe headache, nausea, vomiting, flushing, hypotension, tachycardia, dyspnea, diaphoresis, chest pain, palpitations and confusion. Rarely, it can lead to respiratory and cardiac collapse, unconsciousness, convulsions and death.

Symptoms of disulfiram – alcohol reaction can occur within 5 to 10 minutes to ingestion of alcohol and subsides usually within 2 hours of ingestion of alcohol.

The usual dose of disulfiram is 250 – 500 mg/day in the first week and 250 mg/day subsequently for maintenance treatment. The effects begin within 12 hours of first dose and remains for 7 – 10 days after the last dose.

Contraindications

1. First trimester of pregnancy
2. Coronary artery disease
3. Liver failure, chronic renal failure
4. Peripheral neuropathy, muscle disease
5. History of psychosis in past

Disulfiram therapy is not a cure for alcoholism. It provides a measure of control for the individual who desires to avoid impulsive drinking.

Other Deterrent Agents

1. Citrated calcium carbimide
2. Metronidazole
3. Nitrafezole
4. Methyl tetrazolethiol
5. Charcol
6. Cephalosporins

NURSE'S RESPONSIBILITY IN PSYCHOPHARMACOLOGY

- Teach the clients about side-effects of drugs and if any observed ask them to report to the physician instead of discontinuing the medication
- Teach the clients, the methods of managing and avoiding unpleasant side-effects and maintaining the medication regimen
- Ask the client to take sugar free fluids and eating sugar free hard candy to ease dry mouth
- Avoid calorie beverages and candy to avoid weight gain
- Regular exercise
- Consuming water and bulk form foods in diet to overcome constipation
- Stool softners can be avoided
- Usage of sunscreen lotions to overcome photosensitivity
- Monitor sleeping pattern
- A high fiber diet, increased fluid intake and laxative if needed, help to reduce constipation
- Advise the patient to get up from the bed or chair very slowly to prevent orthostatic hypotension
- Check BP before and after medication is given
- Differentiate between akathesia and agitation and inform the physician. a change of drug may be necessary if side effects are severe. Administer antiparkinsonism drugs as prescribed.
- Observe the patient regularly for abnormal movements.
- Take all seizure precautions
- A patient risk for developing agranulocytosis. Monitor TC, DC essentially in the first few weeks of treatment. Stop the drug if the WBC count drops to < 3000/mm3 of blood. The patient should also tell to report if sore throat or fever develops, which might indicate infection.
- Cyclic compounds should be consumed at night in a single daily dose
- Clients should exercise caution when driving or performing activities requiring sharp, alert reflex until sedative effects can be determined.

- Tyramine-rich foods, e.g. beef liver, chicken liver, fermented sausages, dried fish, chocolate, cheese, pizza, meat, bean curd, over ripe fruit, peanuts, beverages like wine, beer and coffee, etc. have to be avoided by the client who are consuming MAO inhibitors which can result in hypertensive crises..
- Report promptly if occipital headache, nausea, vomiting, chest pain, or other unusual symptoms occur; these can herald the onset of hypertensive crisis.
- Instruct the patient not to take any medications without prescription.
- Caution the patient to change his position to avoid orthostatic hypotension.

9 The Therapeutic Community—Milieu Therapy

The world milieu is French for "middle". The English translation of the word is "surroundings or environment".

DEFINITION

According to **Skinner (1979)** a scientific structuring of the environment in order to effect behavioral changes and to improve the psychological health and functioning of the individual. "A therapeutic community is a drug-free environment in which people with addictive (and other) problems live together in an organized and structured way in order to promote change and make possible a drug-free life in the outside society. The therapeutic community forms a miniature society in which residents, and staff in the role of facilitators, fulfill distinctive roles and adhere to clear rules, all designed to promote the transitional process of the residents"(Ottenberg 1993).

Stuart and Sundeen defined therapeutic community as "a therapy in which patient's social environment would be used to provide a therapeutic experience for the patient by involving him as an active participant in his own care and the daily problems of his community".

OBJECTIVES

- To use patient's social environment to provide a therapeutic experience for him
- To enable the patient to be an active participant in his own care and become involved in daily activities of his own community

- To help patient to solve problems, plan activities and to develop the necessary rules and regulations for the community
- To increase their independence and gain control over many of their own personal activities
- To enable the patient to become aware of how their behavior affects others.

ELEMENTS OF THERAPEUTIC COMMUNITY

- Free communication
- Shared responsibility
- Active participation
- Involvement in decision making
- Understanding of the roles, responsibilities, limitations and authorities

PURPOSES

1. Sets limits on disturbing and maladaptive behavior.
2. Teaches psychosocial skill.

COMPONENTS OF THERAPEUTIC COMMUNITY

a. Daily community meetings
   - These meetings are composed of 60-90 patients. All levels of unit staff are involved, including administrative personnel. Acute patients are not involved in the meetings.
   - Meetings should be held regularly for 60 minutes
   - Discussion should focus mainly on day to day life in the unit
   - During discussion patients feelings and behaviors are examined by other members
   - Frank discussion are encouraged ,these may take place with much out poring of emotions and anger

b. Patient Government or Ward council
   - The purpose of patient government is to deal with practical unit details such as house-keeping functions, activity planning and privileges

- A group of 5-6 patients will have specific responsibilities, such as house keeping, physical exercise, personal hygiene, meal distribution, a group to observe suicidal patients. Staff members should be always available
- All decisions should be feedback to the community through the community meetings

c. Staff meetings or review

A staff meeting should be held following each community meeting (patients are excluded and only staff are present). In this meeting the staff would examine their own responses, expectations and prejudice.

d. Living and learning opportunities

Learning opportunities are provided within the social milieu, which should provide realistic learning experiences for the patients.

LENGTH OF TREATMENT IN A THERAPEUTIC COMMUNITY

In general, individuals progress through drug addiction treatment at varying speeds, so there is no predetermined length of treatment. Those who complete treatment achieve the best outcomes, but even those who drop out may receive some benefit. Good outcomes from TC treatment are strongly related to treatment duration, which likely reflects benefits derived from the underlying treatment process. Individuals who complete at least 90 days of treatment in a TC have significantly better outcomes on average than those who stay for shorter periods.

Traditionally, stays in TCs have varied from 18 to 24 months. Recently, however, funding restrictions have forced many TCs to significantly reduce stays to 12 months or less and/or develop alternatives to the traditional residential model .For individuals with many serious problems (e.g. multiple drug addictions, criminal involvement, mental health disorders, and low employment), research again suggests that outcomes were better for those who received TC treatment for 90 days or more.

In the TC, the level of treatment engagement and participation is related to retention and outcomes. Treatment factors associated with increased retention include having a good relationship with one's counselor, being satisfied with the treatment, and attending education classes. Important attributes linked to treatment retention include self-esteem, attitudes and beliefs about oneself and one's future, and readiness and motivation for treatment. Retention can be improved through interventions to address these areas.

CURRENT STATUS OF THE THERAPEUTIC COMMUNITY

Milieu therapy came into its own during the 1960s through early 1980s. The current focus of inpatient psychiatric care has changed. **Hall (1995)** states care is inpatient psychiatric facilities can now be characterized as short and biologically based. By the time patients have stabilized enough to benefit from the socialization that would take place in a milieu as treatment program.

Components

According to **Gunderson (1978)** described 5 components of therapeutic community.

1. Containment
2. Support
3. Structure
4. Involvement
5. Validation

Factors	*Characteristics*
1. Containment	It provides for the physical wellbeing of the patient like food, shelter, treatment, etc.
2. Support	Help the patient feel better and enhance their self esteem. It includes reduce anxiety, secure, provide comfort, smooth communication, suggestions and education.
3. Structure	It deals with predictable organization of place, time and person. It deals with meeting, group sessions and timing of the therapeutic activity.
4. Involvement	It cover the rules and regulations of therapeutic activity. It helps the activity to attend to their social environment and modify maladaptive interpersonal patterns.
5. Validation	It means that the individuality of each patient is recognized. It deals with individual treatment planning, showing respect for a patients rights, and providing opportunities for the patient to fail as well as succeed.

NURSING IMPLICATIONS

The psychiatric nurse should first identify what each patient needs from the therapeutic milieu. The nurse can then engage aspects of the therapeutic milieu to meet the patient's needs by providing the following.

Factors	*Nurses role*
Containment	Limits and controls
Support	Education about patient's illness and treatment plan
Involvement	Opportunities for social interaction
Validation	Acknowledgement of the patient's feeling.

PROMOTING FACTORS OF THERAPEUTIC COMMUNITY

1. Basic physiological needs are fulfilled.
2. The physical facilities are conductive to achievement of the goals of therapy.
3. A democratic form of self government exists.
4. Responsibilities are assigned according to client capabilities.
5. A structured programme of social and work related activities is scheduled a part of the treatment programme.
6. Community and family are included in the programme of therapy in an effort to facilitate discharge from treatment.

VARIOUS ACTIVITIES FOR THERAPEUTIC MILIEU

Whether in a hospital, nursing home, community or at home the care environment should support effective interventions. These are:

1. Cognitive stimulation – for developing or improving patient cognitive functions.
2. Promote calm and quite.
3. Consistent physical layout – provide consistent room arrangement to avoid physical injuries for the disoriented patients.
4. Structured routine: The daily schedule should be as predictable as possible. Like sleep time, time for meals, breakfast and sneaking time etc.
5. Strength and abilities

According to his/her strength and abilities planning his activities.

6. Minimize demands for complainant behaviour.
7. Minimize challenging behaviour.
8. Providing safety.

TEAM MEMBERS OF THERAPEUTIC COMMUNITY

There are psychiatrist, clinical psychologist, psychiatric nurse, psychiatric social worker, occupational therapist, recreational therapist, music therapist, art therapist, psycho dramatist, dieticians and chaplain.

STAFFING

TCs are often staffed by a carefully chosen group of professionals who receive training in the specifics of the TC model. Experts suggest that program staff should comprise a mix of self-help recovered professionals and other traditional professionals (e.g. nurses, physicians, lawyers, case workers, counselors) 8). An average resident to staff ratio was cited as approximately 15:1.

THE DAILY REGIMEN

A typical TC day begins at 7 am and ends at 11 pm and includes morning and evening house meetings, job assignments, groups, seminars, scheduled personal time, recreation, and individual counseling. As employment is considered an important element of successful participation in society, work is a distinctive component of the TC model.

In the TC, all activities and interpersonal and social interactions are considered important opportunities to facilitate individual change. These methods can be organized by their primary purpose, as follows:

- Clinical groups (e.g. encounter groups and retreats) use a variety of therapeutic approaches to address significant life problems.
- Community meetings (e.g. morning, daily house, and general meetings and seminars) review the goals, procedures, and functioning of the TC.

- Vocational and educational activities occur in group sessions and provide work, communication, and interpersonal skills training.

Community and clinical management activities (e.g. privileges, disciplinary sanctions, security, and surveillance) maintain the physical and psychological safety of the environment and ensure that resident life is orderly and productive.

ADVANTAGES OF THERAPEUTIC COMMUNITY

- Patient develops harmonious relationships with other members of the community
- Gains self–confidence
- Develops leadership skills
- Learns to understand and solve problems of self and others
- Becomes sociocentric
- Learns to live and think collectively with the members of the community
- It provides opportunity to participate in the formulation of hospital rules and regulations that affect patient's personal liberties like bedtime, meal time, weekend permission, control of radio or TV, social activities, late night privileges

DISADVANTAGES OF THERAPEUTIC COMMUNITY

- Role blurring between staff and patient
- Group responsibility can easily become nobody's responsibility
- Individual needs and concerns may not be met
- Patient find the transition to community difficult

THE ROLE OF NURSE

Therapeutic Milieu providing inpatient and outpatient setting. In all setting the nursing process is used for the delivery of nursing care. On going assessment, diagnosis, outcome identification, planning, implementation and evaluation are necessary for this successful management of the therapeutic milieu.

1. She involved in all day-to-day activities.
2. Nurses are responsible for ensuring that clients physiological needs are met.
3. Nurses are responsible for the management of medication administration.
4. Nurse should maintain the one to one relationship which helps grows out of a developing trust between nurse and patient.
5. She is responsible for setting limits on unacceptable behaviour in therapeutic milieu.
6. Teacher role: Nurse must be able to assess learning, readiness of the clients. So she can provide information about medical diagnosis side effect of medication and other management etc.
7. Other cares of safety, structure and support.

10 Psychological Therapy

PSYCHOTHERAPY

Definition

Psychotherapy can be defined (Wolbers) as, the treatment by psychological means, of problems of an emotional nature, in which a trained person (therapist) deliberately establishes a professional relationship with the patient to:

1. Remove, modify or retard existing.
2. Mediate disturbed patterns of behavior and/or
3. Promote positive personality growth and development.

Psychotherapy is the use of techniques that facilitate or allow people to modify their feelings, attitudes and behaviors.

Uses

1. To treat an emotional disorder.
2. To treat chronic disorder.
3. To gain insight and self knowledge.
4. To train people in the helping profession.
5. To promote positive personality.

Major Approaches

1. **Supportive Therapy:**

   Supportive therapy allows the client to express feelings, explore alternative and make decisions in a safe, caring relationship, e.g. guidance, occupational therapy, ventilation.

2. **Re-education therapy:**

   It involves new ways of perceiving and behavior. In client explores alternatives in a planned, systematic way, which may require more than 10 – 25 sessions, e.g.

   1. Client-centred therapy
   2. Directive approaches — confrontation, reality therapy.
   3. Casework therapy
   4. Crisis intervention
   5. Biofeedback.

3. **Reconstructive therapy:**

   Reconstructive therapy, typically involving deep psychotherapy or psychoanalysis was pioneered by Freud, Jung and others, e.g.

   1. Classical psychoanalysis
   2. Ego psychoanalysis.

Individual Psychotherapy

One to one relationship between therapist and patient for the therapeutic purpose.

Stages of Psychotherapy

The three stages of psychotherapy are

1. **Introductory stage:**

   In the introductory stage, the client and therapist meet and begin to work together. This stage usually involves taking a history of the client's life, including any medical problems and current medications.

2. **Working stage:**

   In the working stage, the client is able to become more trusting, to disclose and to begin exploring with the therapist the thoughts, feelings and behaviors to problems.

3. **Termination stage:**

   For this stage, client behavior modified or remove the maladaptive symptoms, if it is not changed, allow the next session for the treatment.

Techinques of psychotherapy

1. Ventilation
2. Abreaction
3. Reassurance
4. Suggestion
5. Persuasian
6. Reinforcement
7. Relaxation.

BEHAVIOR THERAPY

Behavior therapy is a type of psychotherapy, which is based on theories of learning. The principles of behavior therapy based on the classical conditioning and operant conditioning.

Classical Conditioning

Classical conditioning is a process of learning that was introduced by the Russian Physiologist Pavlov. This was an important discovery in terms of how learning can occur. Pavlov found that unconditioned responses (salivation) occur in response to unconditioned stimuli (eating food). He also found that over time, an unrelated stimulus (sound of the bell) introduced with the unconditional stimulus could elicit the same response alone that is the conditional response. The unrelated stimulus is called the conditioned stimulus.

Operant Conditioning

Operant conditioning was introduced by skinner, an American psychologist, stimuli are environmental events that interact with and influence on individual's behaviour. Stimuli may precede or follow a behavior. A stimulus that follows a behavior (or response) is called a reinforcing stimulus or reinforcer. The function is called reinforcement.

When the reinforcing stimulus increases the probability that the behavior all reoccur, it is called a positive reinforcer (positive reinforcement) and increasing the probability that a behavior will recur by removal of an undesirable reinforcing stimulus — called as negative reinforce (negative reinforcement).

Techniques for Modifying Client Behavior

1. **Shaping:**
   In shaping the behavior of another, reinforcement are given for increasingly closer approximations to the desired response. For example, in eliciting speech from an autistic child, the teacher may first reward the child for (a) watching the teacher's lips that (b) for making any sound in imitation of the teacher then (c) for forming sounds similar to the word uttered by the teacher.
2. **Modeling:**
   It refers to the learning of new behaviors by imitating the behavior in others. Role models are individuals who have qualities or skills that and person admires and wishes to imitate.

   (Howard, 2000)

   Modeling occurs in various ways. Children imitate the behavior patterns of their parents, teachers, friends and others.
3. **Time out:**
   It is an aversive stimulus or punishment during which the client is removed from the environment where the unacceptable behavior is being exhibited. This is often used in therapy with children.
4. **Flooding:**
   This technique, sometimes known as impulsive therapy, is also used to desensitize individuals to phobic stimuli. This is a method used in treatment to phobias. Here, the person is directly exposed to the phobic stimulus, but escape is made impossible. Through therapist's guidance and encouragement and therapist's modeling behavior, anxiety decreases.
5. **Systematic desensitization:**
   Systematic desensitization was designed to decrease the avoidance behavior linked to a specific stimulus. The goal of

systematic desensitization is to help the patient change his/her response to a threatening stimulus.

(Kormos, 2003)

It is a technique for assisting individuals to overcome their fear of a phobic stimulus. With systematic desensitization, the patient must first be able to relax the muscles. Next, a hierarchy of the anxiety – provoking or feared situations is constructed. This is based on reciprocal inhibition principle (Wolpe introduced).

6. **Aversion therapy:**

   Aversion therapy helps reduce unwanted but persistent maladaptive behaviours. Aversive conditioning applies an aversive or noxious stimulus when a maladaptive behaviour occurs.

   This is used for the treatment of those conditions which are pleasant but undesirable, e.g. alcohol dependence, transvestism, homosexuality, other sexual disorders.
7. **Token economy**
8. **Role playing**
9. **Social skills training**
10. **Overt sensitization**
11. **Covert sensitization**
12. **Reciprocal inhibition**
13. **Extinction**
14. **Cognitive behavior therapy.**

11 Family Therapy

HISTORY

The origins of family therapy are vague. The beginning of family interventions can be traced to the Child-guidance and marriage counseling movements in early 1900s. Sigmund Freud (1909/1977) was the first among to include a parent in the psychotherapy of a child. Freud explained about marital and family relationships and their possible roles in both individual normal development and psychopathology. Freud's description of unconscious processes like introjection, projection, and identification explained how individual experiences could be transmitted across the generations in a family. Freud's successors, Anna Freud, Melanie Klein, and Donald Winnicott, elaborated and modified his formulations.

THE AIMS OF FAMILY THERAPY

The aim of the treatment is to alleviate the problems hat led to the disorder in the identified patient and improve family functioning. Family therapy is advised not only to resolve problems and difficulties but also to teach the family to solve further impasses by itself, to communicate more clearly with one another, to develop strategies for avoidance of conflicts, to accept another's handicaps and differences without blaming and scapegoating, and to foster functional processes for appropriate balancing of competing values such as family cohesiveness and individuation, balanced separateness and togetherness, stability and flexibility (Bodin, 1984).

MODELS OF INTERVENTION

Many models of family therapy exist, none of which superior to others. Whatever the methods, family therapist have the following goals for the family: (a) improved communication, (b) improved autonomy for each member, (c) improved agreement about roles, (d) reduced conflict, and (e) reduced distress in the member who is the patient.

1. Psychodynamic Methods

These methods use concepts taken from the psychoanalytical treatment of individual patients. it is assumed that current problems in the family originates in the separate past experiences of its individual members, particularly those of the parents. Present problems arise in part from unconscious conflict within individual members. Family members need to gain insight in these conflicts in order to change their behavior. The therapist's goal is to help members to gain these insights into their own unconsciousness, and into the ways in which one person's problems may interlock with those of other. The therapist does this by examining the relationship between himself and the different family members to throw light on the conscious aspects of the problems. The therapist may give interpretations but is not directive.

2. Bowen Model

Murray Bowen called his model family systems. Here the person's differentiation form his family of origin, their ability to be their true selves in the face of familial and other pressures that threaten the loss of love or social position. Problem families are assessed on two levels: the degree of their enmeshment versus the degree of their ability to differentiate and the analysis of emotional triangles in the problem for which they seek help. An emotional triangle is defined as a three-party system arranged so that the closeness of two members expressed as their love or repetitive conflict tends to exclude the third. Emotional cross currents can happen when the excluded person tries to join one of the other. The therapist's role is, first , to stabilise or shift the short triangle and second to work with the most psychologically available family members, individually if necessary, to achieve enough personal differentiation so that the short triangle does not recur. Therapist has to keep his neutrality. Bowen also originated the 'genogram'.

3. Structural Family Model

The term family structure refers to a set of unspoken rules that recognise the ways in which family members relate to one another. Some rules determine the hierarchy in the family. Some rules determine cooperation in the family. Rules also determine the boundaries: sometimes these are broken, for example when an unhappy wife involves her son involves her son in the problems with her husband. In structural family therapy, hypotheses are presented to the family in a paradoxical way: for example, you seem to be very dependent on your wife: what does she do to make you feel less competent?¡¦ Some interventions may increase family tension in the short-term until a new set of rules is established.

4. General Systems Model

It is based on the general systems theory originally developed by Von Bertalanffy (1962). It is the study of the relationships between and among interacting components of a system that exists over time. The family is construed similarly as a system. Families have external boundaries and internal rules. Every member presumed to play a role (spokesperson, persecutor, victim, rescuer, symptom bearer, nurturer), which is relatively stable, but which member each role may change. Some families scapegoat one member by blaming him or her for the families problems. The general systems model overlaps with some of the other models, particularly Bowen and Structural models.

5. Eclectic Methods

Comprehensive review of outcome research suggests that many models equally effective in most situations. But levels of effectives vary with variety of clinical problems. But often a combined approach is used in practice.

Indications for Family Therapy

Family therapy is a mode of psychological treatment, and does not constitute a unitary approach. The problem in relating can involve a couple, a parent-child dyad, siblings, or any member of the family.

Six categories can be listed as indication of family therapy:

1. The clinical problem manifests in explicitly family terms, i.e. family dysfunction. For example, a marital conflict dominates; with repercussions for the rest of the family; or tension between parents and an adolescent child dislocates family life with everyone get involved in the prevailing conflict. Here family therapy is the treatment of choice.
2. The family has experienced a major stressful or disruptive life event, which has led or is leading to dysfunction. These events are either predictable or accidental and include, for instance, accidental or suicidal death, severe financial embarrassment, diagnosis of a serious physical illness, the unexpected departure of a child from the home, and so forth. As such, any family equilibrium that previously prevailed has been disturbed; the ensuing disequilibrium becomes associated with family dysfunction and/or the development of symptoms in one or more members.
3. Continuing demanding circumstances in a family are of such a magnitude as to lead to poor or inappropriate adjustment. The family's resources may be stretched to the tilt; external sources of support may be scanty or unavailable. Typical situations are chronic physical illness, persistent or recurrent psychiatric illness, and the presence in the family of a frail elderly member.
4. An identified patient may have become symptomatic in the context of a poorly functioning family. Symptoms are an expression of that dysfunction. Depression in a mother, an eating problem in a daughter, alcohol misuse in a father, on

family assessment, are adjudged to reflect underlying family difficulties.

5. A family member is diagnosed as having a specific conventional condition such as schizophrenia, agoraphobia, obsessive-compulsive disorder, or depression-the complicating factors are the adverse reverberations in the family stemming from that diagnosis. For example, the son with schizophrenia taxes his parents in ways that exceed their problem-solving' capacity; an agoraphobic woman insists on the constant company of her husband in activities of daily living; a recurrently depressed mother comes to rely on the support of her eldest daughter. In these circumstances, family members begin to respond maladaptively towards the diagnosed relative, which paves the way for deterioration of his condition, manifest as chronicity or a relapsing course.
6. Thoroughly disorganized families, faced by many problems, are viewed as the principal target of help, e.g. one member abuses drugs, another is prone to violence, and a third manifests antisocial behaviour.

Contraindications for Family Therapy

These are more straightforward than indications.

1. The family is unavailable because of geographical dispersal or death.
2. There is no shared motivation for change. One or more family members may wish to participate, but their chances of benefiting from a family approach are likely to be less than if committing themselves to individual therapy. (Need to distinguish here between poor motivation and ambivalence; in the latter, the assessor teases out factors that underlie the ambivalence and may encourage the family's engagement).
3. The level of family disturbance is so severe or long-standing, or both, that a family approach seems prognostically futile. For example, a family that has fought bitterly for years is unlikely to engage in the constructive purpose of exploring their patterns of functioning.

4. Family equilibrium is so precarious that the inevitable turbulence arising from family therapy is likely to lead to decompensation of one or more members; for example, a sexually abused adult may do better in individual therapy than by confronting the abusing relative.
5. The patient is too incapacitated to withstand the demands of family therapy. The person in the midst of a psychotic episode or someone buffeted by severe melancholia is too affected by the illness to engage in family work.

Structure and Composition of Therapy

- Family therapy may be conducted with:
- One patient or client present (e.g. Bowen family systems therapy).
- May be limited to the nuclear family (e.g. behavioral, psychoanalytic), or
- May even be transgenerational (e.g. structural, symbolic-experimental).
- Combined therapies (e.g. individual and family) are more common.
- Most family therapy is conducted by a single therapist, though cotherapy (especially of one male and one female therapist) is somewhat common in training centres, and is even preferred in some family therapy approaches (e.g. contextual, symbolic-experiential).
- The length of family therapy ranges from ideal courses of fewer than ten visits (e.g. Mental Research Institute brief therapy) to up to dozens of visits (e.g. Bowen family systems) or even hundreds (e.g. psychoanalytic) over several years.
- Most family and couple therapy lasting 10 to 20 sessions over a period of less than 6 months.
- Family therapy is typically conducted in private offices and clinics but not uncommonly takes place on hospital wards and even in family homes.

The Process of Family Therapy

Steps in the process of family therapy include: assessment and goal-setting, formulation of hypothesis, working phase, evaluation, termination. These steps may overlap as hypotheses can be formulated during the process of assessment. Similarly, evaluation and assessment can be done anytime during working phase.

Assessment and Goal Setting

Family assessment, an extension of conventional individual psychiatric assessment, adds a broader context to the final formulation. It has four phases.

- History from the patient
- A provisional formulation concerning the relevance of the family
- An interview with one or more family members, and
- A revised formulation.

A. History from the Patient

The most effective way to obtain a family history is by constructing a family tree. Apart from showing the family structure, it allows further information to be added summarising important events and a wide range of family features. Personal details can be recorded for each family member such as age, date of birth and death, occupation, education and illness, as well as critical family events (for example, migration, crucial relationship changes, notable losses, and achievements), and the quality of relationships. Following questions give more information:

- Who knows about the problem?
- How does each of them see it?
- Has anyone else in the family had similar problems?
- Who have you found most helpful, and least helpful thus far?
- What do they think needs to be done?

The presenting problem and changes in the family

Questions aimed at understanding the current context include:

- What has been happening recently in the family?

- Have there been any changes (e.g. births, deaths, illness, losses).
- Has your relationship with other family members changed?
- Have relationships within the family altered?'

B. The Wider Family Context

- Questions about the family's response to major events can be posed: for example, ¡¥How did the family react when your grandmother died? Who took it the hardest?
- Relationships should be explored at all levels, covering those between the patient and other family members and between those other members themselves.
- Conflicted ties are particularly illuminating. Understanding the roles' taken by members is also useful: Who tends to take care of others? Who needs most care? Who tends to be the most sensitive to what is going on in the family?

C. The Family in Problem Maintenance

Interactions revolving around the patient's illness may act to maintain it.

- First, the illness becomes a way of 'solving' a family problem, e.g. Anorexia nervosa in a teenager due to attend a distant university may lead to her abandoning this plan since she feels unable to care for herself. Were she to leave, parental conflict would become more exposed and her mother, with whom the patient is in coalition against her father, would find herself unsupported. The illness therefore keeps the patient at home and enmeshed in the parental relationship, and also provides a focus for shared concerns and an ostensible sense of unity.
- Maintenance of the illness does not solve a family problem, but may have done so in the past.
  - In the previous example, the father's mother died 9 months later. His wife subsequently expressed feelings of closeness, feelings not experienced by him for years; their relationship gradually improved. Both parents, however, continued to treat their daughter as incapable of achieving autonomy,

reinforcing her own uncertainty about coping independently if she were to recover.

D. The Family Interview

- A non-judgemental stance is important.
- Introductions are made in the initial phase.
- Names and preferred modes of address are clarified.
- The therapist then explains the meeting's purpose, details of which may crucially influence future family participation.
- The therapist invites everyone to share their views about the nature and effects of problems they have encountered.
- The therapist may have an idea about how the identified patient's problems relate to family function, and can test it out by asking probing questions and observing interactions.
- This idea is characteristically kept private since it is unhelpful for a hypothesis to be put forward prematurely.
- Triadic relationships can be scrutinized both through questioning (what does A do when B says this to C?) and observation (what does A do when B and C reveal tensions?).
- A third person may be asked to comment on what two others convey to each other when a particular event occurs.
- The discussion then extends to all spheres of family life: beliefs, traditions, rules, and values.
- Concerns are attended to and the members strengths and efforts acknowledged.
- The interview concludes with a summary of what has emerged.
- Arrangements are made for a follow-up session.

E. Revised Hypotheses Formulation

- Since more information becomes available at each level, the initial formulation can be revised as necessary.
- The five observational levels of structure, transitions, relationships, patterns of interaction, and global family functioning are re-examined in terms of the family as reactive, resourceful, or problem-maintaining.

- Appropriate interventions can be planned, at least for a follow-up session. We can now turn to the course of typical family therapy.

Working Phase

Based on the theoretical orientation of the therapist, intensity of the problem and information gathered in the assessment phase, therapy progresses. There can be altercations among the members, but the therapist should intervene only when required. Observation of the interaction of family members help the therapist to verify the information already gathered. Depending on the assessment made in the initial session, therapist can decide on the number of sessions.

Termination

A regular review of goals help the therapist in planning the final phase. If objectives are clear and the process is moving towards the termination is easy. Follow-up may be required on regular basis.

Role of the Family Therapist

Beels and Ferber, among the first observers to consider various roles for family therapists, divided them into 'conductors' and reactors'.

- The therapist as a conductor is represented in the work of practitioners like Satir, Bowen, and Minuchin. Satir emphasises on communication, the family therapist is a teacher who shares expertise in optimal communication by setting goals and the direction of treatment. The therapist is an explicit authority, who intervenes actively in implementing change.
- The therapist as reactor plays a different role by resonating with, and responding to, what the family manifests. Therapists in the psychoanalytical tradition belong to this group. Typically, the therapist shares observations about patterns of interaction and relating that emerge during the sessions. Problems encountered in therapy

- Family treatment does not always succeed. Indeed, deterioration may occur, albeit in a small percentage of cases.
- What common difficulties are encountered?
  - Missed appointments may punctuate the course of therapy, often linked to turbulent experiences between sessions or apprehension about what a forthcoming session may reveal.
  - Like any psychotherapy, drop-out is possible. On occasion, this is appropriate in that the indication for family therapy was misconstrued. In other circumstances, drop-out is equivalent to failure and may derive from such factors as therapist ineptitude, unearthing of family conflict which they cannot tolerate, and inappropriate selection of family therapy based on faulty assessment.
  - The family's dysfunction may be so intractable that it proves impervious to change, the family may lack the psychological sophistication required, members may retreat in the face of change because of insecurity..
  - Dependency becomes a problem as the family discards any vestige of autonomy and encounters a greater security when relying on the authority of the therapist
  - Finally, part of the family may harbor a secret that threatens the principle of open communication between members

12 Occupational Therapy

The word "occupational therapy" means "to occupy" (Occupy – to employ, busy, engage and take up) George–Barton

Definition

Occupational therapy is the application of goal oriented purposeful activity in the assessment of individual with psychological, physical or developmental disabilities — Susan B Fine

Occupational therapy is defined as "an active method of treatment with a profound psychological justification

— Clark(1963).

Major Goals of Occupational Therapy

To enable the patient to achieve a healthy balance of occupations through the development of skills.

Sub – goals are:

i. To remove or minimize behaviours that interfere with occupational performance.
ii. To arouse interest, courage and confidence.
iii. To exercise mind and body in activity.
iv. To reestablish the capacity for social usefulness.

Services of Occupational Therapy

- Independent living skills, self care/self maintenance, e.g. bathing, washing, combing, dressing.
- Task oriented treatment – Crafts, play, socialization, leisure time.

- Work adjustment program:
  Home making : child care/parenting.
- Sensory motor treatment (Neuromuscular)
- Design, fabrication and application of arthotic devices.
- Therapeutic exercise.
- Discharge planning and community re-entry.
- Patient or family education and counseling.

Benefits of Occupational Therapy

i. Diversion of mind
ii. Expression of emotion
iii. Skill building
iv. Helps process of intervention

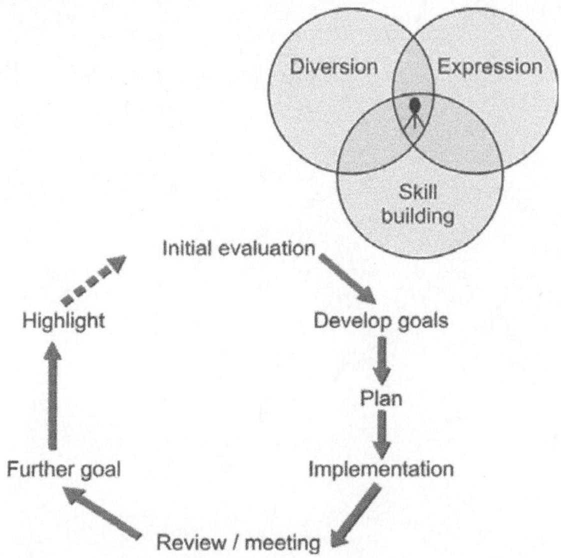

Advantages

1. Diverts the patients attention from himself on to other things.
2. His interests and energies are directed to work.
3. Maintain normal habits of work.
4. Provides an incentive and a goal.
5. Stimulates interest and attention.

6. May teach the patient a new skill/hobby.
7. Feeling of doing something useful.
8. Offers opportunities to explore and re-evaluate self concepts and objects concepts.
9. Helps to make the patient more accessible and more co-operative with other therapy.
10. Enable the patient to have a feeling of achievement when he completes the task.

Adoption Studies

In studies conducted by both American and Danish investigators, adopted children born of schizophrenic mothers were compared with adopted children whose mothers had on psychiatric disorder. It was found that the children who were born of schizophrenic mother were more likely to develop the illness than the comparison control groups **(Black and Andreasen, 2003).**

Biochemical Influences

(i) **The Dopamine Hypothesis**

Schizophrenia may be caused by an excess of dopamine – dependent neuronal activity in the brain. Dopamine is important in responses to stress and has many connections to the limbic system. Dopamine is present in high levels in the brain, when schizophrenia usually appears. Serotonin and Glutamine also cause the schizophrenia.

(ii) **Neurobiology**

Research suggests that the prefrontal cortex and the limbic cortex ma never fully develop in the brains of persons with schizophrenia.

Computed tomography (CT) and Magnetic Resonance Imaging (MRI) studies of brain structure show decreased brain volume in people with schizophrenia. Findings include, larger lateral and third ventricles, atrophy in the frontal lobe, cerebellum and limbic structures and increased size of sulci on the surface of the brain.

Position Emission Tomography (PET) scans usually demonstrate decreased cerebral blood flow to the frontal lobes with schizophrenia.

Psychotic behaviors may be related to – lesions in the frontal, temporal and limbic regions of the brain and dysregulation of neurotransmitter systems connecting these regions.

Viral Theories

Evidence indicates that prenatal exposure to the influenza virus, particularly during the second trimester, may be one of the factors in the etiology of schizophrenia in some people but not in others.

Another research findings revealed that more people with schizophrenia are born in the winter or early spring and in urban setting (Crowded places).

Environmental Influences

(1) **Stressful Events**

There is no scientific evidence to indicate that stress causes schizophrenia. It is known that extreme stress can precipitate psychotic episodes. The stress can be biological, environmental or both. The environmental component can be either biological (e.g. an infection) or psychological (e.g. a stressful family situation). Stressful like events ma be associated with exacerbation of schizophrenic and increased rates or relapse.

Sociocultural Factors

Some therapists proposed that poverty, society and cultural disharmony could cause schizophrenia or that people chose to become schizophrenia to cope with the insanity or the modern world. Research shows that greater numbers of individuals from the lower socioeconomic classes experience symptoms associated with schizophrenia. Other causes of schizophrenia.

- Congested housing accommodations
- Associated with living in poverty
- Inadequate nutrition
- Absence or prenatal care
- Feeling of hopelessness for changing one's life style of poverty.

Assessment

Schizophrenia can identify through history collection, physical examination and mental status examination.

History

Outline of psychiatric history
Name, age , address of patient, name of informant if any and their relationship to the patient
History of present condition
Family history

Personal History

- Early development, health during childhood, nervous problems in childhood, education, occupation, menstrual history, sexual history, marriage,

Past illness

- Past physical illness, medical illness, forensic history

Personality

- Relationships, leisure activities, prevailing mood, character, attitudes and standards, premorbid personality

Drugs, alcohol, tobacco

Mental Status Examination

General appearance and behavior

Deteriorated appearance and manners

Often disheveled with poor personal hygiene

May dress bizarrely

Social withdrawal

Shifting emotional tone or no emotional tone at all

Difficulty establishing rapport

Lack of motivation

Often shows lack of concern about illness

General lack of planning and action

Disorders of thought and speech

Loose associations

Ranges from loosening of logical association to complete incomprehensibility and "word salad".

The individual seems completely unaware that they are incomprehensible.

Thought blocking

Poverty of content

Inability to use abstract concepts

Loss of prosody

Mutism

Neologisms

Stilted language

Echolalia

Loss of ego boundaries

Disorders of affect

Reduced emotional response

Ranges from blunted to completely restricted.

Should be interpreted in appropriate cultural context.

Inappropriate responses

Bizarre emotions

Intensely positive or intensely negative Extreme emotional sensitivity Strong simultaneous ambivalence
Disorders of behavior Stereotyped behavior Stuporous states Catatonia, waxy flexibility Far less common today than 60-70 years ago Eating disorders Self-induced water intoxication Echopraxia Negativism Somatic symptoms Range from plausible and mild to bizarre and severeHowever, some will not complain about even very seriousmedical conditions.
Disorders of perception Hallucinations Auditory are most common but any kind is possible A voice keeping a running commentary or twovoices at one time are especially significant Unusual perceptual sensations Often involves sensory unfamiliarity with normalsurroundings Delusions Usually of the referential, persecutory, orgrandiose variety Neurological signs and symptoms Rapid and frequent blinking Rapid eye movement Some lose of natural gracefulness and fine motorcoordination Poor left-right discrimination Difficulty with rapid oppositional movement Difficulty identifying common objects by touch

PHASES OF SCHIZOPHRENIA

The pattern of development of schizophrenia, which can be viewed in 4 phases.

Phase I: The Schizoid Personality

The DSM – IV TR (APA, 2000) describes these individuals as indifferent to social relationship and having a very limited range of emotional experience and expression. They appear cold and aloof.

However, most schizophrenia patients evidence if having these characteristics in the premorbid condition.

Phase II: The Prodromal Phase

This phase having following symptoms — social withdrawal, impairment in role functioning, peculiar behaviour, neglect of personal hygiene, inappropriate affect disturbances in communication and lack of initiative, interests or energy.

Phase III: Schizophrenia

Here, psychotic symptoms are prominent. According to DSM – IV TR diagnostic criteria for schizophrenia.

1. Two or more of the following, each present for a significant portion of time during a one month period (or less if successfully treated.
   b) Delusion
   c) Hallucinations
   d) Disorganized speech
   e) Grossly disorganized or catatonic disorders
   f) Negative symptoms – affective flattening, alogia/avolition.
2. One or more major areas of functioning such as work, interpersonal relations, or self care are markedly below the level achieved before the onset (or when the onset is in childhood or adolescence, failure to achieve expected level of interpersonal, academic or occupational achievement).
3. Continuous signs of the disturbance persist for at least 6 months.
4. Schizoaffective and mood disorder with psychotic features have been ruled out.
5. The disturbance is not due to the direct physiological effects of a substance or a general medical condition.
6. Relationship to a pervasive developmental disorder.

If there is a history of autistic disorder or other pervasive developmental disorder, the additional diagnosis of schizophrenia is made only if prominent delusions or hallucinations are also present for at least 1 month (or less if successfully treated).

Phase IV: Residual Phase

It is characterized by periods of remission and exacerbation. It usually follows an active phase or the illness.

MANAGEMENT OF SCHIZOPHRENIA

Old:
- Psychoanalysis
- Shock treatment (Insulin, ECT)
- Lobotomy
- Institutionalization

New:
- Antipsychotic drugs, also known as neuroleptic drugs
- ECT
- Psychosocial Treatment- Psychotherapy to help increase functioning and compliance in taking medications
- Psychosurgery-limbic lobotomy.

1. Antipsychotic Medications

Typical Antipsychotics
- Chlorpromazine
- Thioridazine
- Trifluperazine
- Haloperidol
- Pimozide
- Triflupromazine
- Prochlorperazine
- Flupenthixol
- Zuclopenthixol

Side Effects

- Antiadrenergic effects—Sedation, postural hypotension, inhibition of ejaculation

- Extrapyramidal effects: Movement symptoms such as Parkinson's-like shaking (pseudoparkinsonism), dystonia, akathesia and tardive dyskinesia
- Anticholinergic effects: dry mouth, reduced sweating, urinary hesitancy and retention, constipation and blurred vision, precipitation of glaucoma
- Other effects: cardiac arrhythmias, weight gain, amenorrhea, galacorroea, hypothermia
- Work best with type I

Atypical Antipsychotics
- Clozapine
- Resperidone
- Olanzapine
- Quetipine
- Ziprezidone
- Aripiprazole

Side Effects

- Less side effects
- Agranulocytosis
- Weight gain

Depot antipsychotics
- Fluphenazine deconate
- Flupenthixol
- Zuclopenthixol
- Haloperidol

2. ECT

- Catatonic stupor
- Uncontrolled catatonic excitement
- Acute exacerbation not controlled with drugs
- Severe side effects with drugs

3. Psychosocial Treatment

1. Psychoeducation
2. Group psychotherapy

3. Family therapy
4. Milieu Therapy
5. Individual psychotherapy
6. Psychosocial rehabilitation

   Psychotherapy: Addresses coping mechanism, family relationships, social skills

4. Hospitalization, Day Programs may be Necessary

Management in Special Groups

Children, elderly and pregnancy

- Children and elderly are more prone to develop side effects. Elderly may have impaired renal and hepatic function
- Pregnancy- because o the risk of developing teratogenesis
- Breastfeeding mothers- caution

Nursing Management

Nursing Diagnosis: Disturbed Sensory Perception (Specify: Visual, Auditory, Kinesthetic, Gustatory, Tactile, Olfactory

- Change in the amount or patterning of incoming stimuli accompanied by a diminished, exaggerated, distorted, or impaired response to such stimuli.

Assessment

- Hallucinations (auditory, visual, tactile, gustatory, kinesthetic, or olfactory)
- Listening intently to no apparent stimuli
- Talking out loud when no one is present
- Rambling, incoherent, or unintelligible speech
- Inability to discriminate between real and unreal perceptions
- Attention deficits
- Inability to make decisions
- Feelings of insecurity
- Confusion

Expected Outcomes

- Demonstrate decreased hallucinations
- Interact with others in the external environment

- Verbalize knowledge of hallucinations or illness and safe use of medications
- Participate in the real environment
- Make sound decisions based on reality
- Participate in community activities or programs

Nursing interventions	*Rationale*
Be aware of all surrounding stimuli, including sounds from other rooms (such as television or stereo in adjacent areas).	Many seemingly normal stimuli will trigger or intensify hallucinations. The client can be overwhelmed by stimuli.
Try to decrease stimuli or move the client to another area.	Decreased stimuli decreases chances of misperception. The client has a diminished ability to deal with stimuli.
Avoid conveying to the client the belief that hallucinations are real. Do not converse with the "voices" or otherwise reinforce the client's belief in the hallucinations as reality.	You must be honest with the client, letting him or her know the hallucinations are not real.
Explore the content of the client's hallucinations during the initial assessment to determine what kind of stimuli the client is receiving, but do not reinforce the hallucinations as real. You might say, "I don't hear any voices-what are you hearing?"	It is important to determine if auditory hallucinations are "command" hallucinations that direct the client to hurt himself or herself or others. Safety is always a priority.
Use concrete, specific verbal communication with the client. Avoid gestures, abstract ideas	The client's ability to deal in abstractions is diminished. The client may misinterpret your gestures
Avoid asking the client to make choices. Don't ask "Would you like to talk or be alone?" Rather, suggest that the client talk with you.	The client's ability to make decisions is impaired, and the client may choose to be alone (and hallucinate) rather than deal with reality (talking to you).
Respond verbally and reinforce the client's conversation when he or she refers to reality.	Positive reinforcement increases the likelihood of desired behaviors.
Encourage the client to tell staff members about hallucinations.	The client has the chance to seek others (in reality) and to cope with problems caused by hallucinations.
If the client appears to be hallucinating, attempt to engage the client's in conversation or a concrete activity.	It is more difficult for the client to respond to hallucinations when he or she is engaged in real activities and interactions.

Contd...

Contd...

Maintain simple topics of conversation to provide a base in reality.	The client is better able to talk about basic things; complexity is more difficult.
Provide simple activities that the client can realistically accomplish (such as uncomplicated craft projects).	Long or complicated tasks may be frustrating for the client. He or she may be unable to complete them.
Encourage the client to express any feelings of remorse or embarrassment once he or she is aware of psychotic behavior; be supportive.	It may help the client to express such feelings, particularly if you are a supportive, accepting listener.
Show acceptance of the client's behavior and of the client as a person; do not joke about or judge the client's behavior.	The client may need help to see that hallucinations were a part of the illness, not under the client's control. Joking or being judgmental about the client's behavior is not appropriate and can be damaging to the client.

Nursing Diagnosis: **Disturbed Personal Identity**

- Inability to distinguish between self and nonself

Assessment data

- Bizarre behavior, Regressive behavior, Loss of ego boundaries (inability to differentiate self from the external environment), disorientation, disorganized, illogical thinking, flat or inappropriate affect, feelings of anxiety, fear, or agitation, aggressive behavior toward others or property

Expected Outcomes

- Be free from injury
- Not harm others or destroy property
- Establish contact with reality
- Demonstrate or verbalize decreased psychotic symptoms and feelings of anxiety, agitation, and so forth
- Participate in the therapeutic milieu
- Express feelings in an acceptable manner
- Reach or maintain his or her optimal level of functioning
- Cope effectively with the illness
- Continue compliance with prescribed regimen, such as medications and follow-up appointments

appropriate to place the delirious patient in a room close to the nursing station or other workstation.

- Sun downing can be lessened by leaving a radio on in the patient's room
- It has long been recognized that, in certain cases, the hallucinations of delirium can be specifically treated: visual hallucinations by controlled visual stimuli, auditory hallucinations by music and other meaningful external sounds, and olfactory hallucinations by the introduction of odors or scents
- To help the patient perceive the environment accurately, adequate daytime lighting and a night light should be provided
- Hearing aids, eyeglasses and other devices that assist sensory perception should be used whenever possible and should not be put away during a delirious episode.
- One of the most helpful interventions is having family members stay with the patient. Family members should also be encouraged to bring personal effects from home, because some patients with delirium are greatly comforted by the presence of familiar photographs or objects.

Cognitive interventions

Reorientation is one of the most easily accomplished cognitive interventions. The first step is to place a clock and a calendar where the patient can see them easily. The patient should then be verbally reoriented to time and place several times over the course of the day. Repetition is recommended to compensate for memory impairment in the delirious patient.

Psychologic interventions

The delusions expressed by a patient should not be directly disputed. Instead, alternative explanations of events should be offered, and frequent reassurance should be given.

Pharmacologic Interventions

- 100 mg of B_1 IV for thiamine deficiency and IV fluids for fluid and electrolyte imbalances.

- Symptomatic management: as many patients are agitated, emergency psychiatric treatments may be needed. Small doses of benzodiazepines (lorazepam or diazepam) or antipsychotics (haloperidol) may be given orally or parenterally.

Prognosis

Resolution of symptoms may take longer in patients with poor pre- morbid cognitive function, incorrect or incomplete diagnosis of contributing factors, and structural brain diseases treated with large doses of psychoactive medications prior to the onset of acute medical illness.

For some patients, the cognitive effects of delirium may resolve slowly or not at all.

Patient Education

- Educating families and patients regarding the etiology and course of disease is an important role for physicians.
- Educate the patient, family, and primary caregivers about future risk factors.
- Families may worry that the patient has brain damage or a permanent psychiatric illness. Providing reassurance that delirium often is temporary and is the result of a medical condition may be beneficial to both patients and their families.
- Suggest that family members or friends visit the patient, usually one at a time, and provide a calm and structured environment.

Encourage them to furnish some familiar objects, such as photos or a favorite blanket, to help reorient the patient and make the patient feel more secure.

Nursing Management

Assessment

- Client history : from the clients history, nurses should assess the following areas of concern.

  Type, frequency, and severity of mood swings, personality and behavioral changes catastrophic emotional reactions

- Cognitive changes such as problems with attention span, thinking process, problem-solving
- Language difficulties
- Orientation to person, place, date and situation
- Appropriateness of social behavior.

Physical Assessment

Assessment should focus on two main areas:
- Signs of damage to the nervous system
- Evidence of diseases of other organs

Nursing Diagnoses

1. Risk for trauma related to impairment in cognitive and psychomotor function
   Outcome criteria : Client will not experience injury
   Interventions:· Arrange furniture and other items in the room to accommodate clients disabilities
   - Store frequently used items within easy access
   - Do not keep bed in elevated position
   - Assist the client with ambulation
   - Keep a dim light on at night
   - Frequently orient the client to place ,time and situation
   - Soft restraints may be required if client is very disoriented and hyperactive
2. Disturbed thought process related to cerebral degeneration as evidenced by disorientation, confusion, memory deficits and inaccurate interpretation of the environment.
   Outcome criteria: Client will interpret the environment accurately and maintain reality orientation to the best of his or her cognitive ability.
   Interventions:· Frequently orient the client to reality. Use clock and calendars with large numbers that are easy to read:
   - Notes and large bold signs may be used as reminders
   - Keep explanation simple
   - Discourage rumination of delusional thinking

- Talk about real people and real events
- Monitor for medication side effect

3. Self care deficit related to disorientation, confusion and memory deficits as evidenced by inability to fulfill the ADL Outcome criteria: Client will accomplish the ADLs to the best of his or her ability. Unfulfilled activities may be kept by caregivers.
   Interventions:
   - Identify the self care deficits and provide assistance as required
   - Provide guidance and assistance for independent actions
   - Provide a structured schedule of activities that does not change from day to day
   - Provide for consistency in assignment of daily caregivers
   - Perform ongoing assessment of clients ability to fulfill nutritional needs ,ensure personal safety ,follow medication regimen and communicate need for assistance with activities that she or he cannot accomplish independently
   - Involve the family members in the care of the patient

DEMENTIA

Introduction

It is a chronic organic mental disorders. It mainly affect the intellectual abilities and normal functioning. The term dementia is derived from the Latin *demens,* meaning "without mind".

Definition

Dementia is defined as a loss of intellectual abilities of sufficient severity to interfere with social or occupational functions.

— Niraj Ajuha (2006)

It is characterized by the following main features:

1. Impairment of intellectual function
2. Impairment of memory (Predominantly of recent memory, especially in early stages).
3. Deterioration of personality with lack of personal care.

Epidemiology

About 10 to 20% of all persons above age 65 has mild to moderate dementia, Alzheimer's disease is the most common dementia disorder. Dementia is most common in elderly people; it used to be called senility and was considered a normal part of aging.

- About 4-5 million people in the United States have some degree of dementia, and that number will increase over the next few decades with the aging of the population.
- Dementia affects about 1% of people aged 60-64 years and as many as 30-50% of people older than 85 years.

Etiology

Mnemonic- "VINDICTIVE MAD".

A. Degenerative Diseases of the Central Nervous System.

1. Senile dementia
2. Alzheimer's disease
3. Pick's disease
4. Huntington's chorea
5. Parkinson's disease
6. Creutzfeldt-Jakob disease
7. Normal pressure hydrocephalus
8. Multiple sclerosis
9. Lewy body disease.

B. Intracranial Causes

- Space-occupying lesions — Tumors, chronic subdural hematomas, chronic abscesses, aneurysm

C. Vascular Causes

1. Multi-infarct dementia
2. Occlusion of the carotid artery
3. Stroke
4. Hypertension
5. Cranial arthritis

D. Metabolic and Endocrine Disorders

1. Endocrinopathies – Addison's disease, Cushing's syndrome, hyperinsulinism, hypothyroidism, hypopituitarism, hypoparathyroidism, hyperparathyroidism.
2. Hepatic failure
3. Renal failure
4. Renal dialysis
5. Respiratory failure
6. Hypoxia
7. Chronic uremia.
8. Chronic electrolyte imbalance.
9. Hypocalcemia
10. Hypercalcemia
11. Hypokalemia
12. Hyponatremia
13. Hypernatremia
14. Remote effect of carcinoma or lymphoma.

E. Nutritional Causes

1. Sustained lack of B_{12} pernicious anemia
   a) Niacin - Pellagra
   b) Thiamine - Wernicke - Korsakoff's syndrome
2. Vitamin intoxication — vitamin A , vitamin D – Paget's disease

F. Traumatic Causes

1. Severe single head injury
2. Repeated head injuries in boxers and others.

G. Infections and related conditions

1. Encephalitis of any cause
2. Neurosyphilic
3. Chronic meningitis
4. Cerebral sarcoidosis
5. Cysticercosis
6. AIDS and AIDS-related complex.

H. Toxic Causes

1. Alcohol
2. Poisoning with heavy metals — lead, arsenic, thallium, mercury, carbon monoxide.
3. Drug and alcohol withdrawal of anxiolytic sedative drugs, amphetamine.

I. Anoxia

1. Anemia
2. Postanesthesia
3. Cardiac arrest
4. Chronic respiratory failure.

SIGNS AND SYMPTOMS

At the initial stages of dementia, patients show fatigue, difficulty in sustaining mental performance, and a tendency to fail when a task is novel or complex or requires a shift in problem-solving strategy. The inability to perform tasks becomes increasingly severe and spreads to every day tasks, such as grocery shopping as the dementia progresses. Eventually, patients with dementia may require constant supervision and help to perform even the most basic tasks of daily living. The major defects in dementia involve orientation, memory, perception, intellectual functioning and reasoning and all these functions become progressively affected as the disease process advance. Affective and behavioral changes, such as defective control of impulses and liability of mood, are frequent, as are accentuations and alterations of premorbid personality traits.

1. **Intellectual deterioration with failure of:**
   a. **Memory:** Memory impairment is typically an early and prominent feature in dementia, especially in dementias involving the cortex, such as dementia of the Alzheimer's type. Early in the course of dementia, memory impairment is mild and is usually most marked for recent events; people forget telephone numbers, conversations and events of the day. As the course of dementia progresses, memory impairment becomes severe and only the earliest learned information is retained.

b. **Orientation:** In as much as memory is important for orientation to person, place and time, orientation can be progressively affected during the course of a dementing illness. For example, patients with dementia may forget how to get back to their rooms after going to the bathroom. No matter how severe the disorientation seems, how every, patients show no impairment in their level of consciousness.
c. **Language:** Dementing processes that affect the cortex, primarily dementia of the Alzheimer's type and vascular dementia, can affect patient's language abilities. Aphasia is one of the diagnostic criteria of dementia . The language difficulty may be characterized by a vague, stereotyped, imprecise or circumstantial locution, and patients may also have difficulty in naming objects.
d. **Thinking and Judgment:** Thinking becomes slower with reduced flow of ideas and impaired concentration; Judgment is impaired from early on and leads to poor insight; Paranoid thoughts and ideas of reference are common and may develop into delusions.
e. **Comprehension of Learning Capacity:** The brain ability to process incoming information is impaired.
f. **Calculation:** This cognitive skill is usually impaired from early on dementia.
g. **Insight**
h. **Concentration**

2. **Emotional changes:** Emotions become too easily stimulated, and have reduced control over laughter or tears.
3. **Deterioration of personality:**
   a. Increasing tendency to selfishness.
   b. Lack of consideration for other people's feelings.
   c. Personal habits, table manners, toilet, habits and hygiene deteriorate.
   d. Sexual offences may be committed.

   Changes in the personality of a person with dementia are especially disturbing for the families of affected patients. Pre-existing personality traits may be accentuated during the development of a dementia. Patients with dementia may also become introverted and may seem to be less concerned than they previously were about the effects of their behavior on others. People with dementia who have paranoid delusions are generally hostile to family members and caretakers. Patients with frontal and temporal involvement are likely to have marked personality changes ad may be irritable and explosive.

4. **Age-related body system changes**
   a. **Cardiovascular system:**
      - Decreased cardiac output.
      - Diminished ability to respond to stress.
      - Slower heart recovery rate, increased BP.
      - Leads to fatigue with increased activity.

   b. **Respiratory system:**
      - Increase in the residual lung volume
      - Decrease in vital capacity
      - Decreased gas exchange of diffusing capacity
      - Decreased cough efficiency
      - Leads to fatigue and breathlessness with sustained activity, impaired healing of tissue due to decreased oxygenation, difficulty in coughing up secretions.

   c. **Integumentary system:**
      - Decreased protection against trauma
      - Decreased protection against temperature extremes.
      - Diminished secretion of natural oils and perspiration.
      - Thin and wrinkled skin
      - Complaints of injuries bruises and sunburns.
      - Complaints of intolerance to heat.
      - Bone structure is prominent dry skin.

   d. **Reproductive system:**

      Female-vaginal narrowing and decreased elasticity, decreased vaginal secretion
      - Painful intercourse, vaginal bleeding following intercourse, vaginal itching and irritation, delayed orgasm.

Male: Decreased size of penis and testes slower sexual response.

- Delayed erection and achievement of orgasm.

e. **Genitourinary system:**

- Bladder capacity decrease, delayed sensation to void leads to urinary retention and difficulty to voiding.

Male: Benign prostatic hypertrophy

Female: Relaxed perineal muscle frequency and incontinence of urine

f. **Gastrointestinal system:**

- Decreased salivation
- Difficulty in swallowing food
- Complaints of dry mouth
- Delayed esophageal and gastric emptying leads to complaints
- Of fullness, heartburn and indigestion
- Reduced gastrointestinal mobility leads to constipation, flatulence and abdominal discomfort.

g. **Musculoskeletal system:**

- Loss of bone density, muscle strength and size, degenerated joint cartilage leads to height loss, kyphosis, fracture, complaints of backpain, loss of strength, flexibility and endurance and joint pain.

h. **Nervous system:**

- Reduced speed in nerve conduction, increased confusion with physical illness and loss of environmental cues , reduced cerebral circulation causes slower to respond and react , learning takes longer , becomes confused, complaints of forgetfulness and frequent falls.

5. **Special Senses**

Vision: Diminished ability to focus on close objects , inability to tolerate glare, difficulty in adjusting changes of light intensity, decreased ability to distinguish colors. As a result holds objects for away from face, complaints of glare, complaints of poor night vision and confusion color.

Hearing: Decreased ability to hear high frequency sounds Results in inappropriate responses, asks people to repeat words .Strains forward to hear .

Taste and smell: Decreased ability to taste and smell, results in excessive use of sugar and salt.

6. **Hallucinations and Delusions:**

   As estimated 20 to 30 percent of patients with dementia, primarily patients with dementia of the Alzheimer's type, have halluci-nations and 30 to 40 percent have delusions, primarily of a paranoid or persecutory and unsystematized nature, although complex, sustained and well systematized delusions are also reported by these patients. Physical aggression and other forms of violence are common in demented patients who also have psychotic symptoms.

7. **Other Signs and Symptoms:**

   Psychiatric: 40 to 50 percent of patients with dementia are having anxiety and depression , in addition to psychosis and personality changes patients with dementia may also exhibit pathological laughter or crying , extremes of emotions – with no apparent provocation .

   Neurological: In addition to the aphasias in patients with dementia, apraxias and agnosias are common other neurological signs that can be associated with dementia are seizures, seen in approximately 10 percent of patients with dementia of Alzheimer's type and in 20 percent of patients with vascular dementia, and atypical neurological presentations , such as non-dominant parietal lobe syndromes, primitive reflex — such as the grasp , snout , suck , tonic — may be present on neurological examination and myoclonic jerks are present in 5 to 10% of patients..

   Headaches, dizziness, faintness, weakness, focal, neurological signs and sleep disturbance are some of the additional neurological symptoms in-patient with vascular dementia. Cerebrovascular disease pseudobulbar palsy, dysarthria and dysphagia are also more common in vascular dementia than in other dementing conditions.

Catastrophic reaction: Patients with dementia also exhibit reduced ability in abstract attitude patients have difficulty in generalizing from a single instance , in forming concepts and in grasping similarities and differences among concepts. Catastrophic reaction marked by agitation secondary to the subjective awareness of intellectual deficits under stressful circumstances.

Sundown syndrome: This is characterized by drowsiness, confusion ataxia and accidental falls. It occurs in older people who are overly sedated and in patients with dementia who reach adversely to even a small dose of a psychoactive drug. The syndrome also occurs in demented patients when external stimuli, such as light and interpersonal orienting cues are diminished. It most commonly occurs as a result of benzodiazepines.

Types of Dementia

I. As per details of dementia types

1. **Cortical and Subcortical Dementia**

   Dementia may be associated with multiple subcortical or cortical infarcts and clinical features vary according to that.

Distinguishing Features of Subcortical and Cortical Dementia

Non-Alzheimer's dementia basically means subcortical dementia. Some distinguishing features of sub cortical and cortical dementia are as follows:

	Subcortical dementia	*Cortical dementia*
1. Language	No aphasia	Aphasia early
2. Memory	Impaired recall >recognition	Recall and recognition impaired equally
3. Attention and immediate recall and visuospatial skills	Impaired	Impaired
4. Calculation	Preserved until late	Involved early
5. Frontal system abilities (executive function)	Disproportionately affected	Degree of impairment consistent with other involvement

Contd...

Contd...

	Subcortical dementia	*Cortical dementia*
6. Speed of cognitive processing	Slowed early	Normal until late in disease
7. Personality	Apathetic inert	Unconcerned
8. Mood	Depressed	Euthymic
9. Speech	Dysarthric	Articulate until late
10. Posture	Bowed or extended	Upright
11. Co-ordination	Impaired	Normal until later
12. Motor speed and control	Slowed	Normal
13. Adventitious movements	Chorea, tremor, tics, dystonia	Absent (Alzheimer's dementia: some myoclonus).

2. **Reversible Dementia and Nonreversible Dementia.**

Reversible dementia — is a term used in the medical literature to describe a dementia that as a specific treatable cause. In the past, dementia has implied a progressive or irreversible course. Potentially reversible dementia syndromes include those arising from inflammatory processes, e.g. encephalopathy caused by systemic lupus erythematosus (SLE) , infections such as syphilis; or toxic conditions (e.g. Alcohol abuse) that produce memory loss and abnormal frontal lobe functions (Cummings 1987). Metabolic related dementia such as hypothyroidism or hyperthyroidism and nutritional syndromes such as vitamin B_{12} and rotate deficiencies may also be reversible with appropriate therapy. It is estimated that 30% to 40% of persons with memory disturbances have a reversible and there fore treatable dementia. Although most of the patients will have physical disorders, psychiatric disturbances such as depression are a significant challenge in the differential diagnosis. Treatment of such conditions as depression, drug – induced dementia, infections and metabolic disturbances leads to complete restoration off functioning with prompt diagnosis and appropriate treatment the dementia can be reversed.

Non-reversible dementia: When a reversible cause of intellectual impairment can't be identified, the clinical diagnosis is presumed to be a nonreversible dementia many diseases can produce a progressive and nonreversible dementia. Most of these are rare and can affect adults of all ages with older individuals more likely to be affected when dementia does occur in a younger person it have been associated with suicide (Margo and Finkel 1990). The most common nonreversible dementia are Alzheimer's disease, Parkinson's disease, Huntington's disease, pick's disease, Creutzfeldt– Jakob disease and multi – infarct dementia. transient ischomic attack (TIAs) are included in the category because they can lead to a disabling cerebral infarction.

3. **Presenile Dementia and Senile Dementia**

   Presenile dementia: It resembles that of senile dementia except that disorders occurs in younger age group . the onset of disease occurs in people of 40s and 50s and people with this disease live an average 11 years after the onset of disease.

   Senile dementia : It occurs usually after the age of 65 yrs. Due to degenerative bring changes as accompanied by a clinical picture of mental deterioration. The types of senile dementia are already mentioned previously.

II. Types of dementia according to underlying etiology.

A. Dementia in Alzheimer's disease:

Alzheimer's disease was first described by Alois Alzhemer, a German neurologist in 1906. Alzheimer's disease is a primary degenerative cerebral disease of unknown etiology, with characteristic neuropathological and neurochemical features. The onset can be in middle adult life or even earlier but the incidence is higher in later life. In cases with onset before the age of 65-70 years. There is the likelihood of a family history of dementia, a more rapid course and prominence of features of parietal and temporal lobe damage, including dysphasia or dyspraxia, general impairment of higher cortical function.There are characteristic changes in the brain: a marked reduction in the population of neuron, particularly in the hippocampus, appearance of neurofibrillary tangles, neurotic plagues, which consist largely of amyloid. Marked reduction in the enzyme chorine acetyl transference in acetylcholline it self.

Sign and Symptoms

Insidious onset with slow deterioration while the onset usually seems difficult to pinpoint in time, realization by others that the defects exist may come suddenly.Absence of clinical evidence of findings from special investigation, to suggest that the mental state may be due to other systemic or brain disease which can induce a dementia. Absence of a sudden, apoplectic onset, or have neurological signs of focal damage such as hemiparesis, sensory loss, visual field defects, and in coordination occurring early in the illness.

a. **Dementia in Alzheimer's disease with early onset**
   - Dementia in Alzheimer's disease beginning before the age of 65 years
   - Evidence of relatively rapid onset and progression.
   - In addition to memory impairment, there must be rapid deterioration, disorders of the higher cortical functions, Aphasia, Agraphia, alexia and aparaxia occur relatively early onset of dementia.

b. **Dementia in Alzheimer's disease with late onset**
   Dementia in Alzheimer's disease with late on set where the clinically observable onset in after the age of 65 years and usually in the late 70s or there after with a slow progression and usually with memory impairment as the principal feature.

c. **Dementia in Alzheimer's disease, a typical or mixed type.**
   This term and code should be used for dementia that have important atypical features or that fulfill criteria for both early – and late onset types of Alzheimer's disease.

d. **Dementia in Alzheimer's disease unspecified.**

Four A's of Alzheimer's Disease

1. **Amnesia:** Inability to learn new information or to recall previously learned information.
2. **Agnosia**: Failure to recognize or identify objects despite intact sensory function.
3. **Aphasia**: Language disturbances that can manifest in both understanding and expressing the spoken word.
4. **Apraxia:** Inability to carry out motor activities despite intact motor function (e.g. ability to grab a doorknob but not knowing what to do with it.)

B. **Vascular Dementia**

Vascular dementia which includes multiinfarct dementia, is distinguished from dementia in Alzheimer's type by history of onset. There is a history of transient ischaemic attacks with brief impairment of consciousness, fleeting pareses or visual loss. Cerebrovascular accidents cause impairment of memory and thinking becomes apparent. Onset in later life can be abrupt in ischaemic episode or gradual emergences. The dementia is result of infraction of brain due to vascular disease including hypertensive cerebrovascular disease.Vascular dementia is the second commonest type of dementia. This disorder arises earlier between 50 and 60 years of age, but more prevalent between ages 60-70 years. It is slightly more common in male than in females.

Clinical Features

- The patient develops multiple episodes of cerebral ischemia which may or may not be apparent.
- Impairment of cognitive function.
- Memory disturbances.
- Intellectual deficits
- Focal neurological sign changes.
- There may be aphasias, disarthria, and dysphagia.
- There may be headache, dizziness, faintness , weakness, sleep disturbance and personality changes.
- Insight and judgment may be preserved.
- An abrupt onset or a step wise deterioration.·Seizure occurs in 20 percent of cases.

a. **Vascular dementia of acute onset:**

This dementia develops rapidly (i.e. usually within one month but with in no longer than 3 months) after a succession of strokes or a single large infarction.

b. **Multi-infarct dementia:**

This is more gradual in onset than the acute form , following a number of minor ischemic episodes which produce an accumulation of infarcts in the cerebral parencyma.

c. **Subcortical vascular dementia**
   There may be a history of hypertension. There is evidence of foci of ischemic destruction in the deep white matter of the cerebral hemispheres.
   Which can be suspected on clinical groups and demonstrated on computerized cortex is preserved and this contrasts with the clinical picture, which may closely resemble that of dementia in Alzheimer's disease.
d. **Mixed cortical and subcortical vascular dementia.**
   Mixed cortical and sub cortical components of the vascular dementia may be suspected from the clinical features, the results of investigation (including autopsy) or both.
e. **Other vascular dementia**
f. **Vascular dementia, unspecified.**

3. Dementia in Other Disease

Cases of dementia due to cause other than Alzheimer's disease or vascular disease. Onset may be at any time in life, rarely in old age.

a) **Dementia in Huntington's disease**
   Huntington's disease is an autosomal dominant disorder caused by a gene which has been localized to the most distal band of the short arm of chromosome 4. Therefore 50% of the children of one affected parent can develop this disorder. Spontaneous mutations can also give rise to sporadic cases in which there is no known family history.

Pathological Features

Microscopically the brain is usually small with reduced mass and there is marked atrophy of the corpus striatum of the basal ganglia, particularly the caudate nucleus, and of the frontal lobes.

Histological change include neuronal loss in the cerebral cortex, particularly affecting the frontal lobes, and in the corpus striatum, particularly affecting GABA neurons.

Biochemical changes include reduced levels of GABA and glutamic acid decarboxylase, and dopamine hypersensitivity. Huntington disease – the coronal section shows atrophy of caudate nucleus.

Clinical Features

- Males and females are affected equally by Huntington's disease and the average age of onset is in the 30s.
- Insidious onset of involuntary choreiform movement disorder.
- Involuntary choreiform movements in face, hands, shoulder or in the gait.
- Slurring of speech, extra pyramidal rigidity and epilepsy.
- Psychiatric features include depression, increased risk of suicide and schizophreniform and delusional disorders.
- Insight tends to be retained until a late stage.
- Death usually occurs within 15 years of the onset of symptoms.

Although there is no known cure, phenothiazine antipsychotics in low doses may be given to help with emotional disturbance, while depression may be treated with antidepressants. Involuntary movements may be decreased by giving tetrabenzine. This may act by causing dopamine depletion at never endings, but may cause depression to develop, thereby limiting.

b. **Dementia in Pick's Disease**

It occurs in middle life usually between 50 and 60 years, characterized by slowly progressing changes of character and social at deterioration, memory impairment, impairment of intellect and language functions with apathy, euphoria and extra pyramidal phenomena. There will be atrophy of the frontal and temporal lobes, but with out the occurrence of neuritic plaques and neurofibrillary tangus in excess of that seem in normal aging.

Signs and Symptoms

- Onset is slow with steady deterioration.
- A predominance of frontal lobe involvement is evidenced by two or more of the following:
  - Emotional blunting
  - Coarsening of social behaviour
  - Disinhibition
  - Apathy or restlessness
  - Aphasia

– Behavioral manifestations which precede memory impairment.

c. **Dementia in Creutzfeldt-Jakob Disease**
Creutzfeldt– Jakob disease with extensive neurological signs due to specific neuropathological changes that are presumed to be caused by a transmissible agent, onset is middle age or later age typically in the fifth decade, but may be at any adult age. The course is subacute, leading to death within 1-2 years.

Signs and Symptoms

There is very rapid progression of dementia with disintegration of virtually all higher cerebral functions. One or more of the following types of neurological symptoms and signs emerge, usually after or simultaneously with the dementia.

- Pyramidal symptoms
- Extrapyramidal symptoms
- Cerebellar symptoms
- Aphasia
- Visual impairment

d. **Dementia in Parkinson's Disease**
Parkinson's disease is a disorder of a nucleus of norm cell, deep in the centre of the brain, called the substantia nigra. Because of the death of cells in this nucleus there is a reduction in the neurotransmitter dopamine and cause the typical symptoms. The dementia in parkinsonism develop is thought to be due to reduction in acetylcoline and the evidence in affected of cell death in the nucleus of Meynert.

Signs and Symptoms

- Rigidity
- Shuffling gait
- Mask like face
- Mumbling of speech
- Hypokinesia
- Difficulty in co-ordination.

e. **Dementia in Human Immunodeficiency Virus (HIV) Disease**
A disorder characterized by cognitive deficits meeting the clinical diagnostic criteria for dementia. HIV dementia presents with complaints of forgetfulness, slowness, poor concentration and difficulties with problem solving and reading, Apathy, reduced spontaneity and social withdrawal are common and in significant minority of affected disorder, psychosis or seizure. Tremor, impaired rapid, repetitive movements, imbalance, ataxia, hypertonia, generalized, hyper reflexia. Positive frontal release signs and impaired pursuit and saccadic eye movement, children also develop and HIV associated neurodevelopmental disorder characterized by developmental delay, hypertonia, microcephaly and basal ganglia calcification.

f. **Alcoholism Dementia**
Chronic alcoholics develop a specific recent memory loss called Korsakoff's syndrome. This is progressive if the person continues to drink or as after a head injury or stroke, some recovery of function may be possible over months or even years. Since it does not affect the over all functions of the cerebrum, Korsakoff's syndrome is not strictly speaking a dementia. There is evidence that some alcoholics develop a more generalized shrinking of the brain which shows up on CT scanning. This shrinkage is a sign of developing general dementia.

Assessment

1. **Hospitalization**
Clear indication for hospitalization are need for diagnostic procedure. A history of rapidly symptoms, and the rupture of patient, usual support system also indication for hospitalization any adverse changes in symptoms, external behaviour or attitude of support system is sufficient to warrant hospitalization.
2. **History Taking**
This is the baseline from which all other information is judged by history taking information continues to be relevant in other ways throughout the illness. History of both patients and families are very important.

a. **The patient's history.**

The patient's history gives information about the past, which comes from the patient, older and more important memories may be maintained late in dementia because they have been rehearsed often over the years that they are very fixed, because patient returns to these memories when the present and recent past are fading. In the earliest stages she will be able to given quite a full account of her life up to recent times, this information must be checked for memories become incomplete and time sequences muddled. These more or less muddled memories are important in understanding how the patient reacts to her/his illness.

b. **The relative's history**

From relative's history we can obtain more information about patients previous personality, attitudes, level of activity, interests, social functioning and self care it is important to help the relatives separate recent events, from events that happened before dementia. This information will provide clear evidence of how much changes has occurred and also helps in understanding what new problems that family is having to cope with and so helps to explain their reactions.

History taking gives the essential baseline in assessing what support the patient can expect from family and friends, what interests and activities might continue to engage in and what her living conditions are we need to know whether a good supportive relationship has existed in the pass or whether there was animosity or indifference.

3. **The Physical Examination**

A physical examination should be done where indicated and this is particularly important in the following circumstances.

- Where physical symptoms such as weight loss, pain are present.
- Where the patient has a history of potentially relevant physical disorder like a history of endocrine disorder including an appropriately detailed neurological assessment with particular attention to vision and hearing.

Systemic observation should be made of his behaviour provide a scheme for assessing memory for general events, past personal events and recent personal events which gives a useful indication of the severity of intellectual handicap.

Physical Investigation

- Hemoglobin , TLC, DLC,
- Blood sugar – In diabetes
- Blood Urea- For renal disease
- Serum creatinine
- Thyroid function test – Hypo/hyperthyroidism.
- Liver function test – Liver disease
- Serum calcium – Parathyroidism
- VDRL – Neurosyphillis
- Serum copper – Wilson's disease
- HIV – AIDS
- EEG – To find out the focal sign
- ECG – To find out cardiac problems
- CT – Scan
- MRI
- Fundus examination – Evidence of atherosclerosis

4. **Psychological Testing**

   Psychometric tests depends on the patient's cooperation but can be valuable when it is done by experienced tester. They may help in localizing lesion in certain sites. They are of more value in monitoring changes in psychological functioning over time and assessing patterns of disability as a basis for planning rehabilitation. Some of the tests are:

   a. **Wechsler Adult Intelligence Scale (WAIS)**

      This is a well standardized test providing a profile of verbal and non-verbal abilities Analysis of subscores, can provide useful information for diagnosis. Organic impairment is indicated by a discrepancy between performance IQ and verbal IQ.

   b. **Perceptual functions, especially spatial relationship**

      This test is exemplified by the Benton Revised Visual Retention test, which requires the patient to study and reproduce ten designs.

c. **New Learning as a test of memory**

There are many new word learning tasks for example the Walton Black modified word learning test and the paired associated learning test, both of which give a useful quantitative estimate of memory impairment.

d. **Specific test**

This test are the Wisconsin card sorting test for frontal lobe damage and the token test for receptive language disturbance.

e. **Dementia Rating Scale**

In this test 2 types of rating scale is used, the intellectual and behavioral. This scale have been over used in diagnosis and limited value in identifying problems. They are most informative when used to measure the progression of impairments over time and to predict the future care needs of the patient.

5. **Mental Status Examination**

The purpose of the mental state examination is to detect abnormal features in a patient's behavior and state of mind at the time of the assessment. If the abnormal features are found this information contributes to the diagnostic process. The examination consists of systemic observation of the patient during the interview and various aspects of their thinking , feelings , perceptions and cognitive functioning , impairment of memory, orientation and consumption problems.

a. **General appearance and behavior.**

Abnormalities in patient's appearance and behavior may point to organic impairment , in an early dementia or minor dementia or minor delinquency in a confusional state. Rather more specific abnormalities that reflect the patient's failing intellectual powers. In appearance and behavior observe the pt. May restrict his activities to an increasingly limited area within which he is able to cope. He will often repeat things that he has done several times. Apparently without any awareness of what he is doing. It is an inability

to stop one thing and move on to next. Appearance following things to be noted:
- Neatness
- Untidy
- Appropriateness
- Cleanliness
- Apparent age, etc.

b. **Speech**

Speech may show a variety of more or less non-specific anomalies together with restriction of content, difficulty in finding words and naming objects, reduced fluency, repetition, preservation and lastly speech is striking when it occurs again be alert to any neurological abnormalities.

c. **Attitude**

Observe the attitude of the patient whether it may:
- Co-operative
- Hostile
- Suspicious
- Fearful
- Evasive, etc.

d. **Mood**

Organic mood change is an impoverishment of mood. The patients emotional response lack of depth and are poorly sustained. They may show more specific changes:
- Emotional incontinence
- Excessive laughing or crying initiated by frivol stimuli and then continuing unchecked.
- Threshold effects: No apparent response up to level of stimulation and then a sudden excessive reaction.
- Incongruous emotion
- Failure to respond to significant stimuli but excessive respond to trivial stimuli.
- Catastrophic reaction
- A sudden explosive outburst of rage and distress often prompted by the recognition of falling powers. This is the first signal of early organic impairment .

e) **Cognitive function**

Organic states such as toxic confusional states and dementia's are not difficult to diagnose once they are well established cognitive impairment may indicate organic etiology, cognitions are:

- Orientation
- Memory
- Concentration and attention

If any impairment in these cause may lead to dementia.

Orientation

Orientation is tested in time, place and person. A patient is fully oriented if he/she known,

what time it is?

where he is ?

who are the people around him ?

Disorientation for time is not necessarily sign of organic impairment. Distress are being in unfamiliar surroundings is enough to cause a greater or lesser degree of disorientation. Ask the patient the day of the week and the date. Find out if the patient knows qualitatively, where he is in time. A patient who is merely distressed and unfamiliar surroundings, is unlikely to have lost tract of time to point where he no longer knows even qualitatively where he is in time.

Testing orientation for place, ask the patient where he is, if patients is not able to tell then organically impaired. Testing orientation for person, if the patient knows who you and who other people around him are.

Memory

Memory is tested as recent and remote recent memory is tested with new learning, It is the ability to retain and recall new information remote memory is tested that the ability to recall.

- **Recent memory:** To test for recent memory ask to patients, what did you eat for lunch ? (Verify)

- **Remote memory**: For testing remote memory ask him:
  - Birth date
  - Stories from childhood
  - Current Indian President
- **Retention of memory**: For testing this ask the patient to repeat the names of 3 items that you list (immediately and in 5 minutes).

Concentration

Concentration is the capacity for sustained attention, it is tested both in its own right, and because normal concentration is condition of adequate performance in any other test. The serial seven test. In this ask the patient to take seven away from a hundred, until he/she gets down to naught – write down what patient says as he says it, marking any errors and the time is taken, with this we can fine the patients concentration other test also can applied for concentration like counting forwards or reciting the days of the week forwards.

Intelligence

In intelligence test IQ test is done. It is verbal and performance, Verbal IQ is concerned with language function and performance IQ with arithmetic and visuospatial functions.

In dementia there is a fall in full scale. This may be difficult to assess at an early stage. It has to be judged against previous academic and employment achievements. Verbal IQ is more dependent than performance IQ on long established skill and therefore relatively protected in early dementia. A performance IQ is more than 20 points below verbal IQ may be significant.

f. **Thought content**

   The content of the patient's thought like their behavior and speech, reflects the decline in their intellectual functions in being impoverished may also show concrete thinking. This can be tested by asking the patient to explain the meaning of a common proverb, e.g. ask to explain "Do not cry over split milk" or "Astilch in time", etc.

g. **Judgment**
It can be tested by asking "what would you do with a stamped, addressed letter that you find out on the side walk "or why are criminals put in to prison".

h. **Delusions**
Organic delusion is characterized by their form. They are poor quality delusion, a product of combined intellectual and emotional impoverishment functional delusions are poorly sustained coming and going in a few hours or days, simple rather than elaborate, lacking in emotional intensity.

i. **Hallucinations**
Where organic delusions are poor quality delusions but organic hallucinations are good quality hallucinations. Organic hallucinations are visual formed being of people animals and things, coloured moving often show size distortion, etc.

j. **Rapport**
At the end of the examination the examiner should evaluate how friendly and open the relationship with the patient was, whether the patient was frank, hostile or guarded, evasive and negative. The patient's responses to both the examination and examiner are important factor in the overall quality of the mental status examination.

Management of Dementia

The dementia in these conditions may be reversible or partially reversible, even if the underlying disease or damage is not.

1. Basic Investigations

Complete blood count, urinalysis, blood glucose, serum electrolytes, renal function tests, thyroid function test, serum biz and arterial PO_2 and PCO_2, X-ray chest, X-ray skull, EEG, lumbar puncture, RT scan/MRI scan of brain.

2. Treatment of Underlying Causes If Treatable

Some underlying causes of dementia are treatable (Reversible dementia)

Treatment – HT – for MID
Thyroxine – Hypothyroid for Hypothrome Dementia
Levodopa – Parkinsonism.

Care of Dementia

1. *Head injury:* The resulting damage of brain cells can lead to dementia.
2. *Infections:* Infections of brain structures, such as meningitis and encephalitis, are primary causes of dementia. Other infections, such as HIV/AIDS and syphilis, can affect the brain in later stages. In all cases, inflammation in the brain damages cells.
3. *Normal pressure hydrocephalus:* If fluid builds up in the ventricles, the fluid pressure remains normal ("normal pressure hydrocephalus"), but brain tissue is compressed from within.
4. *Simple hydrocephalus:* Simple hydrocephalus may cause typical dementia symptoms or lead to coma. In normal pressure hydrocephalus, people have trouble walking and become incontinent (unable to control urination) at the same time they start to lose mental functions, such as memory. If normal pressure hydrocephalus is diagnosed early, the internal fluid pressure may be lowerable by putting in a shunt. This can stop the dementia, the gait problems, and the incontinence from getting worse.
5. *Brain tumors:* Tumors can cause dementia symptoms in a number of ways. A tumor can press on structures such as the hypothalamus or pituitary gland, which control hormone secretion. They can also press directly on brain cells, damaging them. Treating the tumor, either medically or surgically, can reverse the symptoms in some cases.
6. *Toxic exposure:* People who work around solvents or heavy metal dust and fumes (lead especially) without adequate protective equipment may develop dementia from the damage these substances can cause to brain cells. Some exposures can be treated, and avoiding further exposure can prevent further damage.

7. *Metabolic disorders:* Diseases of the liver, pancreas or kidneys can lead to dementia by disrupting the balances of salts and other chemicals in the blood. Often, these changes occur rapidly and affect the person's level of consciousness. This is called delirium. Although the person with delirium, like the person with dementia, cannot think well or remember, treatment of the underlying disease may fully reverse the condition. If the underlying disease persists, however, brain cells may die, and the person will have dementia.
8. *Hormone disorders:* Disorders of hormone-secreting and hormone-regulating organs such as the thyroid gland, the parathyroid glands, the pituitary gland, or the adrenal glands can lead to hormone imbalances, which can cause dementia if not corrected.
9. *Poor oxygenation (hypoxia):* The most common causes of hypoxia are lung diseases such as emphysema or pneumonia. Cigarette smoking is a frequent cause of emphysema. It can worsen hypoxic brain damage by damaging the lungs and also by increasing the levels of carbon monoxide in the blood. Heart disease leading to congestive heart failure may also lower the amount of oxygen in the blood. Sudden, severe hypoxia may also cause brain damage and symptoms of dementia.
10. *Drug reactions, overuse, or abuse:* Some drugs can cause temporary problems with memory and concentration as side effects in elderly people. The most common culprits are sleeping pills and tranquilizers. Other drugs that cause dry mouth, constipation, and sedation ("anticholinergic side effects") may cause dementia or dementia symptoms. Illegal drugs, especially cocaine (which affects circulation and may cause small strokes) and heroin (which is very anticholinergic) may also cause dementia, especially in high doses, if taken for long periods, or in older people. The withdrawal of the drug usually reverses the symptoms.
11. *Nutritional deficiencies:* Deficiencies of certain nutrients, especially B vitamins, can cause dementia if not corrected.

12. *Chronic alcoholism:* Dementia in people with chronic alcoholism is believed to result from other complications such as liver disease and nutritional disorders, etc.

Medical care should focus on optimizing the individual's health and quality of life while helping family members cope with the many challenges of caring for a loved one with dementia. Medical care depends on the underlying condition, but it most often consists of medications and nondrug treatments such as behavioral therapy.

Correcting Drug Doses and/or Withdrawing Misused Drugs

Many require ongoing medications for chronic conditions such as heart failure, high blood pressure, high cholesterol, diabetes, prostate enlargement, and many others.

Reviewing these medications can reveal incorrect doses, drug interactions, side effects, or poor compliance (taking drugs inappropriately or not at all) that could be responsible for part or all of the person's dementia symptoms.

Slowing Progression of Dementia

Dementia due to some conditions, such as Alzheimer's disease, can sometimes be slowed in the early-to-intermediate stages with medication. The medications that have worked the best so far are the cholinesterase inhibitors.

Cholinesterase is an enzyme that breaks down a chemical in the brain called acetylcholine. Acetylcholine acts as an important messaging system in the brain.

Cholinesterase inhibitors, by stopping the breakdown of this neurotransmitter, increase the amount of acetylcholine in the brain of a person with dementia and improve brain function. These drugs not only improve or stabilize mental functions, they may also have positive effects on behavior and activities of daily living.

They are not a cure, and in many people the effect is fairly modest. In others, these drugs do not have much of a noticeable effect. Moreover, the effects are temporary, since these drugs do not change the underlying medical condition.

Another drug, memantine (Namenda), which works in a different way, is showing promise in certain types of dementia.

Medications

Except for the cholinesterase inhibitors, the US Food and Drug Administration (FDA) has not approved any drug specifically for dementia. The drugs listed here are some of the most frequently prescribed from each class.

Cholinesterase inhibitors - Tacrine (Cognex), donepezil (Aricept), rivastigmine (Exelon), galantamine/galanthamine (Reminyl).

Antidepressants/anxiolytics - Fluoxetine (Prozac), sertraline (Zoloft), paroxetine (Paxil), citalopram (Celexa).

Antipsychotics – Haloperidol (Haldol), risperidone (Risperdal), quetiapine (Seroquel), olanzapine (zyprexa), ziprasidone (Geodon).

Anticonvulsants - Valproic acid (Depakote), carbamazepine (Tegretol) gabapentin (Neurontin), lamotrigine (Lamictal).

Noortropics: Piracetam, Oxiracetam, Aniracetam derivatives of GABA are postulated to have neuroprotective effect on CNS against hypoxia

Ergoloidmesylate: Hydergine is currently used for the non-specific cognitive impairment.

Aspirin and NSA ID: Data suggests that it protect against the development of disease due to its anti-inflammatory properties

Estrogen Therapy: Estrogen therapy in postmenopausal women might help in the delaying the development of dementia.

Sabeluzole: This substance shown to protect neuronal cells against gutamate induced and hypoxia induced injury and may potentiate the tropic effect of nerve growth factor. It may improve long term memory of elderly patient.

Rivastigmine: Rivastigmine in the dose of 6 to 12 mg/day was given to two groups. One group of patient was Alzheimer's disease with vascular risk factor as hypertension and other group was without risk factor. After 26 weeks of trial vascular risk factor group showed significant improvement. Rivastigmine in diffuse Lewy body dementia had shown improvement in cognition particularly attention and in psychiatric symptoms.

Nitrendipine: Elderly people who were suffering from systolic hypertension when treated with nitrendipine, a calcium channel blocker occurrence of dementia was less in this group.

Gingko Biloba, Ginseng: It is also helpful in demented patient.

All drugs cause side effects. In prescribing a drug, doctors weigh whether the benefits of the drug outweigh the side effects. Seniors are especially likely to experience drug side effects. People with dementia who are taking any of these drugs must be checked often to make sure that the side effects are tolerable.

Surgery: No accepted surgical treatment can manage dementia. Surgery is reserved for specific conditions underlying dementia that might improve the condition, such as removal of a brain tumour or drainage of excess cerebrospinal fluid.

Other Therapy

- Occupational therapy may help persons with dementia with activities of daily living such as feeding oneself.
- Physical therapy may improve mobility by teaching patients to use canes or walkers properly and showing them how to get in and out of chairs or beds.
- Music and art activities may be soothing and rewarding for some people with dementia.
- Respite care, having a person with dementia go temporarily to a nursing home, is another important source of help for family caregivers.

Psychotherapy

The specific psychotherapy treatments divided in to 4 broad of range: Behavior-oriented, emotion-oriented, cognition- oriented and stimulation-oriented, behavior approached can be effective in lessening or abolishing problem behaviour, e.g. aggression, incontinence emotion oriented intervention include supportive psychotherapy reminiscence therapy sensory integration and stimulated presence therapy.

a. *Behavior-oriented approaches:* It can be effective in lessening or abolishing where it occurs, how often it occurs have to be determined. The next step is an assessment of specific antecedents and consequences, which will often suggest specific strategies for intervention. Precipitants should be avoided whenever possible.

Whatever intervention, it is critical to match the level of demand on the patients with his or her current capacities, to modify the environment in so far as possible to compensate for deficits and capitalize on the patient's strengths.

b. *Emotion-oriented approaches:* The intervention includes supportive psychotherapy, reminiscence therapy, validation therapy, sensory integration and simulated presence therapy.
   - Reminiscence therapy, which acme to stimulate memory and mood in the context of the patient's life history is associated with modest short lived gain in mood.
   - Validation therapy, aims to restore self-worth and reduce stress by validating emotional ties to the post.
   - Simulated presence therapy may be helpful in diminishing problem behavior with social isolation.
   - Supportive psychotherapy may be helpful in mildly impaired patients to adjust to their illness.

c. *Cognition-oriented approaches:* These techniques include reality orientation and skills training. The aim of these treatments is to redress cognitive deficits, often in a classroom setting. There is some evidence of transient benefit from cognitive redemption and from skills training but here have been report of frustration in patients and depression in caregivers associated with the type of intervention.

d. *Stimulation-oriented approaches:* These treatments include activities or recreational therapies (crafts, gene, and pets) and are therapies (music, dance, art). They provide stimulation and enrichment and thus mobilize the patient's available cognitive resources. There are evidences that, while they are in use, these interventions decrease behavioral problems and improved mood.

Psychotherapy can be given to family members as well as patient's psychotherapy is not very useful for patients. It will be helpful for family members to encourage them to take care of patients family members can be taught to take care of the patients which will help to improve patient's self esteem, and make the patient independent oriented as much as possible.

Family members should not neglect the patient but should help in humanitarian way.

Physiotherapy

It will help to organic and structure their daily activities such as muscle and joint exercises, breathing exercises, speech therapy to improve blood circulation etc.

Physiotherapy is helpful for chronic encephalitis, meningitis and general paresis of insane. It is also helpful to remove contracture of limbs, deformities of extremities or embolities.; It improves physical health. Appetite, digestion elimination, circulation, muscle tone and body temperature.

Social Relationship

Dementia patient become isolated from community. So community member should be in a sympathetic manner. Talking to them and asking ordinary questions also help the patient. More deterioration will take place when there is nothing to talk, to think or to work. The social approach plays a great role in psychiatric illness. The patient must learn or relearn how to assume responsibility for the welfare of himself and others for social relationship.

Day Centers

Day centers are run by the social work department. These have been developed partly because larger day centres are usually not organized to cope with dementia. The core of the large day centre's work concerns older people who wish to meet other people and engage in activities. It is assumed that they will be able to select their friends and select their activities, will take an active part in what goes and in most cases, make their own way to and from centre.

The need for day centres to cater for dementia suffers. Day care is needed who are the physically and the mentally impaired attending together and involving a mice of services.

Nursing management:

Nursing management of patients with dementia

Nursing care should be given according to its cause, onset of illness and severity. The main aim of nursing care is to make the patients life easier and pleasant. There is no effective treatment of cerebral pathology but we can help the patient in adjustment to life and coping with stress.

1) **Maintenance of Optimal Cognitive Functions**
   a) **Reduce environmental confusion**
      - Approach patient in a pleasant, calm way.
      - Introduce yourself to the patient and greet him/her
      - Keep the environment simple and pleasing, remove all unwanted utensils from the room.
      - Maintain a regular daily living schedule, so that the patient will get touch with the daily living activities.
      - Provide memory device like, lists of activities, reminding notes, labels on items; pictures, diagrams, etc. will assist the patient to remember.

   b) **Increased environmental cues.**
      - (It will enhance orientation to time place and person by filling memory gaps and serving as reminders)
      - Identify yourself when interacting with the patient
      - Address patient by name facilitate orientation to self.
      - Offer environmental cues for orientation to time, place and person.
      - Bring the patient near the window and shows him the surroundings.
      - Interpret environmental stimulation as part of the conversation. e.g. Prior to switch on the light late in the evening, tell the patient that the day is going to be over and we need light, hence switch on the light

2) **Maintenance of Physical Safety**
   a) **Control of environment**
      - Approach patient in a pleasant, calm way.
      - Introduce yourself to the patient and greet him/her
      - Keep the environment simple and pleasing, remove all unwanted utensils from the room.
      - Maintain a regular daily living schedule, so that the patient will get touch with the daily living activities.
      - Provide memory device like, lists of activities, reminding notes, labels on items; pictures, diagrams etc. will assist the patient to remember.

   b) **Monitor medication regimen**
      - Administer drug at appropriate time and dose, should not leave the medicine by the patient.

   c) **Monitor the temperature of food.**
      - Patient is protected from burning his mouth with warm food.

   d) **Permit maximum independence and freedom.**
      - Allow freedom to move around in the safe environment will give a sense of autonomy and relaxation

Contd...

Contd...

- Avoid use of restraints (restraints may increase agitation)
- Keep identification tag on patient will facilitate a safe return to the ward.

3) **Maintenance of an optimal level of psychological functioning.**
   a) **Reduce anxiety provoking situations in daily routine.**
      - Keep reality orientation, non-threatening but acceptable to the patient – repeat the answer if the patient asks again and again.
      - Be patience with forgetfulness.
      - Maintain a daily, regular routine so that the client is able to recall the daily activities.
      - Simple structured stimuli are easiest to interpret, for example call the patient by name just before lunch, tell him the exact time and about the lunch.
      - Be with the patient and listen to him what he/she actually wish to communicate with you.
      - Avoid situation that have upset patient in the past.
      - Do not try to reason with the patient (Patient is unable to conduct abstract thinking)

   b) **Enhance the quality of life.**
      - Offer multiple opportunities for fulfillment like light music, walks, exercises, old hobbies watching TV, etc. if the patient is able to perform such activities.

   c) **Encourage positive feeling of self.**
      - Treat the person as an individual with feelings (acceptance is the great inner support)
      - Should not under estimate the patient.
      - Openly discuss his feelings of anxiety and encourage him for further emotional ventilation when ever he needs and teach him relaxation methods , to reduce anxiety.
      - Praise appropriately for expected behavior.
      - When skills are lost do not try to restrain deterioration of the cognitive process makes loss of skills inevitable.

4) **Attainment of an optimal exchange of ideas between the patient and others.**
   a) **Implement strategies to promote the patient's interpretation of messages.**
      - Be calm, pleasant, and unhurried.
      - Keep verbal message short and simple.
      - Use non-verbal messages along with words.
      - Be consistent in conversation.
      - Simple message are easiest to interpret.
      - Write down simple instructions and lists.
      - Observe patient's expression for signs that he understands.
      - Talk to the patient even if he givens little or no response.

Contd...

Contd...

b) **Develop strategies to improve the patient's ability to express messages.**
   - Supply forgotten words when possible. This will allow to express his needs and feelings.
   - Guess the message and confirm with the patient (Active listening will minimize frustration)
   - Ignore mistakes
   - Allow adequate time for conversation
   - Encourage short, simple sentences.
   - Ask "Yes/No" questions unhurried attitude will enhance communication.
   - Provide alternative methods for communication pointing, describing with pictures, etc.
   - Acknowledge frustration in conversation that the patient is experiencing. It facilitate confidence.

5) **Maintenance of maximum independence in activities of daily living.**

a) **Develop plan to facilitate daily performance of activities.**
   - Maintain a regular daily schedule at a time convening with the patient.
   - Provide adaptive devices like lengthy brush for bath. Keep the instruction simple and divide the tasks in to small parts and do it first then ask the patient to do if further as much as he can. Stay with the patient till the task is over. Remind him if he stops in between because of confusion or short attention span.
   - Monitor functions of body system supervision will promote optimal function and help to detect early problems.

b) **Provide specific safe guards of safety in bathing.**
   - Monitor bath water temperature
   - Help the patient to take his bath completely and safely.
   - If we leave the patient alone for bath he may pour few mugs of water and come off, sometimes he may loose connection with what is being done ? why he is in the bath room ?
   - Encourage use of safety measures in the bathroom like hand rails , rubber mats to prevent bath room falls

c) **Provide specific measures to remember places.**
   - Provide accessibility to bath room. Indicate bathroom with colored pictures, visual stimuli reinforces recognition.
   - Remind the patient about toilet, where it is , it is in the north/south? Confused or disoriented patient may pass motion in an odd place thinking that is toilet.
   - Use clothing that open easily.
   - Maintain toileting schedule every two hourly (This help to maintain normal elimination)
   - Encourage adequate fluid and fiber rich food and activity for regular bowel movement.
   - Restrict fluid in evening hours. (This may interfere with sleep)

Contd...

Contd...

6) **Maintenance of optimal level of nutrition**
   a) **Monitor food intake and observe food habits.**
      - Note weight loss or gain
      - Provide regular mealtime schedule.
      - Encourage adequate fluid intake.
      - Provide balanced diet. If the client is unable to feed himself, feed the patient; during feeding narrate short stories which stimulate appetite as well as concentration.
      - Maintain a calm and pleasant atmosphere.
      - Offer a menu choice if possible.
      - Offer familiar food. (Pleasant mealtime C favorite and familiar food, the client will eat well with enjoyment).
   b) **Promote regular mouth care.**
      - Encourage care of gums and teeth after meals.
      - Assist and encourage the patient to maintain clean mouth
7) **Maintain optimum personal hygiene**
   a) **Promote healthy skin**
      - Keep the skin clean and dry.
      - Massage the extremities and back it will helps to improve muscle tone and circulation.
      - Lubricate the skin it is dry.
      - Assist with back, buttock and foot, care to prevent bedsore.
      - Provide clean and dry under clothing's.
   b) **Promote healthy hair and scalp.**
      - Wash hair weekly twice. Comb the hair daily , apply oil if needed and massage the scalp.
      - Prevent pediculosis.
   c) **Encourage nail care.**
      - Maintain clean and short nails of both extremities.
      - Provide soap and water to wash hands after each toiler visit.
8) **Maintenance of a balance of sleep and activity.**
   - Reduce nighttime distractions such as noise, nursing procedures or for mid-night medications, etc.
   - Take measurement to increase safety.
   - Provide adequate night-lights.
   - Enhance comfort if awake at night.
   - Avoid use of restraints
   - Design a balanced schedule of activity/sleep
   - Increase daytime wakefulness and encourage short rests than long time rest.
   - Encourage regular exercise and activity programs to mobilize joints (Daily activity and exercise reduce agitation and produce soothening and a calming effect.

Contd...

Contd...

9) **Enhancement of socialization and fulfillment of intimacy needs.**
   - Encourage visits from family and friends.
   - Use touching to maintain contact with patient. Tactile stimulation is easiest to interpret.
   - Introduce the family members and friends using names which is familiar to the patient.
   - Address the patient with his designation e.g.: Daddy, Uncle, and Granny, etc.
   - Share feelings honestly and openly with patient simultaneously holding his/her hands or touching on his/her shoulder. (He client continuous to need love and affection from his own people)
   - Limit numbers of visitors one or two at a time, to avoid confusion and to maintain single stimuli.
   - Accept the patient despite negative interactions.

10) **Provide Rehabilitation**
   - Support and retrain the existing skills.
   - Provide Physiotherapy if the client has difficulty in walking.
   - Provide hearing aids, if the hearing is impaired.
   - Speech therapy and cognitive retraining in the case of aphasia (expressive aphasia)
   - Impaired vision, provide big lettered books/schedule
   - Reading glass if necessary
   - Bladder and bowel training if incontinence is present.

SELF-CARE AT HOME

1. Many individuals with dementia in the early and intermediate stages are able to live independently.

   With regular checks by a local relative or friend, they are able to live without constant supervision.

   Those who have difficulty with activities of daily living require at least part-time help from a family caregiver or home health aide.

   Visiting nurses can make sure that these individuals take their medications as directed.

   Housekeeping help is available for those who cannot keep up with household chores.

2. Other affected individuals require closer supervision or more constant assistance.

   Round-the-clock help in the home is available, but it is too expensive for many.

Individuals who require this level of assistance may need to move from their home to the home of a family caregiver or to an assisted-living facility.

Many families prefer these options because they give the individual the greatest possible independence and quality of life.

3. For individuals who are able to remain at home or to retain some degree of independent living, maintaining a familiar and safe environment is important.

   The individual must be comfortable and safe if he or she is to continue to function independently.

   Minor modifications of the home may be needed. Most important is to prevent falls and accidents. Getting rid of area rugs and putting grab bars in the shower and mats in the tub are easy important steps to make the environment safe. Sometimes, disabling the stove or using child proof knobs may be necessary to prevent cooking accidents.

   The balance between safety and independence must be assessed often. If necessary, changes must be made to keep the individual safe.

4. Individuals with dementia should remain physically, mentally, and socially active.

   Daily physical exercise helps the body and mind function and maintains a healthy weight. Exercise can be as simple as a daily walk.

   - The individual should engage in as much mental activity as he or she can handle. Mental activity is believed to slow the progress of some types of dementia. Puzzles, games, reading, and safe hobbies and crafts are good choices.
   - Social interaction is stimulating and enjoyable for most people with dementia. Most senior centers or community centers have scheduled activities, such as parties and clubs that are suitable for those with dementia.

5. A balanced diet that includes low-fat protein foods and plenty of fruits and vegetables helps maintain a healthy weight and prevent malnutrition and constipation. An individual with dementia should not smoke, both for health and safety reasons.

Prevention

- No known way to prevent irreversible dementia or even many types of reversible dementia exists. The following may help prevent certain types of dementia.
- Maintaining a healthy lifestyle that includes a balanced diet, regular exercise, moderate use of alcohol, and no smoking or substance abuse .
- Taking precautions to prevent infections.
- Using protective equipment such as a seat belt or motorcycle helmet to prevent head injury.

Problems of the Carer

The carer, often a spouse is likely to also be elderly and possibly with poor physical health. If the carer is a child they may have family responsibilities such as dependent children, producing divided loyalties and some times marital conflict. The carer may live a distance away and suffer financial problems from travel expenses. There may be embarrassment caused by the reversal of roles, especially if caring for the personnel hygiene of a parent of the opposite sex. Lack of insight and knowledge of the progress of dementia, which symptoms can be modified and how to obtain help, can all be remedied by introducing the carer to a support group such as Age concern and the Alzheimer's Disease society.

Help of Carer

Carer giving is hard work and is usually considered a professional activity. Amateur careers are untrained so it is not surprising they makes mistakes such as using restrain to prevent behavior (e.g. locked doors or request for sedation) rather than environmental or Psychological management. Brodaty (1992) suggests that, training should be comprehensive, tailored to Individual needs, and continuing through the different phases of the illness. A joint report by the RCP (1989) suggests that for the massive issue of dementia, the emphasis should be on support of carer. Attention should be given to "Those aspects which wear careers down such as restlessness, aggression, disturbed nights and in continence "together with complicating problems such as depression in patient of career. The report describes the role of the community Psychiatric Nurse as monitoring and support, counseling, helping with practical, financial and emotional difficulties and advocacy on behalf of the patient and families. How ever one must beware the tendency for paternalistic control. Where a patient is in capable of consent, relatives should be consulted closely at every stage of treatment. But when a patient is capable of making certain decisions. It is both unnecessary and stigmatizing to wish to confirm the decision with a relative (Murphy 1986).

1) **In the Home:** The home help service can reduce the amount of work necessary in the house, leaving the carer more time to spent with the patient. Some district run schemes where paid or voluntary carers come to the house and stay with the demented patient while the carer with the demented patient while the career goes out, or take the patient out for some hours giving the career since alone in the home.
2) **Outings:** Many voluntary and statutory groups are able to arrange outings, either day trips or even holidays, for the carer and patient, to give interest and stimulation to them both.
3) **Day Care:** Social service department and voluntary service run day care scheme in all areas. It is usually possible for transport to collect and return the patient, although sometimes a carer may do this, if there are major problems with physically dependency or behaviour such as aggression day care may be provided by the psycho geriatric day hospital, which has a higher number of staff, including nurses to deal with such problems.

ORGANIC AMNESTIC SYNDROME

Is characterized by the following clinical features:

1. Impairment of memory due to an underlying organic cause.
2. No disturbance of consciousness and attention.
3. No disturbance of global intellectual function, abstract thinking, personality.

According to ICD – 10, the following features:

1. Recent memory impairment; anterograded retrograde amnesia.
2. No impairment of immediate, retention and recall, attention, consciousness and intellectual functioning.
3. Historical or objective evidence of brain disease or injury.

Etiology

1. Thiamine deficiency: also called as the Wernicke – Korsakoff syndrome – acute phase of delirium.
2. Any other lesion involving bilaterally the inner core of limbic system.
   a. Head trauma – surgical procedure
   b. Hypoxia – posterior cerebral artery stroke – sol.

Management

1. Treatment of the underlying cause, e.g. thiamin in Wernicke – Korsakoff syndrome.
2. Supportive care.

Other types of OBS

- Organic delusional disorder
- Organic hallucinosis
- Organic catatonic disorder
- Organic mood disorder
- Organic anxiety disorder
- Organic personality disorder
- Organic dissociative disorder
- Organic emotionally labile
- Organic mild cognitive disorder.

15 Mood Disorders

DEFINITION

This group of disorders is characterized by a disturbance of mood, accompanied by a full or partial manic or depressive syndrome, that is not due to any other physical or mental disorder.

INTRODUCTION

Hippocrates coined the term "melancholia" kurl Ludwig kahlbaum – said that these episodes are different stages of the same disease process, which called "Cyclothymia". Emil Kraepelin – called "Manic depressive psychosis".

EPIDEMIOLOGY

Recently, the *World Health Organization (WHO, 2001)* has identified unipolar depression as the 4th cause of DALY (Disability Adjusted Life Years) in all ages and 2nd cause in the age group of 15 to 44 yr. Unipolar depression is also the 1st cause of years of life lived with disability in all cases.

WHO (WHR, 2001) estimates that there are 121 million people world wide suffering from depression.

CLASSIFICATION

According to the ICD –10, the mood disorders are classified as follows:

1. Manic episode
2. Depressive episode

3. Bipolar mood disorder
4. Recurrent depressive disorder
5. Persistent mood disorder (including cyclothymia and dysthymia)
6. Other mood disorders (including mixed affective episode and recurrent brief depressive disorder).

MANIC EPISODE

The life time risk of manic episode is about 0.3 – 1%. This disorder tends to occur in episodes lasting usually 3 – 4 months, followed by complete clinical recovery.

Clinical Features

1. A distinct period of abnormally and persistently elevated, expansive or irritable mood.

   Euphoria [mild elevation of mood] Stage I
   ↓
   Elation [Moderate elevation of mood] Stage II
   ↓
   Exaltation [Severe elevation of mood] Stage III
   ↓
   Ecstasy [Very elevation of mood] Stage IV
2. During the period mood disturbance, at least three of the following symptoms have persisted.
   a - inflated self esteem or grandiosity
   b - decreased need for sleep
   c - more talkative than usual
   d - flight of ideas
   e - distractibility (attention to early drawn to unimportant)
   f - increased in goal – directed activity or psychomotor agitation.
3. Psychomotor activity
   - Over activeness and restlessness
   - Manic excitement where the person is "on-the-toe-on-the-go".

4. Speech and thought:
   - More talkative than usual
   - Pressure of speech
   - Rhyming, joking and teasing and speaks loudly
   - Flight of ideas
   - Grandiosity
5. Other features
   Sleep is usually reduced with decreased need for sleep.
   Appetite – may be increased but late there is usually decreased food intake due to over activity.
   - Insight into the illness is absent
   - Delusion, hallucination and grandiosity.

Triad Symptoms

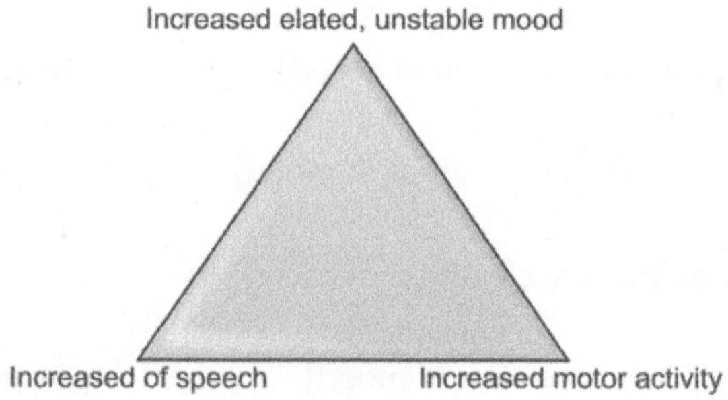

Types of Mania

1. Hypomania
2. Acute mania
3. Delusional mania
4. Bell's mania or Delirious mania

DEPRESSIVE EPISODE (UNIPOLAR)

The life time risk of depression in males is 8 – 12% and in females is 20 – 26%. However, the life time risk of major depression is about 8%.

Clinical Features

1. Depressed mood

The most important feature is the sadness mood or loss of interest/ pleasure in almost all activities (pervasive sadness), present throughout the day (persistent sadness).

In severe depression, there may be complete anhedonia (inability to experience pleasure).

2. Depressive ideation/cognition

Sadness of mood is usually associated with pessimism, which can result in 3 common types of depressive ideas.

1. Hopelessness [there is no hope in the future].
2. Helplessness [no help is possible now].
3. Worthlessness [feeling of inadequacy and infirmity].

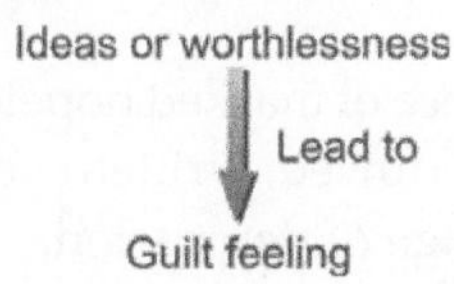

3. Psychomotor Activity

Retardation is more common slow thinking and activity, decreased energy. In a severe form, the patient can become stuporous (depressive stupor). In the older patients, agitation is commoner. It often presents with marked anxiety, restlessness.

4. Physical Syndrome

Multiple physical symptoms (like heaviness of head, vague body aches) are particularly common in elderly depressives and depressed patients from the developing countries.

Hypochondriacal features may be present in up to a quarter of depressive presentis for treatment.

Another common symptom is the complaints of reduced energy and easy fatigability.

5. Biological Functions

Disturbance of biological functions is common, with insomnia, loss of appetite, and weight and loss of sexual drive.

When the disturbance is severe, it is called as melancholia – It cause somatic syndrome, it means decrease in appetite or weight, early morning awakening atleast 2 (or more) hours before the usual time of awakening. Diurnal variation, with depression being worse in the morning, loss of interested lost of reactivity to pleasure stimuli.

It often also implies a good response to somatic methods of treatment.

6. Psychotic Features

About 15 – 20% of depressed patients have psychotic symptoms like delusion, hallucination, grossly inappropriate behavior/stupor.

7. Suicide

More common in presence of marked hopelessness, males; age >40, unmarried divorced/widowed, written/verbal communication of suicidal intent, early stage of depression.

TRIAD

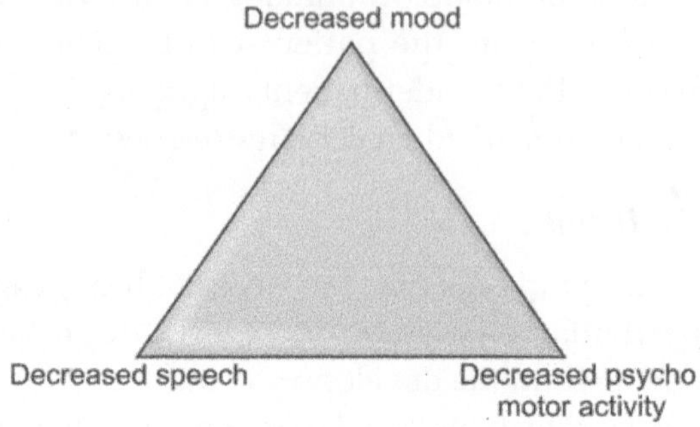

Classification of Depression

1. Unipolar and bipolar mood disorders
2. Psychotic versus neurotic
3. Endogenous versus exogenous

1. **Unipolar:** At least 3 separate episodes of psychotic depression, complex remission in between and no episode of mania.
   Bipolar: At least one episode of depression and one of mania; where repeated mania episodes occur, the disorder is also classified bipolar.
2. **Psychotic:** Presence of delusions and hallucinations.
   Neurotic: No presence of delusions and hallucinations
3. **Endogenous and exogenous**

Endogenous	*Exogenous*
• Otherwise called psychotic, autogenous	• Neuotic reactive
• Biological factors more important.	• Environmental factors
• Insomnia late stage	• Early stage
• More sad during morning	• More said during evening
• Psychomotor retardates, suicidal tendencies, delusion, etc	• Psychomotor agitation and other psychotic feature uncommon
• Relapses common	• Psychotherapy + antidepressants
• Management ECT + antidepressants	

Etiology

Etiology of mood disorders is not known currently, despite several theories having been propounded.

1. Biological Theories

The following findings point towards a biological basis of mood disorders.

a) **Genetic hypothesis:**
   i. First degree relatives: Bipolar mood disorders – 25% recurrent depressive disorder patients is 20%.
   ii. One parent with bipolar mood disorder is 27%.
   iii. Both parents with bipolar mood disorder is 74%.

iv. Monozygotic twins – Bipolar disorders is 65%.
v. Dizygotic twins – Bipolar disorders is 20%.
vi. Unipolar disorder for monozygotic twins – 46%
vii. Unipolar disorder for dizygotics twins – 20%

b) **Biochemical theories:**

The monoamine hypothesis suggests an abnormality in monoamine system in the CNS at one or more site. (catecholamine – Norepinephrine and dopamine).

i. Functional increase or decrease of amines at the synaptic cleft now appear simplistic, through urinary and ESF levels of amine metabolites indicate decreased norepinephrine or 5 HT function in depression and increased norepinephrine in mania.
ii. Severe depression with suicidal intent – to have a marked decrese in serotonergic function, evidenced by decreased urinary and plasma – 5 – HIA and levels and post – mortem studies.

c) **Neuroendocrine theories:**

Mood symptoms are prominently present in many endocrine disorders, like hypothyroidism, Cushing's disease and Addison's disease.

Endocrine function is often disturbed in depression, with cortisol dexamethasone challenge blunted TSH response to TRH, and blunted growth hormone (GH) production during sleep.

d) **Sleep studies:**

Sleep abnormalities are common in mood disorders (e.g. decreased need for sleep in mania, insomnia and frequent awakening in depression).

e) **Brain imaging:**

In mood disorders, brain imaging studies (CT/MRI of brain, PET scan and SPECT) have yielded inconsistent, yet suggestive findings.

These findings include ventricular dilatation, white matter hyper intensities and changes in the blood flow and metabolism in several parts of brain.

2. Psychosocial Theories

(i) **Psychoanalytic theories:**

In depression:

Introjection of lost object

↓

Fixation in the oral sadistic phase of development

↓

Craving for self-love

↓

Depression

Mania

Reaction formation

↓

Mania

(ii) **Stress:**

Increased number of stressful like events before the onset or relapse have a formative rather than a precipitating effect in depression though they can serve a precipitant role in mania.

3. Cognitive and Behavioral Theories

Depressive negative cognition, learned helplessness and anger directed inwards.

Management

I. Somatic Treatment

1. Antidepressants:

Antidepressants are the treatment of choice for a vast majority of depressive episodes. Some of the commonly used antidepressants with their usual stage of therapeutic dose.

Drug	Starting dose	Increased upto
Imipramine	75 – 150 mg	300 mg

Tricyclic antidepressants (TCA)

- Imipramine, antitriptyline, newer antidepressants like selective serotonin reuptake inhibitors.

- Fluoxetine, sertraline, citalopram, serotonin norepinphrine reuptake inhibitors (SNRIS) – renlafaxine, duloxetine.

3 main phases of treatment:

1. Acute treatment: [till remission occurs]
2. Continuation treatment [from remission till end of treatment].
3. Maintenance treatment [to prevent further recurrences].

The treatment choice is:

1. An antidepressants only
2. An antidepressants with ECT
3. An antidepressants with antipsychotic or
4. An antidepressants with lithium.

2. ECT

i. Severe depression with suicidal risk.
ii. Severe depression with stupor, severe psychomotor retardation or somatic syndrome.
iii. Severe treatment refractory depression.
iv. Delusional depression – Psychotic depression.

Several depression with suicidal risk in the first and foremost indication for use of ECT.

ECT method: In most clinical situations usually 6 – 8 ECTs are needed, given 3 times a week.

First 3 ECT - First week
First 2 ECT - 2nd week
First 1 ECT - Third week

ECT also be used for acute manic excitement, if it is not adequately responding to antipsychotic and mood stabilizers.

3. Lithium (Li)

Lithium has traditionally been the drug of choice for the treatment of manic episode as well as for prevention of further episodes in Bipolar mood disorder.

The usual therapeutic dose range is 900 – 1500 mg of lithium carbonate/day.

Therapeutic blood lithium = 0.8 –1.2 mEq/L
Prophylactic blood lithium = 0.6 – 1.2 mEq/L

A blood lithium level of more than 2.0 mEq/L is often associated with toxicity, while a level or more than 2.5 – 3.5 mEq/L may be lethal.

4. Antipsychotics

Antipsychotics are an important adjunct in the treatment of mood disorder. The commonly used drugs include risperidone, olanzapine, quetiapine, halperidol and chlorpromazine.

It is customary to use the atypical antipsychotic first, before considering the older typical antipsychotics.

5. Other Mood Stabilizers

(i) **Sodium valproate:**

Dose range is usually 1000 – 3000 mg/day.

- Therapeutic blood levels are 50 – 125 mg/day
- It is faster action than lithium.
- Acute treatment of mania and prevention of BMD.

(ii) **Carbamazepine and Oxcarbazepine:**

- Treatment for mania and prevention of BMD.
- Dosage range of carbamazepine is 600 – 1600 mg/day [Therapeutic blood levels 6 - 12 mg/day]
- Oxcarbazepine – narrow evidence base and its use in BMD is quite recent.

(iii) **Benzodiazepines:**

Lorazepam and clonazepam are used for treatment of manic episode alone rarely.

T3 and T4 are adjuncts for the treatment of rapid cyclic mood disorders and resistant depression.

6. Other Treatments

Psychosurgery: is an extremely rarely used method of treatment.

Procedures of surgery:

(i) Stereotactic subcandate tractotomy

(ii) Stereotactic limbic leukotomy

II. Psychosocial Treatment

1. **Cognitive behavior therapy:**
   Aims:
   - Correcting the depressive negative cognitions (ideations).
   - Replacing them by new cognitive and behavioural responses.

   Use:
   Mild to moderate, non-bipolar depression and used along with somatic treatment.
2. **Interpersonal therapy:**
   Attempts to recognize and explore interpersonal stressors, role disputes and transitions.
   Uses:
   Mild to moderate unipolar disorder with or without antidepressants.
3. **Psychoanalytic psychotherapy:**
   Aim:
   Changing the personal itself rather than just ameliorating the symptoms.
4. **Behavior therapy:**
   This includes the various short-term modalities like social skill training, problem solving techniques, assertiveness, training, self control therapy, decision making technique.
   It useful for mild depression.
5. **Group therapy:**
   - Useful in mild cases of depression.
   - Psycho education for bipolar and depressive disorder.
6. **Family and marital therapy:**
   The main purpose is to ensure continuity of treatment and adequate drug concordance.

BIPOLAR MOOD (AFFECTIVE) DISORDER

This disorder, earlier known as manic depressive psychosis (MDP), is characterized by recurrent episodes of mania and depression is the same patient at different times.

These episodes can occur in any sequence. The patients with recurrent episodes of mania (unipolar mania) are also classified here as they are rare and often resemble the bipolar patient in their clinical features.

Subtypes of Bipolar Disorder

Bipolar I: Characterized by episodes of severe mania and severe depression.
Bipolar II: Characterized by episodes of hypomania and severe depression.

Recurrent Depressive Disorder

- Recurrent (at least 2) depressive episodes (unipolar depression).
- Current episode in recurrent depressive disorder is specified as one of the following.
  1) Mild
  2) Moderate
  3) Severe with psychotic syndrome
  4) Severe with psychotic symptoms
  5) In remission

Persistent Mood Disorder

Persistent disorder symptoms which last for more than 2 yr but are not severe enough to be labeled as even hypermania or mild depression episode.

If the symptoms consist of persistent mile depression, the disorder is called as dythymia. If symptoms consist of persistent instability of mood between mild depression and mild elation and the disorder is called a cyclothymia.

Other Mood Disorder

- Rapid cycles: More than 4 or more/year.
- 70 – 805 of all rapid cycles are women

Ultrarapid Cyclers

When phases of mania and depression alternate by rapidly (in matter of hours or days).

16 Neurosis

In ICD – 10 neurotic, stress-related and somatoform disorders have been classified into the following type:

1. Phobic anxiety disorder
2. Other anxiety disorder
3. OCD
4. Reaction to stress and adjustment disorders
5. Conversion Dissociative disorders
6. Somatoform disorders
7. Other neurotic disorder.

ANXIETY

Anxiety states are among the most common neurotic syndromes. Anxiety neurosis has been known by many names viz., cardiac neurosis, Dacosta's syndrome, neurosis exhaustion, neuro-circulations, asthenia, soldier's heart.

The term anxiety neurosis was first used by Sigmund Freud in 1895.

Epidemiology

Prevalence of about 2-4% in normal population. This constituted about 25-30% of psychiatric outputs.

Types

1. **Trait anxiety:** This is a habitual tendency to be anxious in general (a trait) and is exemplified by, I often feel, anxious.

2. **State anxiety:** This is the anxiety self at present cross – section moment (state) and is exemplified by, I feel, anxious how'.

Symptoms

I. **Physical Symptoms:**
   (a) **Motoric Symptoms:** Tremors restleonem muscles twitches, fearful facial expression.
   (b) **Autonomic and visceral symptoms:** Palpitations, tachycardia, sweating, flushes, dyspnea, hyperventilation, dry mouth, dizziness, diarrhea.

II. **Psychological Symptoms:**
   (a) Cognitive symptoms:
   Poor concentration, distractibility, hyperarousal.
   (b) Perceptual symptoms:
   Derealization, depersonalization
   (c) Affective symptoms:
   Diffuse, unpleasant, fearfulness, inability to relax, irritability.
   (d) Other symptoms:
   Insomnia, increased sensitivity to noise.

1. Generalized Anxiety Disorder

Persistent anxiety of at least one month duration without the specific symptoms that characterize phobic disorders or OC disorders.

- Insidious onset
- Symptoms should last for atleast a period of 6 months.

Cardinal feature of almost all psychiatric disorders, it is important to exclude other diagnosis.

2. Panic Disorders

Recurrent anxiety attack that occur at times unpredictable through certain situation (e.g.) driving a car.

- Discrete episode of acute anxiety.
- Sudden onset, last for a few minutes and is characterized by very severe anxiety.
- Classically symptoms – "out-of-the blue".
- It can present either alone/with agoraphobia.

Causes

1) Biological theory:

Genetic evidence:

15 – 20% of first degree relatives of patients.

80% - high for monozygotic twins of patients.

20% - high for dizygotic twins of patients.

Biological factors – hereditary, constitution, abnormalities in endocrine disturbance, metabolic and bio chemical are not considered most important causes.

Environmental factors are rated as more important causes.

1. Age

Childhood, adolescence and involution are the periods most susceptible to this illness.

2. Personality

Anxious personality type, obsessive types personality are most susceptible to anxiety disorder.

3. Sex

Both gender involved equal distribution some point of view it more in one sex than another.

- Frustration in sexual aim is considered causes of anxiety disorders.
- Physical, psychological, psychosocial stress of a moderate to severe degree even in well adjusted personalities triggers off the illness.

Treatment

1. Hospitalization is necessary for actual reactions.
2. Pharmacology:

   Chlordizepoxide, diazepam, alprazolam and meprobamate are most common anxiolytics.

   Small dose of neuroleptics like chlorpromazine hydrochloride, trifluorerazine and haloperidol also good results.

3. Psychotherapy:

   Supportive and short-term therapy also very useful. psychotherapy. Deep analytical psychotherapy is needed for chronic maladjusted personalities.

   - Abreactive therapies like IV injection of sodium pentothal, hypnosis helps in those patients.
   - Social casework and counseling.
   - Psychophysiological therapy (PPT)
     - Yoga – meditation.
     - Muscle relaxation techniques.

PHOBIC DISORDERS

Definition

Phobia is defined as an irrational fear of a specific object, situation or activity, often leading to persistent avoidance of the feared object, situations or activity.

Marks (1987) has defined phobia as the following:

1. The fear is out of proportion to the demands of the situation.
2. It cannot be explained on reasoned away.
3. It is beyond voluntary control.
4. The fear leads to an avoidance of the feared object phobias as very common mental disorder. onset of phobia is usually in childhood and adolesecnce. Approximately 5 to 10% of the population is often by phobias common in women.

Main Features of Phobia

a. Persistent, irrational fear attached to an object, situation that objectively does not pose of significant danger.
b. The fear is out of proportion to the dangerous perceived.
c. If recognize the irrational fear.
d. It is unable to control.
e. It develops to persistent avoidance of feared object, situation or activity.
f. Final resulting of phobia, marked disturbance of the freedom of mobility.

Etiology

The cause of phobias is unknown. Various theories exists that may often insight into the cause.

1. Psychodynamic Theory

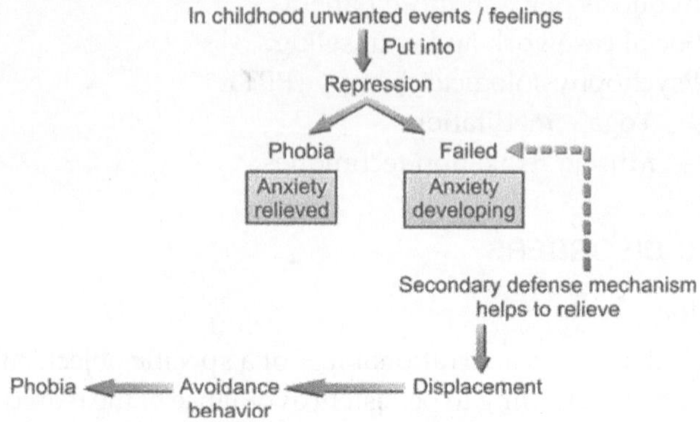

Anxiety is usually relieved with repression defense mechanism. When repression failed the other secondary defense mechanism of ego come into action. In phobia, this secondary defense mechanism is displacement. By this, anxiety is transferred from a really dangerous or frightening object to a neutral object. The neutral object chosen unconsciously is to one which can be easily avoided in day-to-day activity, in contrast to the frightening object.

2. Behavioral Theories

Phobia developed through as a conditional reflex. Early condition, the individual anxiety provoked by a naturally dangerous object occur in contiguity with a second neutral object becomes a conditional stimulus for causing anxiety.

This theory not fully explained all the features of phobia.

3. Biological Theories

Genetic factors in specific phobias acting vital causes like agoraphobia family studies shows that very close for social phobia causes.

Early experience may set the stage for phobic reaction later life. Temperament also one of the influencing factor for phobia.

Types

The common types of phobia are

a. Agoraphobia
b. Social phobia
c. Specific/simple phobia

a. Agoraphobia

Persistent, irrational fear of situations is more commonest type in clinical practice.

Characteristics

1. Irrational fear of being in places away from familiar setting of home.
2. Fear of where there is no easy escape to a safe place.

Patient is afraid of all the places on situation from where escape may be difficult or help may not be available.

Signs and Symptoms

Panic attack, dizziness or falling depersonalization or derealization, loss of bladder and bowel control, tachycardia, disturbed normal activity.

This symptoms may classified

a) Agoraphobia with panic disorders
b) Agoraphobia without panic disorders

b. Social Phobia

Persistent irrational fear of activities or social interactions.

Characteristics

1. Irrational fear of performing activities in the presence of other people or interacting with others.
2. Patient is afraid of his own (activities) actions being viewed by others critically.

Signs and Symptoms

Fear of blushing (erythrophobia), eating, public speaking, public performance, participating in groups, writing in pulse and urinating in a public lavatory (shy bladder).

c. Specific (Simple) Phobia

1. Persistent, irrational fear of objects situations characteristics.
2. Irrational fear of specific objects/situation.
3. Persistent avoidant behavior leads to panic attacks.

Signs and Symptoms

- There is marked distress and for disturbance in daily functioning.
- Panic — palpitation, sweating, dizziness and difficult breathing.

Classification of Specific Phobias:

Acrophobia	:	Fear of high places
Zoophobia	:	Fear of animals
Xenophobia	:	Fear of strangers
Algophobia	:	Fear of pain
Clustro phobia	:	Fear of closed places
Trichophobia	:	Fear of hair
Pyrophobia	:	Fear of fix
Mysophobia	:	Fear of dirt, germs
Numerophobia	:	Fear of numbers
Ophidiophobia	:	Fear of snakes

Management

The management approach is usually multi-model.

1. Psychotherapy

Insight-oriented psychotherapy and supportive psychotherphy. helps the patient to understand the origin of the phobia, the phenomena of secondary gain and role of rest.

3. Supportive psychotherapy helps to adjunct to behavior therapy and drug treatment.
4. Cognitive behavior therapy can also to prevent the anxiety patterns of phobic disorder.

2. Behavior Therapy

Behavior therapy aims at changing maladaptive behavior and substituting it with adaptive behavior. Some of the important behavioral techniques are:

Systematic desensitization, flooding, social skill training – modeling and role playing and relaxation technique.

3. Drug Treatment

The drugs used in phobias,

i. Benzodiazepines — to reduce the anticipatory anxiety, e.g. Alprazolam – Lorazepam, clonazepam and diazepam.
ii. Antidepressants, e.g. Imipramine – (TCA), phenelzine (MAOI), SSRIs – Fluoxefine and Sertraline.

OBSESSIVE-COMPULSIVE DISORDER

Obsessions are defined as unwanted, intrusive, persistent ideas, thoughts, impulses or images that cause marked anxiety or distress. It is recognized as irrational and absurd (insight is present). Patient tries to resist against it but is unable to and failure to resist leads to marked distress.

The most common ones include repeated thoughts about contamination, repeated doubts and sexual imagery.

An obsession is usually associated with a compulsion.

A compulsions are defined as, unwanted repetitive behavior patterns or mental acts that are intended to reduce anxiety. It usually follows obsessions. The behavior is not realistic and performed with sense of subjective compulsion. Insight is present, realizes the irrationality of compulsion.

Epidemiology

It is more common in unmarried males and it is more common from upper social class and high intelligence. Onset is late third decade. Prevalence of obsessive-compulsive disorder is 2 – 3%.

Clinical Types

ICD 10 classifies OCD into 3 clinical subtypes:

1. Predominantly obsessive thoughts or ruminations.
2. Predominantly compulsive acts and
3. Mixed obsessional thoughts and acts.

Clinical Syndromes

Depression is very commonly associated with OCD. Four clinical syndromes are common in OCD.

1. **Washers:**

   Obsession is of contamination with dirt, germs, body excretions etc.

   Compulsion is washing of hands or whole body repeatedly many times a day. For example,
   - Washing of clothes
   - Washing of bathroom/bedroom, door knobs
2. **Checkers:**

   In this type, individual have multiple doubts. Checking repeatedly to remove the doubt. For example,
   - Door has not been locked.
   - Kitchen gas has been left open.
   - Counting of money way no exact etc.
3. **Pure obsessions:**

   It having repetitive intrusive thoughts, impulses or images which are not associated with compulsive acts. Here, they preoccupation with thoughts.
4. **Primary obsessive slowness:**

   More severe obsession and compulsions type. It make absence of anxiety. So, the individual leads to slowness in daily activities.

Etiology of OCD

Exact cause is unknown. Some theories explained causes through theories.

1. Psychodynamic Theory

In early childhood period, disturbed anal phase it fixed with reaction formation. So, child will develop repetition of ideas about the incidence/event. This leads to obsessional personality.

Eventhough, some incidence provoked anxiety in anal phase, the individual put into regression mind. Later reinforced of anal or aggressive impulses, need secondary defense mechanism like isolation of affect. Undoing feeling/act and displacement and so they failed it may develop obsessive thoughts, compulsive acts and phobias respectively.

2. Behavior Theory

Obsessions ← Conditional stimuli to anxiety.

Compulsions ← Learned behavior ¬ Obsessions

↓

Decrease anxiety

3. Biological Theory

- Secondary illness of neurology like – encephalitis, basal ganlia lesions, Tourette syndrome and hypothalamic lesions.
- 5 HT – levels decreased lead to OCD.

Treatment

1. **Psychotherapy:**
   - Psychoanalytic psychotherapy
   - Supportive psychotherapy
2. **Behavior therapy:**
   - Modification of behavior thrush, though stopping, response prevention, systematic desensitization and modeling.

3. **Psychopharmacology:**
   - Anti anxiety drug is benzodiazepine mild dose helps to reduce anxiety.
   - Antidepressants: Serotonin reuptake inhibitors (SSRIs), especially clomipramine, are very effective drugs for OCD. Other drugs are: fluoxetine, broxetine and sertraline are also effective drugs.
   - Anti psychotics: Low doses in the treatment of severe, disabling anxiety patients, e.g. haloperidol.
4. **Electroconvulsive therapy:**
   It is not the treatment of first choice in OCD. It needed when patient suffering severe depression with OCD.
5. **Psychosurgery:**
   It needed when, which has become intractable, not responding to other methods of treatment. Techniques are:
   i. Steriotactic limbic leucotomy
   ii. Stereotactic subcaudate tactotomy

DISSOCIATIVE AND CONVERSION DISORDERS

The word hysteria has been removed from DSM IV as well as ICD –10. ICD 10 replaced by "dissociative (conversion) disorders" and DSM IV by conversion and dissociative disorder.

Hysteria (Consists of conversion, dissociation and summarization disorder) constitutes 6 – 15% of all OPD diagnosis and 14-20% of all neurotic disorders. Females usually most common.

1. Conversion Disorder

It is a psychoneurotic disorder in which repressed inner conflicts are unconsciously converted or transformed into, physical symptoms that have no organic basis.

Characteristics

1. Sudden onset.
2. Two types of disturbance in conversion disorder – motor and sensory.

3. Symptoms develops when the presence of a significant psychosocial stressors.
4. It is used for primary gain, that is the patient gets relief from anxiety.

A. Classification of Conversion Disorder

1. **Dissociative Motor Disorders:**
   The motor disturbance involves either paralysis or abnormal movements.
   The paralysis may be a monoplegia, paraplegia or quadriplegia.
   The abnormal movements range from tremors, choreform movements, and gait disturbances (astasia abasia).
   Examination shows normal CNS function and motor functions.
2. **Sensory disorders:**
   I love and stocking anesthesia, blindness, deafness.
3. Dissociative convulsions (hysterical fits).

Causes:

a. Conversion secondary defense mechanism produced somatic symptoms with symbolic representation and leads to conversion disorders.
b. **Behavioural theory:** It says that conversion and dissociation are learned responses in the stress. Through this behavior, they get secondary gain and avoidance of stress.
c. **Biological theory:** Some physical illness predisposing factors for dissociative disorder, and epilepsy patients are frequently seen with conversion symptoms.

B. Classification of Dissociative Disorders

1. Dissociative amnesia
2. Dissociative fugue
3. Multiple personality (Dissociative Identity Disorder)
4. Trance and possession disorders.

Treatment

1. Behavior Therapy

Certain methods useful for dissociative/convention disorder.

Techniques are:

- Strong suggestion for return to normal.
- Aversion therapy
  - Liquor ammonia, electric stimulus, pressure just above eye balls or tragus of ear, nosing nose and mouth.
  - Hypnosis, free associative, narcoanalysis with suggestion.

2. Psychotherapy with Abreaction Like

- Hypnosis
- Free association
- Intravenous thiopentone/diazepam

3. Supportive psychotherapy:
4. Psychoanalysis
5. Drug therapy
   - Short-term benzodiazepines needed for anxiety condition of patient.
   - Thiopentone/amytal/diazepam in abreaction treatment method.

SOMATOFORM DISORDERS

The somatoform disorders are repeated presentation with physical symptoms which do not have any adequate physical basis and request for investigations and treatment by treating doctors.

In ICD- 10 somatoform disorders are divided into the following:

1. Somatization Disorder

It have multiple somatic symptoms in the absence of any physical disorder. It present at least 2 years duration, and there is frequent change of treating doctor.

Treatment

Supportive psychotherapy, relaxation therapy with physical exercise, drug therapy like antidepressants – benzodiazepines.

2. Hypochondriasis

Defined as a persistent preoccupation with a fear or belief of having one or more serious disease based on person's own interpretation of normal body function or a minor physical abnormality.

Etiology

1. Narcissistic personality ® Narcissistic libido
2. Masked depression ® Hypochondriasis

Treatment

1. Supportive psychotherapy
2. Treatment of associated or underlying depression/anxiety, if present

3. Somatoform Autonomic Dysfunction

"According to ICD-10, this disorder symptom, are presented by the patients as if they were due to physical disorder of an organ system that is predominantly under autonomic control, e.g. heart and CVS (palpitations), upper G I tract (aerophagy and hiccough), low GI tract, irritable bowel, flatulence, respiratory system (hyperventilation), genitourinary system (dysuria) and other organ system.

Treatment

1. Supportive psychotherapy.
2. Drug therapy–Benzodiazepine and antidepressants (Imipramine).

4. Persistent Somatoform Pain Disorder

Persistent severe and distressing pain is the main feature which is either grossly in excess of what is expected fro physical finding or central nervous system. Repeated change of doctors is common. It is more common in females.

Treatment

1. The patients usually refuse psychiatrist intervention.
2. Drug therapy should be avoided, Because it is risk for abuse.
3. In the absence of other modes of successful treatment and supportive relationship with doctor will prevent doctor-shopping.

5. Other Somatoform Disorders

In ICD-10, somatoform not classified in the previous 4 categories, e.g. 'globus hystericus'-psychogenic torticollis, psycogenic pruritus, teeth-grinding, psychogenic dysmenorrhea.

Other Neurotic Disorders

In ICD-10, other neurotic disorders are:

1. **Neurasthenia:** Either persisting and distressing complains of increased fatigue/body weakness after mental effort. Feeling of muscular aches and pains, dizziness, tension head aches, sleep disturbances, irritability and dyspepsia.
2. **Depersonalization disorder:** Alteration in the perception of self, so that the feeling of one's own reality is temporarily changed or lost.

   Derealization— which alteration in the perception of external world, so that the feeling of reality of external world is temporarily changed or lost.

Treatment

a. Supportive psychotherapy.
b. Psychopharmacology amphetamines/antipsychotics.

3. Other Specific Neurotic Disorders

This category including miscellaneous disorders. These are called culture-bound syndromes, for example, dhat syndrome, koro, latah, whitigo, piblokto, and amok.

A. Dhat Syndrome

'Dhat' is a whitish discharge passed in urine and believed to be semen by the patients leads to anxiety, depressive and sexual disturbance.

Treatment

1. Counseling.
2. Symptomatic treatment-anxiety depression and sexual disturbance.

B. Amok

Sudden unprovoked episode of page, in which the affected person runs about and indiscriminately injuries or kills any person who is encountered on the ways.

C. Coro

The affected male persons has the belief that his penis is shrinking and may disappear into his abdominal wall and he may die.

REACTING TO STRESS AND ADJUSTMENT DISORDERS

This category in ICD-10 consists of those disorder which are temporally related to an stressful life event or a significant life change immediately before the ones it.

1. **Acute stress reaction:**
   It is an immediate and clear temporal relationship between and exceptional stressor. The symptoms slow a mixed and changing picture, e.g.
   Death of a loved one, natural catastrophes, rape, accident, etc.
   Symptoms: Anxiety, depression, anger, despair, over activity or withdrawal.
   Treatment: Environment removal and anti anxiety drugs.
2. **Post-traumatic stress disorder (PTSD)**
   According to ICD-10, this disorder arises as a delayed and response to an exceptionally stressful or catastrophic life event or situation which in likely to cause pervasive distress in almost any person.

Causes

Disasters, war rape, accident.

Symptoms

Recurrent and intensive recollection of stressful event either flash back and dreams. Marked symptoms of anxiety and increased arousal.

The other clinical features include partial amnesia for some aspects of the stressful event, feeling of numbness and anhedonia.

PTSD

Treatment

1. Prevention:
   Prevent the event through proper management (e.g.) disaster management.
2. **Supportive disorders**
3. **Drugs therapy**
   Antidepressant and antianxiety (benzodiazepan).
4. **Adjustment disorder:**
   One of the most common psychiatrics disorders. It is most common in adolescents and women. According to ICD-10, the disorder is characterized by these disorder which occur within month of a significant life change.

This disorder mainly due to pour coping skills or personality factors. The duration of disorders less than 6month.

Subtypes

1. Brief depression reaction
2. Prolonged depression reaction
3. Mixed anxiety and depressive reaction.
4. Mixed disturbance of emotions and conduct.
   The most of them recover with in 3 months.

Treatment

1. Supportive PT
2. Crises intervention.
3. Stress management training.
4. Copping skills training.
5. Drug treatment: Benzodiazepan and antidepressant.

17 Child Psychiatry

DEFINITION

Psychological disturbance in childhood is an abnormality of emotions, behavior or relationships which is sufficiently severe and persistent to handicap the child in his social or personal functioning and or to cause distress to the child, his parents or to people in the community (Peter Hoare, 1993).

CAUSES OF CHILD PSYCHIATRIC DISORDERS

1. Constitutional Including Genetic Factors

Constitutional factors those which operate from the time of birth may be divided as follows:

a. Genetic factors
b. The effect of chromosome abnormalities
c. The results of birth injuries
d. Intrauterine damage or disease

a. Genetic Factors

Few child psychiatric disorders due to specific stringle genetic factors, through such factors are responsible for certain forms of mental retardation. The most common of these is phenylkenuria an inborn error. Polygemic influences combined with environmental factors are believed to play significant role in the causation of many child psychiatric disorders, as well as in determining intelligence levels. They have made it in recent years have been great advances in genetics.

b. Chromosomal Abnormalities:

Observable abnormalities of the chromosomes may cause physical abnormalities many of which are severe or fatal that they may affect intelligence and they may contribute to psychological problems.

e.g. i. Trisomy 21 or down syndrome [21, × × ×]

ii. Fragile syndrome or linked mental retardation.

c. Premature Birth and Injury at Birth

Babies who are small for their gestational age at births tend to less developmentally advanced and to show behavioral differences when compared with children of normal birth weight. Injuries at birth due to instrumental delivery, obstructed labor, procedure like amniocentesis, some medical conditions like placental preuria, hydramnios, preeclampsia, etc.

d. Intrauterine Damage or Disease

The recent decades a common tragic cause of fetal damage seems to have been an increase, namely the abuse of drug including alcohol, by pregnant women. The fetal alcohol syndrome may follow severe alcohol abuse during pregnancy. It comprises growth deficiency, mental retardation, the thin upper lip, short palprebral fissures and abnormalities of the nose also affects adversely the development of the fetus and is associated with low birth weight and poor adjustment to school age.

2. Physical Disease and Injury

Brain disease and injury may produce impairment of intelligence, loss of particular motor or sensory functions, epilepsy or (probably) specific forms of abnormal behavior such as motor hyperactivity. Brain damage may be caused by injury, infections, metabolic disorders, minor's a wide variety of degenerative disorders and severe malnutrition in early life. Head injuries are common in childhood and many brain injured children are found to have behavioral or emotional problems. Chronic conditions such as blindness, congenital heart disease, asthma and various forms of dwarfism may cause emotional problems through their physical handicapping effects. Injuries especially serious ones like burns and also can have similar effects.

3. Temperature Factors

In a longitudinal studies in New York, Thomas et al , (1984) found that certain temperamental factors detected before the age of 2 years might predispose later psychiatric disorders.

4. Environmental Factors

The child personality and adjustment in society are the result of the interactions between genetic inheritance and biological make up one hand and the environment on the other changes of family caretakers, as when children are repeatedly placed in and out of the care of child welfare agencies, or are moved frequently one home to another can be damaging and impair seriously the process of personality development. Many are burdened by problems such as feelings of insecurity poor self esteem, unresolved anger and difficulty engaging in trusting, loving relationship with others. School influences are important factors in the development of children. Rates of child psychiatric referral and delinquency vary between schools as it is a social environment.

PSYCHIATRIC DISORDERS IN CHILDREN (ICD – 10) (1992)

I. **Disorders of psychological development:**
   1. Specific developmental disorders of speech and development.
      a. Speech articulation disorders
      b. Expressive language disorders
      c. Receptive language disorders
   2. Disorders of scholastic skills
      a. Specific reading disorder
      b. Specific spelling disorder
      c. Disorder of arithmetic skills
   3. Pervasive developmental disorders:
      a. Childhood autism
      b. Rett's syndrome
      c. Asperger's syndrome

II. **Behavioral and emotional disorders with onset – usually occurring in childhood and adolescent.**

1. Hyperkinetic disorder
2. Conduct disorders
   a. Confined to family content
   b. Unsocialized conduct disorder
   c. Socialized conduct disorder
3. Emotional disorders with onset specific to childhood
   a. Separation anxiety disorder
   b. Phobic anxiety disorder
   c. Social anxiety disorder
   d. Sibling rivalry disorder
4. Disorder of social functioning
   a. Elective mutism
   b. Reactive attachment disorder
   c. Tie disorder
5. Other behavioral and emotional disorder
   a. Nonorganic enuresis
   b. Nonorganic encopresis
   c. Feeding disorder
   d. Pica
   e. Suffering

III. **Other psychiatric disorder with onset in childhood and adolescence:**

1. Psychiatric substance use disorder
2. Schizophrenia
3. Mood disorders
4. Obsessive – compulsive disorders
5. Post-traumatic stress disorders
6. Dissociative disorder
7. Somatoform disorder
8. Anorexia nervosa
9. Bulimia nervosa

IV. **Mental Retardation**

1. Mild mental retardation
2. Moderate mental retardation

c) Severe mental retardation
d) Profound mental retardation

I. DISORDER OF PSYCHOLOGICAL DEVELOPMENT

1. Specific Developmental Disorders of Speech and Language

These are disorders in which normal pattern of language acquisition are disturbed from early stages of development. The conditions are not directly attributable to the neurological or speech mechanism abnormalities, sensory impairment mental retardation or environmental factors. The child may be better able to communicate or understand to certain very familiar situations than in others but language ability in every setting is impaired.

a. Specific Speech Articular Disorder

A specific development disorder in which the child's use of speech sound is below the appropriate level of his or her mental age, but in which there is a normal level of language skills. Normally at the age of four years, error in speech sound production are common. By the age of 6 – 7 years most of the speech sound will be acquired. Though difficulties may be with certain sound combination these should not result in any problems of communication.

Signs and Symptoms

Abnormal development occur when the child's acquisition of speech sounds is delayed or deviant, leading to disarticulation him/ her omissions, distortions or substitutions of speech sounds and in consistencies in the occurrence of sound.

b. Expressive Language Disorder

A specific developmental disorders in which the child's ability to use expressive spoken language is marked by below the appropriate level for his or her mental age, but in which language comprehensive is with in normal limits. There may not be abnormalities in articulation.

Signs and Symptoms

- Absence of single words by the age of 2 years.
- Failure of generate two word phrases by 3 years.
- Restricted vocabulary development.
- Over use of small set of general words.
- Difficulties in selection appropriate word and word substitution.
- Short utterance length.
- Immature sentence structure.

c. Receptive Language Disorder

A specific developmental disorder in which the child's understanding of language is below the appropriate level of his or her mental health. In almost all cases expressive language is markedly disturbed and abnormalities is word sound production are common.

Signs and Symptoms

- Failure to respond to familiar names by the first birthday.
- Inability to identify at least few objects by 18 months.
- Failure to follow simple routine instruction by the age of 2 years.
- Inability to follow or unclastained grammatical structures.
- Lack of understanding of more subtle aspects of language.
- Hyperactivity, inattention, social ineptness, isolation from peers, anxiety, sensitivity and undue shyness are all relatively frequent.

However they differ from autistic children in usually showing normal social reciprocity, normal make, believe play, normal use of parents for comfort, near normal age of gesture and only mild impairment in non verbal communications.

To confirm diagnosis of specific developmental disorders of speech and language clinicians should have the child tested with standardized receptive/expressive language and non verbal intellectual tests. Observations of the child's verbal and sign language pattern in various setting and during interactions with other children.

Treatment of speech and language disorders.

- Speech and language therapy
- Supportive parental counseling
- Psychotherapy.

2. Specific Developmental Disorders of Scholastic Skills

These are disorders in which the normal patterns of skill acquisition are disturbed from the early stages of development of the disorders are thought to stem from abnormalities in cognitive processing that desire largely team some type of biological dysfunctions, the conditions are substantially more common in boys than girls.

Signs and Symptoms

- There must be a clinically significant degree of impairment in the specified scholastic skill.
- The impairment must be specified in the sense that is most solely explained by mental retardation only lesser impairment in general intelligence.
- The impairment must be developmental in the sense that it must have been present during the early years of schooling and not acquired later in the educational process.
- There must be no external factors that could provide a sufficient reason for the scholastic difficulties.

a. Specific Reading Disorders

In the early stages of learning as alpha, beta script, there may be difficulties in reciting the alphabet, in griming the correct names of letters, in griming simple rhymes for words and in analyzing or categorizing sounds. Later there may be errors in oral reading skill such as shown by errors in oral reading skill such as shown by

Signs and Symptoms

- Omissions, substitutions, distortions or addition as of words or parts of words.

- False starts, long hesitation or loss of place in test and inaccurate phrasing.
- Reversal of words in sentences or letters with in words.
- An inability to recall facts read.
- Inability to draw conclusion or inferences from material read.
- Associated emotional and/or behavioral disturbances are also common during the school age period. How self esteem and problems in school adjustments and in peer relationship are also frequent.
- Performance is best assured by means of individually administered standardized and test of reading accuracy.

b. Specific Spelling Disorders

The main feature of the disorder is a specific and significant impairment in the development of spelling skills, in the absence of a history of specific reading disorders. The ability to spell orally and to write out words correctly are both affected.

Signs and Symptoms

- The child's spelling performance should be significantly below the level expected on the basis of his or her age general intelligence and school placement and is best assessed by individually administered standardized test of spelling.
- There should be no history of previous significant reading difficulties.

c. Specific Disorders of Arithmetical Skills

The child's arithmetical performance should be significantly below the level expected on the basis of his or her age, general intelligence and school placement, and is best assessed by means of an individually administered, standardized test of arithmetical.

Signs and Symptoms

- Failure to understand the concepts underlying particular arithmetical operations.
- Lack of understanding of mathematical terms or signs.

- Failure to recognize numerical symbols.
- Difficulty in carrying out standard arithmetical manipulations.
- Difficulty in understanding which numbers are relevant to the arithmetical problem being considered.
- Difficulty to properly aligning numbers or in inserting decimal points or symbols during calculations.

Treatment of Development Disorder of Scholastic Skill

- Treatment of choice is remedial educational approach.
- Co-existing emotional and behavioral problems should be treated by appropriate psychotherapeutic means.
- Computers and electronic calculators can lighten the burden of children who have mathematical learning difficulties.
- Parental counseling.

3. Pervasive Developmental Disorders

These are a group psychiatric conditions in which expected social skill, language development and behavioral report are either do not develop appropriately or are lost in early childhood. In general the disorders affects multiple areas of development are manifested early in life and cause persistent dysfunction.

a. Childhood Autism

This condition was described by **Leo Kanner (1943)** also suggested the name infantile autism. A pervasive developmental disorder defined by the presence of abnormal and or impaired development that is manifest before the age of 3 years, characterized by abnormalities of communication, abnormalities of social development and a restriction of behavior and interests.

Clinical Features

The four main areas of functioning which are affected are:

1. Social interaction
2. Communication
3. Behavior, the range of which is restrictive and repetitive
4. Cognitive functions.

1. **Social interaction:** Inadequate appreciation of socio emotional are as shown by inability to make warm emotional relationship with people. Autistic children do not respond to their parents affectionate behavior.

   Poor use of social signals and weak integration of social, emotional and communicative behavior. They tend to do their own things regardless of who is around or what is happening in the environment as their children. A related behavior is gaze avoidance and failure to make eye to eye contact with people.

2. **Impairments in communication:**
   - Failure to develop normal or sometimes any speech, also failure to communicate by gestures body movements or facial expressions.
   - Lack of social usage of whatever language skills are present.
   - Impairment in make – believe and social imitative play.
   - Lack of creativity and fantasy in thoughts process.
   - May exhibit echolalia.

3. **Behavioral abnormalities:**
   - Characterized by restricted repetitive and stereotyped patterns of behavior interests and activities.
   - Tendency to impose rigidity and routine an a wide range of aspects of day to day functioning.
   - Gets very upset by minor changes in routine or the moving of furniture in their house, wearing different clothes or even change in the order in which books are placed in a book care.
   - Difficulty in generalizing newly learned skills to new situations or tables.
   - Stereotyped and repetitive play, lack of symbolic play.
   - Ritualistic behavior, e.g. checking and touching rituals and dressing in particular ways. When their rituals are interrupted these children may became anxiety or angry.
   - Rocking twirling head banging and similar repetitive behavior are often seen especially in mentally retarded autistic children.
   - Over activity, disruptive behavior and temper tantrums which may occur for little or no obvious reasons.
   - Rear or phobias, eating and sleeping disturbances.

4. **Cognitive abnormalities**
   These are complex and extensive **(Rutter 1983)** and extend well beyond the problems with the use of language mentioned earlier.
   - These children are poor at symbolization, understanding, abstract ideas and grasping theoretical concepts.
   - Memory may be excellent, that they may be preoccupied with things like brain or bus timetables or the different models of cars or airplanes.

Treatment

- Structured classroom training in combination with behavioral methods is the most effective treatment method for many autistic children.
- Careful training of parents in the concepts and the skills of behavior modification and the resolutions of the parents concern may yield considerable gain in the child's language, cognitive and social areas of behavior.
- Administration of haloperiodol reduces behavioral symptoms and accelerates learning.
- Naltrexone an opiate antagonistic is being invested in the hope that blocking and genus opioids will reduce autistic symptoms.
- Insight oriented psychotherapy has proved to be effective.

b. Rett's Disorder

In 1965, Andreas Rett's, an Australian physician identified this syndrome a condition of unknown cause, so for reported only in girls, which has been differentiated on the basis of a characteristic onset, course and pattern of symptomatology.

Diagnostic Guidelines

- Apparently normal or near normal early development.
- Onset as between 7 and 24 months of age.
- Loss of purposive hand movements and acquired fine motor manipulative skills.
- Loss, partial loss of lack of development of language.

- Distinctive, stereotyped totous evengling or hand washing movements with the events flexed in front of chest or chin.
- Often episodes of hyper ventilation.
- Failure to gain bowel and bladder control.
- Excessive dialing and protrusion of tongue.
- Loss of social engagement.
- Stance and gait tend to become broad based hypotonic muscles and poorly co-coordinated tremble movements.
- Rigid spasticity may develop in adolescent or adult hood.
- Epileptic fits occur in a majority of cases.

c. Asperger's Disorders

In 1944 Hans Asperger an Austrian Physician described a syndrome that be named autistic psychopathy. His original description was of persons with normal intelligence who exhibile a qualitative impairment in reciprocal social interaction and behavioral oddities without delay in language development. Since that time persons with mental retardation but without language delay have received diagnosis of Asperger's disorders. The disorders is more common in boys than in girls children with Asperger's syndrome an distant, aloof and lacking in empathy and in there respects resemble autistic children but differs from autism promiscuity in than there is no general delay or retardation in language or cognitive development.

II. BEHAVIORAL AND EMOTIONAL DISORDERS WITH ONSET USUALLY OCCURRING IN CHILDHOOD AND ADOLESCENCE

1. Hyperkinetic Disorders (Attention Deficit Hyperactivity Disorder)

Attention deficit or hyperactivity disorder (ADHD) is characterized by a developmentally inappropriate poor attention span of age–inappropriate features of hyperactivity and impulsivity or both. Hyperkinetic disorders are several times more frequent in boys than in girls. The characteristic behavioral problems should be of early onset.

Diagnostic Guidelines

The cardinal features are impaired attention and over activity, both are necessary for the diagnosis and should be evident in more than one situation.

- Impaired attention is manifested by primarily breaking off from tasks and learning activities unfinished. The children change frequently from one activity to another seemingly loosing interest in one task because they become diverted to another.
- Over activity implies excessive restlessness, especially in situations requiring relative calm. It may depend upon the situation involve the child running and jumping around, getting up from seat when he was supposed to remain seated, excessive talkativeness and noisiness.

  They are often reckless and impulsive, prone to accidents and find themselves in disciplinary trouble because of unthinking breaches of rules.

- The standard of judgment should be that the attention deficit and activity is excessive in the context of what is expected and by comparison with other children of same age and IQ.
- Cognitive impairment is common and specific delays in motor language development are disproportionately frequent.

Treatment

- Pharmacotherapy

  CNC Stimulants — e.g. Dextroamphetamine, methyl phenidate

  Antidepressants — e.g. Imipramine

  Psychotherapy
- Behavior modification
- Parent counseling

2. Conduct Disorders

Conduct disorders are characterized by a repetitive and persistent pattern of dissocial, aggressive or defiant conduct. Such behavior when at its most extreme for the individual should amount to major violations of age appropriate social expectations and is therefore more severe than ordinary childish mischief or adolescent rebelliousness.

Diagnostic Guidelines

Judgement concerning the presence of conduct disorder should take into account the child's development level.

Examples of the behavior in which the diagnosis is based include excessive levels of fighting or bullying, cruelty to animals to others people. Severe destructiveness to property, fire setting, stealing, repeated lying, truancy from school and running away from home, unusually frequent and severe temper tantrums, defiant provocative behavior and persistent severe disobedience. Anyone of these categories of marked is sufficient for the diagnosis but isolated dissocial acts are not.

The main categories of conduct disorders are:

(a) **Conduct disorder confined to the family context:**
This category comprises conduct disorders involving dissocial aggressive behavior in which the abnormal behavior is entirely or almost entirely, confined to the home and or to interactions with members of the nuclear family or immediate household.

(b) **Unsocialized conduct disorder:**
This type of conduct disorder is characterized by the combination of persistent dissocial or aggressive behavior occurring in individuals who are generally well integrated into their peer group.

(c) **Oppositional defiant disorder:**
It is defined by the presence of marked by defiant disobedient provocative behavior and by the absence of more severe dissocial or aggressive act that violate the law or the rights of others. This type of conduct disorder is characteristically seen in children below the age of 9 to 10 years.

Treatment

Treatment is mainly directed to the family usually takes the form is social care work or family therapy.

- Parent training programs – these programs use behavior modification principles. Parents are taught how the child's antisocial behavior may be reinforced unintentionally by their attention to it. Parents are also taught how to reinforce normal behavior by praise or rewards and how to set limits and abnormal behavior.
- Anger management – Anger management program seek to correct inappropriate behavior by talking how to inhibit sudden appropriate responses to angry feelings and how to reappraisee the intentions of other people and use socially acceptable forms of self assertion.
- Group Therapy of the child by using peer pressures to reduce antisocial behavior.
- Individual psychotherapy oriental toward improving problem solving skills can be useful.
- Mediation – overt explosive aggression responds to antipsychotics (e.g. haloperidol or lithium).

3. Emotional Disorders with Onset Specific to Childhood

(a) **Separation Anxiety Disorder of Childhood:**

Some degree of separation anxiety is a universal phenomenon and it is in expected part of a child's normal development. Separation anxiety disorder, however, is present when developmentally inappropriate and excessive anxiety emerges concerning separation from the major attachment figure the anxiety may take form of:

- An unrealistic preoccupying worry about possible harm be falling major attachment figure or a fear that they will leave and nor return.
- Persistent reluctance or refusal to go to school because of fear about separation.
- Persistent reluctance or refusal to go to sleep without being near or next to a major attachment figure.
- Persistent inappropriate fears of being alone, or otherwise without the major attachment figure at home during the day.

- Repeated occurrence of physical symptoms on occasions that involve separation from a major attachment figure, such as learning home to go to school.
- Excessive, recurrent distress following separation from a major attachment figure.
- Repeated nightmares involving the theme of separation.

Treatment

A multi modal treatment approach–including psychotherapy family education and family therapy is recommended for separation anxiety disorder. Family therapy helps the parents understand the need for consistent, and the importance of preparing for any important change in life, such as illness, surgery or geographic relocation. Specific cognitive strategies and relaxation exercise may help the child control the anxiety, pharmaco therapy is also useful, e.g. tricyclic Imi-piramine (antidepressant).

(b) **Phobic Anxiety Disorder:**

Children like adults can develop fear that is focused on wide range or objects or situations. Minor phobic symptoms are common in childhood they usually concern animals, insects, the dark school and death. Most child of the phobias improve without specific treatment provided that the parents adopts a firm and reassuring approach. For phobias that do not improve simple behavioral treatment can be combined with reassurance and support. The child is encouraged to encounter feared situations in a graded way.

(c) **Social Anxiety Disorder of Childhood:**

Children with this disorders show a persistent or recurrent fear and avoidance and strangers. These children are marked anxious in the presence of strangers and avoid them. The fear, which may be mainly of adults or if other children interferes with social functioning its is associated with a normal degree of scheme attachment to parent or to other family persons. According to ICD – 10 this category should be used only for disorders that wise before the age of 6 years. Treatment includes simple behaviors method combined with reassurance ad support.

(d) **Sibling Rivalry Disorder:**

A high proportion or even a majority of young children show a degree of emotional disturbance following the birth of a young sibling certain children show extreme jealously or other signs of rivalry of a sibling, starting during months following the birth of that sibling. The child may regress in behavior losing previously learned control of bladder or bowel. There is usually opposition to the parents and behavior intended to obtain their attention often with temper tantrums. There may be sleep disturbance and problems at bedtime.

4. Disorders of Social Functioning with Onset Specific to Childhood and Adolescence

A. **Elective Mutism:** The condition as characterized emotionally determined selecting in speaking such that the child demonstrates his or her language competence in same situations but fails to speak such that the child demonstrates his or her language competence in same situations but fails to speak in other situation. Associated with parental over protection, parental ambivalence, communication disorders, shyness and oppositional behaviors.

Treatment

Can include a conformation of behavior and family therapy techniques to promote communication and the use of speech, individual psychotherapy also will help failure to improve by the age of 10 years is a poor prognostic sign.

B. **Reactive Attachment Disorder of Childhood:** This disorder occurs in infants and young children is characterized by persistent abnormalities in the child's pattern of social relationships which are associated with emotional disturbance and reactive to change in environment circumstance fearfulness and hypervigilence that do no respond to conforming, poor social interaction with peers, aggression towards the self and others and misery are characteristics. The attachment disorders may also be accompanied by a failure to thrive physically and by impaired physical growth.

Treatment

- Psychotherapeutic interventions including individual psychotherapy family therapy and psychotropic mediations.
- Educational counseling services for parents and child, counseling in increase awareness and understanding of the child's needs to increase parenting skills.
- Close monitoring of the progression of the patients emotional and physical well being.
- If close intervention be inadequate or fail placement with relativeness or in foster care, or residential treatment facility must be considered.

C. **Tic Disorders:** The predominant manifestation in these syndromes is somatoform tic. A tic is an involuntary, rapid recurrent, non-rhythmic motor movement or vocal production that is sudden onset and serves no apparent purpose. Tics tend to be irresistible but they can usually be suppressed for varying period of time.

Both motor vocal tic may be classified as either simple or complex. Common simple motor tics includes eye blinking, neck jacking, shoulder shrugging and facial grimacing. Common simple vocal tics include throat clearing, sniffing and hissing, common complex motor tics include hitting one self, jumping one self, jumping and hopping, common complex vocal ties include the repetition of particular words and sometimes the use of socially unacceptable words and the repetition on one's own words or sounds. The major feature distinguishing tics from the other motor disorders are the sudden rapid transient and circumscribed nature of the movements, together with lack of evidence of underlying neurological disorders their repetitiveness usually their disappearance during sleep and the ease with which they may be voluntarily reproduced or suppressed.

Transient tic disorder is a commonest form of tic and is most frequent about the age of 4 – 5 years and do not persist for longer than 12 months. The tics usually take the form of eye blinking, facial grimacing or head jerking, chronic motor or vocal tic disorder may be either single or multiple and last for more than a year.

Tourette's Disorder

George Gilles Dela Tourette described this form of tic disorder in which there are or have been multiple motor tics and one or more vocal tics. Onset is a almost always in-childhood or adolescence. A history of motor tics before a development of vocal tics is common. The symptoms frequently worsen during adolescence and it is common for the disorder to persist into adult life. As with motor tics, the vocal tics may be voluntarily suppressed for short periods, be exacerbated by stress and disappear during sleep.

Treatment of the Disorders

Whether the tics will disappear spontaneously progress or become chronic is unclear in the beginning focusing attention on tics may exacubate them. So the clinician of the beginning recommends that at first the family disregard the tics as much as possible. But if the tics are so severe that they impair the patient or if they are accompanied by significant emotional disturbances, complete psychiatric and pediatric neurological examination are recommended.

Psychotherapy may be indicated to minimize the secondary emotional problems caused by the tics. Behavioral techniques particularly habit reversal treatment have been effective treating chronic motor or vocal tic disorders. Psychopharmacology is not recommended unless the symptoms are unusually severe and disabling.

Haloperidol appears to be most effective at relatively low dosages for Tourette's disorders. For children between 3 and 12 years the recommended total daily dosage is between 05 and 0.075 mm per kg administered in divided dosage either 2 or 3 times a day. Patient and their parents must be made aware of the drugs possible immediate and long term adverse affects.

5. Other Behavioral and Emotional Disorders with Onset Usually Occurring in Childhood and Adolescence

a. **Nonorganic enuresis:**

A disorder characterized by involuntary voiding of urine day by day and or by night, which is abnormal in relation to the individuals mental age and which is not a consequence of a lack of bladder control due to any neurological disorder, to epileptic attacks or to any structural abnormality of the urinary tract. Enuresis would not voluntarily be diagnosed in a child under the age of 5 years or with mental age of 4 years. The enuresis may constitute a monosymptomatic condition or it may be associated with a more wide spread emotional or behavioral disorder. Emotional problems may arise as a secondary consequence of the distress or stigma.

Treatment

- Exclude any organic cause.
- Appropriate toilet training with parental reinforcement should have been attempted.
- Behavior therapy – positive reinforcement for dry night is a successful treatment. Encouragement or reward for delaying micturition for increasing length of time during waking hours can be used.
- Psychotherapy may be useful in dealing with the co existing psychiatric problems, emotional and family difficulties.

Pharmacotherapy

Drug should rarely be used to treat enuresis and then only as a last resort in intractable cares causing serious socioemotional difficulties for the sufferer. Imipramine is effacious and has been approved for use in treating childhood enuresis.

b. **Nonorganic Encopresis:**

Encopresis is the repeatedly in voluntary passage of facies, usually of normal or near normal consistency in places not appropriate for that purpose in the individuals own sociocultural setting. The condition may represent an abnormal continuation of normal infantile incontinence. It may involve a loss of incontinence following the acquisition of bowel control or it may involve the deliberate deposition of faces in inappropriate places in spite of normal physiological bowel control. In some instances the encopresis may be accompanied by smearing of faces ever the body or over the external environment. There is usually some degree of associated emotional or behavioral disturbance.

Encopresis can reflect a poor parent-child relationship and as a response to stressful situation children with encopresis have usually been subjected to coercive and obsessional toilet, training practices and the encopresis is seen as a reaction, often of anger and aggression, toward this practices.

Treatment

- Exclude physical causes of chronic constipation.
- Family tension regarding the symptom must be reduced and a non-punitive atmosphere must be created. Parental guidance and family therapy often is needed.
- Behavior techniques have been used with great success including such behaviiuor reinforces as star charts in which the child places a star on a chart for dry or continent nights.
- Individual psychotherapy to gain the cooperation and trust of the child.

c. **Pica of infancy and childhood:**

Persistent eating of non-nutritive substances. Pica may occur as one of many symptoms of a more widespread psychiatric disorder or as a relatively isolated psychopathological behavior. This phenomenon is most common in mental retardation. However, pica may also occur in children of normal intelligence.

Treatment

Includes parental guidance to keep the child away from the non nutritive substances. Aversive conditioning is also necessary.

Medical complications that develop secondary to pica should be treated.

d. **Feeding disorder of infancy and childhood:**
It generally involves refusal of food and extreme faddiness in the presence of an adequate food supply and reasonably competent care giver and the absence of organic disease. There may or may not be associated rumination. Disorder should be diagnosed only if the difficulties are clearly beyond the normal range, if the nature of the eating problem is qualitatively abnormal in character or if the child fails to gain weight or loses weight over a period of atleast 1 month.

Treatment

Involves parental guidance to improve the child's psychosocial environment. Behavioral techniques have also been used effectively. Aversive conditioning involves administering mild electric shock or squirting an unpleasant substance, such as lemon juice in the month whenever rumination occurs.

e. **Sluttering or Stammering:**
Speech that is characterized by frequent repetition or prolongation of sounds or syllables or words, or by frequent hesitations or pauses that disrupt the rhythmic flow of speech. Minor dysrythmias of this type are quite common as a transient phase in early childhood, minor but persistent speech feature in later childhood and adult life. They should be classified as a disorder only if their severity is such as markedly to disturb the fluency of speech. There may be associated movements of the face and or other parts of the body that coincide in time with the repetitions, prolongations or pauses in speech flow.

III. OTHER PSYCHIATRIC DISORDERS WITH ONSET IN CHILDHOOD AND ADOLESCENCE

1. Mental and behavioral disorders due to psychoactive substance use
2. Schizophrenia

3. Mood disorders
4. Obsessive-compulsive disorder
5. Post-traumatic stress disorder
6. Dissociative (conversion) disorders
7. Somatization disorders
8. Anorexia nervosa
9. Mental retardation.

18 Personality Disorders

Personality disorders result when these personality traits become abnormal, i.e. become inflexible and maladaptive and cause significant social or occupational impairment or significant subjective distress.

PERSONALITY

- Refers to "the aggregate of the physical and mental qualities of the individual's as these interact and function in characteristic fashion with his environment".

  — Taylor
- Also described as the unique pattern of traits with characterize the individual.

Approaches or Theory of Personality

1. Trait approach
2. Psycho analytic approach

a. The Trait Approach

Traits are characteristics of a person that lead him to behave more or less in distinctive and consistent ways in the given situation.

Sheldon described personality according to physique of individual:

Physique	*Psychopathology*
Endomorphic Soft and round people	Severe mood changes (Depression)

Contd...

Contd...

Physique	*Psychopathology*
Mesomorphic Muscular built strong and athletic type	These types of people have severe types of mood alteration.
Ectomorphic Thin body built, slender and very delicate and fragile	Sensitive and delicate intellectual, more religious • Schizophrenia

According to **Eretschmer:**

Physique	*Psychopathology*
Pyknic (Fat and round and graceful people)	Mood alteration – MDP (Manic depressive psychosis)
Atheletic (Muscular built and strong skeleton)	Schizophrenia Mood changes
Asthenic Thin body build, tall and skin is dry.	Schezoid and schizophrenia

Carl Jung: described two traits in personality; Introverts and Extroverts.

Physique	*Psychopathology*
Introvert Thin built individuals	Schizophrenia, depression
Extrovert Fat, muscular	Mood alteration

b. Psychoanalytic Approach

(i) Levels of consciousness (ii) Subsystems of personality

(i) Levels of Consciousness

(1) Conscious level: It relates to the awareness of an individual to his environment.
(2) Preconscious level: It is described as that part of mind in which ideas and reactions are stored and partially forgotten.
(3) Unconscious level: It is largest part of mind. It is the storehouse for all the memories, feeling and responses experienced by individual during his entire life.

(ii) Subsystems of Personality

It is also called as agencies of mind.

They are, ID, ego and superego.

ID: Latin word of ID is "IT". ID is the original source of personality which is present in a newborn. ID is present in deepest level of the unconscious, ID is completely selfish. ID operates on the basis of the pleasure principle. In other words, it is referred to as a primary process thinking.

Ego: The Latin word of Ego is "I" which means "Self". Ego is functionally the executive of personality. Ego acts as a mediator or balances between the demands of ID and Superego. Ego is based on the reality principle. It is secondary process thinking. Ego waits for the right moment for the satisfaction of desire, whereas ID satisfies desires immediately.

Super Ego: Latin word of super ego is "Higher Self". Super ego is developed over a period of time. Moral principle is based for Super Ego.

Factors Influencing the Development of Personality

1. **Heredity:**
   Physical characteristics, mental characteristics also be passed into person by the family.
2. **Environment:**
   Environment influencing in shaping the personality of an individual. The child may be born with many potentialities and abilities, but the use of these abilities will be shown by the person according to the environment in which he is growing.
3. **Self:**
   I or self is the integrated care of the personality. The components of self are: knower, striver and doer. Self means "I" concept means what ideas I have about me.

Stages of Development According to Freud

(a) *Oral stage 0 to 18 months:* During the first year of life month is principle organ.

(b) *Anal stage 18 months to 3 yr:* Membranes of anal region provide pleasure. Not passing fecal matter also gives pleasure to the child.
(c) *Phallic stage 3 to 6 yr:* Sexuality repressed, focus on relationship with same sex peers.
(d) *Latency stage of 6 to 12 yr:* Sexuality repressed, focus on relationship with same sex peers.
(e) *Genital (13 ˘ 20 yr):* Begins with puberty. Libido reawakened as genital organs mature, focus on relationship with members of the opposite sex.

Psychosocial Theory by Eric Erickson

Age	*Developmental task*
0 – 18 months (Infancy)	Trust vs Mistrust
18 months – 3 yr (Early childhood)	Autonomy vs Sham/doubt
3 – 5 yr middle (Childhood)	Initiative vs Guilt
5 – 12 yr (Late childhood)	Industry vs Inferiority
13 – 19 yr (Adolescence)	Identity vs role diffusion
20 – 40 (Early adulthood)	Intimacy vs Isolation
40 – 65 yr (Middle age)	Generativity vs Stagnation
65 – Death – Old age	Ego Integrity vs Despair

Prevalence

The prevalence of personality disorders in the general population is 5-10%.

In DSM – IV, the personality disorders are coded on Axis II and have been divided into three clusters.

In ICD – 10, the personality disorders are listed under section on "Disorders of adults personality and behavior".

According to ICD – 10 CDDG, the diagnostic guidelines for specific personality disorder include conditions not directly attributable to gross brain damage or disease or to another psychiatric disorder, meeting following criteria:

1. Markedly disharmonious attitudes and behavior involving usually several areas of functioning, e.g. affectivity, arousal,

impulse control, ways of perceiving and thinking and style of relating to others.

2. The abnormal behavior pattern is enduring of long standing and not limited to episodes of mental illness.
3. The abnormal behavior pattern is pervasive and clearly maladaptive to a broad range of personal and social situations.
4. The above manifestation always appear during childhood or adolescence and continue into adulthood.
5. The disorder leads to considerable personal distress but this may only become apparent late in its course.
6. The disorder is usually, but not invariably, associated with significant problems in occupational and social performance.

CLUSTERS: DSM IV – TR

1. Cluster A (Odd and Eccentric)
   Schizophrenic – continuum
   1. Paranoid PD
   2. Schizoid PD
   3. Schizotypal PD
2. Cluster B (Dramatic, emotional and erratic)
   Psychopathic continuum
   1. Antisocial PD
   2. Historic PD
   3. Narcissistic PD
   4. Borderline PD
3. Cluster – C(Anxious and Fearful)
   "Introversion"
   1. Avoidant PD
   2. Dependent PD
   3. Obsessive – Compulsive PD

1. Paranoid Personality Disorder

According to ICD – 10,

1. Excessive sensitiveness to setbacks and rebuffs.
2. Tendency to bear grudges persistently, i.e. refusal to forgive insults and injuries or slights.

3. Suspiciousness and a pervasive tendency to distort experience by misconstruing the natural or friendly actions of others as hostile or contemptuous.
4. A combative and tenacious sense of personal rights, out of keeping with actual situation.
5. Recurrent suspicious, without justification, regarding sexual fidelity of spouse or sexual partner.
6. Tendency to experience excessive self-importance, manifest in a persistent self-referential attitude.
7. Preoccupation with unsubstantiated "conspiratorial" explanations of events, both immediate to the patient and in the world at large.

Psycho dynamically, the underlying defense mechanism is projection.

Treatment

1. Individual psychotherapy
2. Supportive psychotherapy

2. Schizoid Personality Disorder

1. Few, if any, activities, provide pleasure.
2. Emotional coldness, detachment or flattened affectively.
3. Limited capacity to express either warm, tender feeling or anger towards others.
4. Apparent indifference to either praise or criticism.
5. Little interest in having sexual experienced with another person.
6. Almost invariable preference for solitary activities.
7. Excessive preoccupation with fantasy and introspection.
8. Lack of close friends or considering relationship and of desire for such relationships.
9. Marked insensitivity to prevailing social norms and conventions.

Psychodynamically, it is supposed to result from "cold and aloof" parenting in a child with introverted temperament.

Treatment

1. Individual psychotherapy
2. Psychoanalysis
3. Gradual involvement in group psychotherapy

3. Schizotypal Disorder

Characterized by eccentric behavior and anomalies of thinking and affect which resemble those seen in schizophrenia, though no definite and characteristic schizophrenia anomalies have occurred at any stage. Following symptoms – continuously or episodically for a period of atleast 2 yr.

1. Inappropriate or constricted affect (the individual appear cold and aloof.
2. Behavior or appearance that is odd, eccentric or peculiar.
3. Poor rapport with others and a tendency to social withdrawal.
4. Odd beliefs or magical thinking, influencing behavior.
5. Suspiciousness or paranoid ideas.
6. Obsessive ruminations without inner resistance, sexual or aggressive contents.
7. Unusual perceptual experiences including somatosensitivity or other illusive, depersonalization or derealization.
8. Vague, circumstantial, metaphorical, over elaborate, or stereotyped thinking manifested by odd speech.
9. Occasional transient quasi-psychotic episodic with intense illusions, auditory or other hallucination and delusion.

Treatment

1. Psychoanalysis
2. Individual psychotherapy
3. Drug therapy: Antipsychotics

4. Antisocial/Dissocial Personality Disorder

This disorder is synonymous with psychotherapy and sociopathy but does not always mean criminal behavior.

1. Callous unconcern for the feeling or others.
2. Gross and persistent attitude of irresponsibility and disregard for social norms, rules and obligation.
3. Incapacity to maintain enduring relationships though having no difficulty in establishing them.
4. Very low tolerance to frustration and a low threshold for discharge of aggression.
5. Incapacity to experience guilt and to profile from experience, particularly punishment.

There may also be persistent irritability as an associated feature. Conduct disorder during childhood and adolescence, though no invariably presence may further support the diagnosis.

Divided into 4 clinical types namely,

1. Aggressive psychopath
2. Inadequate psychopath
3. Creative psychopath
4. Sexual psychopath.

Treatment

1. Individual psychotherapy
2. Psychotherapy
3. Group psychotherapy and self-help groups
4. Drug therapy: Pericyazine (Antipsychotic)

5. Historic Personality Disorder

1. Self-dramatization, theoretically, exaggerated expression of emotions.
2. Suggestibility, easily influenced by others or by circumstances.
3. Shallow and labile affectivity.
4. Continual seeking for excitement, appreciation by others and activities in which the person is center of attention.
5. Inappropriate seductiveness in appearance/behavior.
6. Over – concern with physical attractiveness.

Associated features may include egocentricity, self-indulgence, continuous longing for appreciation, feeling that are easily hurt, and persistent manipulative behavior to achieve own needs.

This disorder is more common in females. Psychodynamically, there are intense dependency needs. The defense mechanism used most often are acting out and dissociation.

Treatment

1. Psycho analysis
2. Psycho analytic psychotherapy

6. Narcissistic Personality Disorder

A relatively new concept, this disorder is characterized by:
1. Ideas of grandiosity ad inflated sense of self-importance.
2. Preoccupation with fantasies of unlimited success.
3. Attention seeking, dramatic behavior, needs constant praise and unable to face criticism.
4. Lack of empathy with others, with exploitative behavior.
5. Shaky self-esteem, underlying sense of inferiority, easily depressed by minor events.

Treatment

Individual psychotherapy

7. Emotionally Unstable Personality Disorder

Emotionally unstable personality disorder is described as a disorder in which there is a marked tendency to act impulsively without consideration of consequences together with affective instability. This disorder is further classified into two types: Impulsive and borderline type.

Impulsive type: Emotional instability and lack of impulse control. Outbursts of violence or threatening behavior are common. Particularly in response to criticism by others.

Borderline type: Emotional instability, in addition, patient's own self-image, aims and internal preferences are often unclear or disturbed. There are usually chronic feelings of emptiness.

The borderline type is also known as borderline personality disorder.

1. Significant and persistent disturbance of identity of self.
2. Unstable and intense interpersonal relationship patterns.
3. Impulsivity.
4. Unstable emotional responses, with rapid shifts. Anger outbursts may occur.
5. Chronic feeling of boredom or emptiness.
6. Deliberate self harm is common in the form of self-mutilation, suicidal gestures.

Treatment

1. Psychoanalytic psychotherapy
2. Supportive psychotherapy
3. Drug therapy: Anti depressants, ECT, antipsychotics, Lithium, Carbamazepine.

8. Anxious (Avoidant) Personality Disorder

1. Persistent and pervasive feelings of tension and apprehension.
2. Belief that one is socially incept, personally unappealing, or inferior to others.
3. Excessive preoccupation.
4. Unwillingness to become involved with people.
5. Restrictions in life style because of need to have physical security.

Treatment

1. Individual PT
2. Group PT
3. Behavior therapy

9. Dependent Personality Disorder

1. Encouraging or allowing others to make most of one's important life decisions.
2. Subordination of one's own needs to those of others on whom one is dependent and undue compliance with their wishes.
3. Unwillingness to make even reasonable demands on the people one depends on.

4. Feeling uncomfortable or helpless when alone.
5. Preoccupation with fears of being abandoned by a person with whom one has a close relationship.
6. Limited capacity to make everyday decision without an excessive amount of advice and reassurance from others.

Treatment

1. Individual PT
2. Group PT
3. Behavior PT

10. Obsessive-Compulsive (Anankastic) Personality Disorder

1. Feeling of excessive doubt and caution.
2. Preoccupation with details, rules, lists, order, organization and schedule.
3. Perfectionism that interferes with task completion.
4. Excessive consciousness, scrupulousness.
5. Excessive pedantry and adherence to social conventions.
6. Rigidity and stubbornness.
7. Intrusion of insistent and unwelcome thoughts or impulses.

Psychodynamically, this disorder is believed to result from fixation at and sadistic phase, with the employment of reaction formation as a defense mechanism.

Treatment

1. Psychoanalysis
2. Group therapy

11. Passive-aggressive Personality Disorder

1. Significant and persistent passive resistance of demands for adequate social and occupational performance.
2. Stubbornness, intentional inefficiency, procrastination, unjustified protests, forgetfulness and dawdling are used to achieve the purpose.

Passive resistance is viewed as expression of "covert anger" or "retroflexed anger".

An overlap with dependent personality disorder is common. Secondary depression may develop.

Treatment

1. Supportive psychotherapy
2. Behavior therapy
3. Group therapy
4. Drug therapy: Antidepressants

19 Psychophysiological Disorders

Any of a large group of mental disorders that is characterized by the dysfunction of an organ or organ system controlled by the autonomic nervous system and that may be caused or aggravated by emotional factors. The disorders are named and classified according to the organ system involved, such as cardiovascular, respiratory, musculoskeletal, and GI. Also called **psychosomatic illness or psychosomatic reaction.**

Psychosomatic or Somatoform disorders are among the most common psychiatric disorders found in general practice. It is a condition of dysfunction or structural damage in bodily organs through inappropriate activation of the involuntary nervous system and the glands of internal secretion.

Psychosomatic disorder is mainly used to mean a physical disease which is thought to be caused, or made worse, by mental factors. Some physical diseases are thought to be particularly prone to be made worse by mental factors such as stress and anxiety.

Psychophysiology is the branch of physiology that is concerned with the relationship between mental (psyche) and physical (physiological) processes; it is the scientific study of the interaction between mind and body. The field of psychophysiology draws upon the work of physicians, psychologists, biochemists, neurologists, engineers, and other scientists.

HISTORY

The American Psychiatric Association's Diagnostic and Statistical Manual of Mental Disorders *(DSMIV)* classifies psychosomatic illnesses under "Psychological Factors Affecting Physical Conditions." Physicians have been aware that people's mental and emotional states influence their physical wellbeing since the time of Hippocrates. In the twentieth century, the discoveries of psychologists have shed new light on how the mind and body interact to produce health or illness. **Sigmund Freud** introduced the idea that **unconscious** thoughts can be converted into physical symptoms (**conversion reaction**). The formal study of psychosomatic illnesses began in Europe in the 1920s, and by 1939, the journal *Psychosomatic Medicine* had been founded in the United States. Eventually, sophisticated laboratory experiments replaced clinical observation as the primary method of studying psychosomatic illness. Researchers in the field of psychophysiology measured such responses as blood pressure, heart rate, and skin temperature to determine the physiological effects of human behavior. Animal research has also contributed to the growing body of knowledge about psychosomatic disorders.

CAUSES

Three theories have been particularly popular in explaining why certain persons develop psychosomatic disorders and what determines the forms these illnesses take. One theory contends that psychological **stress** affects bodily organs that are constitutionally weak or weakened by stress. Another links specific types of illness with particular types of stress. Still another theory suggests that physiological predispositions combined with psychological stress to produce psychosomatic illness.

The parts of the body most commonly affected by psychosomatic disorders are the gastrointestinal and respiratory systems. Gastrointestinal disorders include gastric and duodenal ulcers, ulcerative colitis, and irritable bowel syndrome. (**Anorexia** nervosa and **bulimia** are sometimes considered psychosomatic disorders, but they also appear under the category of "anxiety disorder—eating disorders" in *DSM-IV*.) Respiratory problems caused or worsened by psychological factors include asthma and hyperventilation syndrome. Cardiovascular complaints include coronary artery disease, hypertension, tachycardia (speeded-up and irregular heart rhythm), and migraine headaches. Psychosomatic disorders also affect the skin (eczema, allergies, and neurodermatitis) and genitourinary system (menstrual disorders and **sexual dysfunction**).

Probably the most well-known psychosomatic connection is that of stress and coronary heart disease. The term "Type A" has been used for over twenty years to describe the aggressive, competitive, impatient, controlling type of person whom researchers have found to be more prone to heart disease than people who are more easygoing and mild-mannered and less hostile and concerned with time. In 1981, a panel appointed by the National Heart, Lung, and Blood Institute found that Type A behavior poses a greater risk of coronary heart disease and myocardial infarction (heart attack) than do cigarette smoking, age, hypertension, or a high serum cholesterol count.

Emotional stress can also affect the immune system, raising the risk to the body from such foreign invaders as bacteria, viruses, and cancer cells. People under stress are more likely to develop infectious diseases, including those stemming from the reactivation of latent herpes viruses. It is known that several of the body's reactions to stress, including the release of cortical, adrenaline, and other **hormones**, suppress the activity of the immune system. A special field, psychoneuroimmunology, studies how the interaction of psychological and physiological reactions affects the functioning of the immune system.

SIGNS AND SYMPTOMS

According to the DSM II classification it has listed 10 categories of psychophysiologic disorder:

1. Skin disorders
2. Muscoskeletal disorders
3. Respiratory disorders
4. Cardiovascular disorders

5. Genitourinary disorders
6. Endocrine disorders
7. Disorders of organ of special sense — Chronic conjunctivitis
8. Disorder of other types — Disturbances in the nervous system in which emotional factors play a significant role, such as multiple sclerosis.

Sometimes a physical symptom is a metaphor for the person's psychologic problem, as when a person with a "broken heart" experiences chest pain. Other times, a physical symptom reflects identification with another person's pain.

Some people also use the term psychosomatic disorder when mental factors cause physical symptoms, but where there is no physical disease. For example, a chest pain may be caused by stress, and no physical disease is can be found.

A psychophysiological disorder is characterized by physical symptoms that are partly induced by emotional factors. Some of the more common emotional states responsible in forming illness include anxiety, stress, and fear. Common psychosomatic ailments include migraine headaches, attention deficit hyperactivity disorder), arthritis, and heart disease.

DIAGNOSIS

The field of psychophysiology is leading the way to an ongoing investigation into the intricacies of the mind/body relationship. Applied psychophysiology focuses on the effects of emotional states on the central nervous system, by observing and recording data on such physiological processes as sleep rhythms, heart rate, gastrointestinal functioning, immune response, and brain function. Techniques used to measure such factors include electroencephalograms (EEGs), magnetic resonance imaging (MRI), and computerized axial tomography (CAT) scans.

When stresses, traumas, or debilitating emotional states are present, individuals may experience physiological unrest. For example, if an individual with a known allergy to bee stings receives such a sting, the natural reaction could be panic. As a result of this psychological response, blood pressure and heart rate increase, digestive functions decrease, and the person become dizzy. If emotional stresses or traumas of this kind remain in the body/ mind for extended periods of time, an imbalance in the healthy system may eventually manifest, as when individuals under chronic stress succumb to illness or disease.

Illness can be due to many factors. It can occur as a result of social or environmental factors. It may also happen as a result of genetic or hereditary reasons: a tendency for a certain condition to run in families. Some families also tend to suppress feelings: any emotion then tends to be expressed by physical symptoms. Children can learn this behavior which may continue to adult life. Some people think that it is our personality that is a major factor in determining which illness we develop. For example, people with what is known as Type a personality tend to be ambitious, impatient, and set themselves high standards. They seem more likely to develop heart attacks. Quiet, introverted individuals, who tend to conceal their feelings and fears and to suppress emotions, may be more likely to develop cancers.

Condition in which psychological stresses adversely affect physiological (somatic) functioning to the point of distress. It is a condition of dysfunction or structural damage in bodily organs through inappropriate activation of the involuntary nervous system and the glands of internal secretion. Thus, the psychosomatic symptom emerges as a physiological concomitant of an emotional state. In a state of rage, for example, the angry person's blood pressure is likely to be elevated and his pulse and respiratory rate to be increased. When the anger passes, the heightened physiologic processes usually subside. If the person has a persistent inhibited aggression (chronic rage), however, which he is unable to express overtly, the emotional state remains unchanged, though unexpressed in the overt behavior, and the physiological symptoms associated with the angry state persist. With time, such a person becomes aware of the physiological dysfunction. Very often he develops concern over the resulting physical signs and symptoms, but he denies or is unaware of the emotions that have evoked the symptoms.

TREATMENTS

Treatments for psychosomatic illnesses are being synthesized from both the allopathic and alternative medical worlds. Methods vary from drug therapy and biofeedback to the use of meditation, yoga, and massage therapy. In general, treatments are selected if they complement and strengthen an individual's awareness of the body/mind relationship.

Such practices are most effective in achieving overall states of health when addressing the mind to affect the body, and vice versa. For example, two disciplines that have proven effective in establishing this awareness are meditation, a mind-centered activity, and Rolfing, a form of therapeutic bodywork. Treatments that simultaneously work with both the physiology and the psychology are highly beneficial. This thorough approach may be achieved by pairing modalities that complement one another. Examples include combining psychotherapy with bodywork, and certain drug therapies with meditation, visualization, and yoga.

People suffering from psychosomatic disorders have been helped by treatment of their physical symptoms, the underlying psychological causes, or both. If the disorder is in an advanced stage (such as in severe asthma attacks, perforated ulcers, or debilitating colitis) symptomatic treatment must be undertaken initially as an emergency measure before the emotional component can be addressed.

Psychological approaches range from classic **psychoanalysis**, which addresses a person's early traumas and conflicts, to **behavior therapy** that focuses on changing learned behaviors that create or increase anxiety. Medications such as tranquilizers or **antidepressants** may be effective in relieving symptoms of psychosomatic disorders. **Hypnosis** has successfully been used to treat hyperventilation, ulcers, migraine headaches, and other complaints. Today, psychologists commonly treat psychosomatic ailments with the aid of such relaxation techniques as progressive relaxation, autogenic training, transcendental meditation, and yoga. **Biofeedback** has been used in treating a number of different clinical problems, including tachycardia, hypertension, and both tension and migraine headaches.

20 Psychosexual Disorders

The sexual disorders can be classified into 4 main types:
1. Gender identity disorders
2. Psychological and behavioral disorders associated with sexual development and maturation
3. Paraphilias (disorders of sexual preference)
4. Sexual dysfunction.

I. GENDER IDENTITY DISORDERS

Characterized by disturbance in gender identity, e.g. the sense of one's masculinity or feminity is disturbed. This group includes:
A. Transexualism: Male and female; primary and secondary
B. Gender identity disorder of childhood
C. Dual-role transvertism
D. Intersexuality.

A. Transsexualism

It is characterized by following clinical features: (1) Normal anatomic sex, (2) Persistent and significant sense of discomfort regarding one's anatomic sex and a feeling that it is inappropriate to one's perceived gender, (3) Marked preoccupation with the wish to get rid of one's genitals, (4) Diagnosis is made after puberty.

It is of two types: 1. Primary 2. Secondary

1. Primary

Onset is early childhood and has a stable course overtime. There are two types:

(i) Male – Primary transexualism (Male to Female)
(ii) Female – Primary transexualism (Female to Male)

2. Secondary

It has an onset later in life. A majority of these patients are more transsexuals (Male – to – Female).

Prevalence

1:1,00,000 in Males and 1:4,00,000 in Females.

Treatment

1. Reconciliation with anatomic sex: psychotherapy and behavior therapy.
2. Sex change to desired gender (SES) – Sex reassignment surgery.

B. Dual Role Transvertism

Characterized by wearing of clothes of the opposite sex in order to enjoy the temporary experience of membership of the opposite sex, but without any desire for a more permanent sex change.

C. Gender Identity Disorder of Childhood

This is a disorder similar to transexualism, with a very early age of onset (2 – 4 yrs of age).

D. Intersexuality

The patients with this disorder have gross anatomical or physiological aspects of the other sex. It can be in

i) Chromosomes – Turner's syndrome, Klinefelter's Syndrome.
ii) Hormonal disturbances
iii) Internal sex organs.

II. PSYCHOLOGICAL AND BEHAVIORAL DISORDERS ASSOCIATED WITH SEXUAL DEVELOPMENT AND MATURATION

A. Sexual Maturation Disorder

- Usually begins in adolescence.

- It is characterized by uncertainty regarding the gender identify or sexual orientation.
- It leads to anxiety and depression.

B. Egodystonic Sexual Orientation

It is sexual orientation disorder. The individual wishes to change the orientation because of associated distress and psychological symptoms. This disorder is seen most commonly in homosexuality.

Homosexuality

The sexual relationship between persons of the same sex. It is of 2 types. Male homosexuality and female homosexuality. Female homosexuals are also called as lesbians/sapphic. Male homosexuals are also called as gay.

Prevalence

In USA – 4 – 6% of males and 1 – 2% of females.
5 – 10% - show bisexual orientation.

Treatment

1. For seeking a change in sexual orientation:
   a. Psychoanalytic psychotherapy
   b. Behavior therapy
   c. Supportive therapy
   d. Androgen therapy
2. For seeking removal of distress only
   a. Psychotherapy
   b. Drug therapy — antidepressants/benzodiazepines

C. Sexual Relationship Disorders

The GID or disorder of sexual preferences leads to difficulties in establishing or maintaining sexual relationships.

III. PARAPHILIAS (DISORDERS OF SEXUAL PREFERENCE)

Background

Paraphilia is a rare disorder, and the best criteria for diagnosis come from the Diagnostic and Statistical Manual of Mental Disorders, Fourth Edition, Text Revision (DSM-IV-TR)[1] or the International Statistical Classification of Diseases, 10th Revision (ICD-10). The disorder is characterized by a 6-month period of recurrent, intense, sexually arousing fantasies or sexual urges involving a specific act, depending on the paraphilia.

Paraphilia is a means for some people to release sexual energy or frustration. The act commonly is followed by arousal and orgasm, usually achieved by masturbation and fantasy. These disorders are not well recognized and often are difficult to treat for several reasons. Often, people who have these disorders conceal them, experience guilt and shame, have financial or legal problems, and can (at times) be uncooperative with medical professionals.

Some psychiatrists discuss whether paraphilias are a part of the impulse control disorders or if they fall within the spectrum of obsessive-compulsive disorders. The more common paraphilias include voyeurism and frotteurism, and the most rare paraphilia is zoophilia. In this age of computer technology, individuals can easily access information about paraphilias from any computer, thus fueling a disorder that already is difficult to control.

Definition

A paraphilia is a sexual problems where the sexual arousal is in response to objects or stimuli not associated with normal sexual behavior patterns and that may interfere with the establishment of normal sexual relationships.

> Paraphilias referred sexual deviations or sexual perversions. Disorder of sexual preference in which sexual arousal occurs persistently and significantly in response to objects which are not a part of normal sexual arousal – like non-human objects, suffering or humiliation of self or sexual partner, with children or non-consenting person.

The American Psychiatric Association's Diagnostic and Statistical Manual of Mental Disorders (DSM-IV-TR), the prevailing resource for diagnostic criteria of paraphilias, describes the essential feature of paraphilias as recurrent, intense, sexual urges and sexually arousing fantasies generally involving nonhuman objects, the suffering or humiliation of oneself or partner, or children or other non consenting persons. The DSM-IV-TR describes the more commonly observed paraphilias and makes reference to several other examples. People who experience one paraphilia may also experience other paraphilias. Commonly, people who manifest paraphilias also exhibit personality disorders, drug abuse, alcohol abuse, and other substance abuse problems, or affective disorders.

Pathophysiology

Many theories exist regarding the etiology of paraphilias, including psychoanalytical, biological, and sociobiological theories; however, none are conclusive. This subject requires additional research.

Psychoanalytical Theory

According to psychoanalytical theory, several possible factors may contribute to the origin of paraphilias. Freud and his colleagues suggested that some paraphilias may be attributed to possible distortion of the courtship phases. Normal courtship behavior is what brings males and females together for the purpose of mating. It usually occurs during adolescence and may or may not involve sexual intercourse at this early stage of sexual development. Courtship is composed of 4 definitive phases.

1. Location of a potential partner: The initial phase of courtship.
2. Pretactile interaction: Talking or flirting with a potential partner.
3. Tactile interaction: Usually consists of touching, hugging, hand holding, etc (This could also be considered foreplay).
4. Effecting genital union: More commonly known as sexual intercourse.

According to this particular literature, distortions of the courtship behaviors are only associated with the first 3 phases.

Certain paraphilias are associated with distortions of courtship behaviors.

- *Voyeurism:* This is the distorted view of the initial courtship phase. Normally the initial courtship phase is known as locating a potential partner. Psychoanalysts postulate that voyeurism may be attributed to a child witnessing episodes of his or her parents engaged in sexual intercourse.
- *Exhibitionism:* Psychoanalysts consider exhibitionism a distortion of the pretactile interaction of the courtship phase. Psychoanalytical theory is based on the theory that gender identity for little boys requires psychological separation from the mother, so that he will not identify with her as a member of the same sex as do little girls. Exhibitionists regard their mothers as rejecting them on the basis of their different genitalia. The act of exhibitionism forces women to accept them by forcing them to look at their genitals. The act of self-exposure is also a way for the exhibitionist to compensate for his introversion and lack of assertiveness. The act of exposing oneself may give the exhibitionist a false sense of power, and the danger of discovery may further reinforce this feeling. Therefore, this leads to his search for other unsuspecting victims to fulfill his insatiable need for admiration. The exhibitionist is sometimes compared to an actor on stage who desires an audience, but does not want to participate in the act.
- *Toucherism and frotteurism:* These are considered exaggerations of the tactile interaction of the courtship phase. These paraphilias provide a sexual outlet without the risk of rejection. Toucherism tends to occur in conjunction with other paraphilias.

Behavioral Theory

Behavioral theory attributes the development of certain paraphilias to the process of conditioning. Actually, paraphilias are a result of accidental conditioning. If nonsexual objects are frequently and repeatedly associated with a pleasurable sexual activity, then the object becomes sexually arousing.

Conditioning does not always involve positive reinforcement. Negative reinforcement may occur as well. If an individual experiences unpleasant consequences with normal sexual activity, an aversion to sex may occur, resulting in the development of deviant behavior. An example of this would be a young boy who is humiliated and punished by his parents for proudly displaying his erect penis. As the boy matures he may associate guilt and shame with normal sexual behavior.

Certain atypical sex acts, such as exhibitionism and voyeurism, that provide intense sexual arousal may lead to individual preference of that behavior. Pedophiliacs, exhibitionists, and voyeurs may be driven by risk-taking behaviors. Therefore, the constant threat of discovery may be as arousing to them as the act itself.

Conditioning is not the only contributing factor in the development of paraphilias. These individuals usually experience low self-esteem, which may lead to difficulty in forming person-to-person sexual relationships.

Sociobiological Theory

An article of particular interest in explaining possible etiologies of paraphilias is *A Theory about the Variety of Human Sexual Behavior*, written by Richard A Gardner . Gardner's article combines a couple of theories. These theories are Dawkins's theory of gene transmission and Darwin's well-known survival of the fittest theory. In a sense, this could be considered a sociobiological theory.

Dawkin's Theory

1. Dawkins's theory of **gene transmission** is used in developing a theory regarding the variations in human sexual behavior. These variants in sexual behavior, even atypical sexual behavior (paraphilias), are seen as survival of the species. According to this view, the different paraphilias may be responsible for enhancing society's level of sexual excitation. In turn, this would increase the likelihood of people engaging in sex acts that would ultimately lead to procreation.

Darwin's theory of survival of the fittest relates more directly to reproductive capacity. Each species produces more offspring than could possibly survive; therefore, those who are more capable of adapting to their environment are more likely to survive and perpetuate the species. In general, those species that are less adaptable to their surroundings are more likely to become extinct.

2. **Quantity and quality** are 2 of the operative factors in Darwinian Theory. As already mentioned, the quantity of offspring produced in an environment is far greater than what can actually survive. Therefore, the quality of offspring that is most adaptable to the environment will survive. Each of the sexes is designated to provide either quantity or quality. The male is the species physically able to produce the greatest amount of offspring. Since a female producing a greater quantity of offspring than the male is biologically impossible, she is the one responsible for quality control. As discussed earlier, the woman tends to be selective in the process of choosing a mate. The mate of choice is one that will be the best in providing for and protecting the family. The female will also ultimately take on the responsibility of child rearing.
3. A biology professor at Louisiana State University in Shreveport once said, "Sperm are cheap and eggs are expensive." This pretty much sums it up. If a man devoted his whole life to the procreation process, he could possibly father or produce 30,000 offspring. On the other hand, if a woman were to devote her entire fecund life to procreation, she could only possibly produce 40-45 babies. Child rearing may be the most important of these life activities. If protection is not provided for the young, the babies would be unable to survive. Therefore, to devote one's life to the sole purpose of manufacturing babies without the potential for survival would be senseless. Also, women must try and select the mate that will remain around after impregnation and serve the role as protector and gatherer. In order to have the ability to assess a proper mate, women were more cautious in regards to their

impulsivity regarding sexual gratification. Women with inhibited sexual arousal were more likely to select a proper mate and increase their likelihood of survival. Also, once aroused, a woman is more likely to attempt an ongoing relationship with her mate.

Shanor (1978) conducted a study that found men aged 12-40 years think of sex approximately 6 times an hour. However, we need to determine the distribution by age ranges. Males aged 12-19 years think of sex an average of 20 times per hour or once every 3 minutes. In males aged 30-39 years, this slows down to approximately 4 times per hour. This may be one reason in explaining that paraphilias usually occur in males aged 15-25 years.

Women are more susceptible to caressing, tenderness, and the reassurance of a man's commitment. This commitment ensures that he is emotionally invested in this union and will remain around to supply food and protection for her and their offspring. This may explain one of the reasons that men are more likely to be sexually aroused by visual pornography.

Frequency

Paraphilias are considered rare, affecting only a small percentage of the US population. Researchers have a difficult time trying to determine a specific percentage of involved individuals because many of the acts are illegal and reporting methods (i.e. self-reporting) typically are unreliable.

International

International percentages of patients with paraphilias are difficult to discern because these disorders are rare.

Mortality/Morbidity

Determining the morbidity or mortality of paraphilias depends on the act practiced, the comorbidity involved, the patient's cooperation with the therapist, and whether or not the legal system is involved. Paraphilias can be transient, as demonstrated by experimentation during the teenage years, or can remain a lifelong problem involving legal, financial, interpersonal, occupational, academic, and other problems. Death may occur in some circumstances, through acts such as autoerotic asphyxiation.

Race

Patients typically are white.

Sex

Patients typically are men.

Age

Most patients are aged 15-25 years; this disorder rarely occurs in individuals older than 50 years. The information on paraphilia in older individuals is limited.

CLINICAL DIAGNOSTIC CRITERIA

DSM-IV-TR criteria include the following:

- Exhibitionism
  - Over a period of at least 6 months, patients have recurrent, intense, sexually arousing fantasies, sexual urges, or behaviors that involve exposing their genitals to unsuspecting strangers.
  - The fantasies, sexual urges, or behaviors cause clinically significant distress or impairment in social, occupational, or other important areas of functioning.
  - Exhibitionism typically involves men exposing themselves to women (not a DSM-IV-TR criterion).
- Fetishism
  - Over a period of at least 6 months, patients have recurrent, intense, sexually arousing fantasies, sexual urges, or behaviors involving nonliving objects.
  - The fantasies, sexual urges, or behaviors cause clinically significant distress or impairment in social, occupational, or other important areas of functioning.

  - Patients do not limit the fetish objects to articles of female clothing used in cross-dressing or to devices designated for the purpose of tactile genital stimulation.
  - Patients may have a particular pathological displacement of erotic interest and satisfaction for their entire lives (not a DSM-IV-TR criterion).
- Frotteurism
  - Over a period of at least 6 months, patients have recurrent, intense, sexually arousing fantasies, sexual urges, or behaviors involving rubbing against and touching a nonconsenting person.
  - The fantasies, sexual urges, or behaviors cause clinically significant distress or impairment in social, occupational, or other important areas of functioning.
  - Patients typically practice this behavior in crowded places (not a DSM-IV-TR criterion).
- Pedophilia
  - Over a period of at least 6 months, patients have recurrent, intense, sexually arousing fantasies, sexual urges, or behaviors involving sexual activity with a prepubescent child or children.
  - The fantasies, sexual urges, or behaviors cause clinically significant distress or impairment in social, occupational, or other important areas of functioning.
  - The patient must be aged 16 years or older and at least 5 years older than the child or children involved.
- Sexual masochism
  - Over a period of at least 6 months, patients have recurrent, intense, sexually arousing fantasies, sexual urges, or behaviors involving the act of being humiliated, beaten, bound, or otherwise made to suffer.
  - The fantasies, sexual urges, or behaviors cause clinically significant distress or impairment in social, occupational, or other important areas of functioning.
  - This variant is named for the activities of Leopold von Sacher-Masoch (not part of the DSM-IV-TR criterion).

Sacher-Masoch was born in Lemberg, Austria in 1836. As an author he is most known for his book Venus in Furs. This writing is reportedly based on true events from his life.

- Sexual sadists
  - Over a period of at least 6 months, patients have recurrent, intense, sexually arousing fantasies, sexual urges, or behaviors involving the acts in which psychological or physical suffering of the victim is sexually exciting to the patient.
  - The fantasies, sexual urges, or behaviors cause clinically significant distress or impairment in social, occupational, or other important areas of functioning.
  - This variant is named for the activities of the Marquis de Sade (not part of the DSM-IV-TR criterion).
- Transvestic fetishism
  - Over a period of 6 months, heterosexual male patients have recurrent, intense, sexually arousing fantasies, sexual urges, or behaviors involving cross-dressing.
  - The fantasies, sexual urges, or behaviors cause clinically significant distress or impairment in social, occupational, or other important areas of functioning.
  - Typically, patients derive sexual gratification from wearing clothes usually worn by the opposite sex, and patients typically are heterosexual married males (not a DSM-IV-TR criterion).
- Voyeurism
  - Over a period of at least 6 months, patients have recurrent, intense, sexually arousing fantasies, sexual urges, or behaviors involving the act of observing an unsuspecting person who is naked, in the process of disrobing, or engaging in sexual activity.
  - The fantasies, sexual urges, or behaviors cause clinically significant distress or impairment in social, occupational, or other important areas of functioning.
  - Patients derive sexual gratification from seeing sex organs and sexual acts; scopophilia is a synonym for voyeurism (not a DSM-IV-TR criterion).

- Paraphilia not otherwise specified: This category is included so physicians can code paraphilias that do not meet the criteria for any of the other specific categories.
  - Scatologia involves making obscene phone calls.
  - Necrophilia involves an erotic attraction or sexual interest in corpses. This paraphilia is rare and seldom reported to the police. Patients typically work in mortuaries and funeral parlors. This also involves dangerous situations where the individual could actually acquire infections from the corpse.
  - Partialism is sexual interest exclusively focused on a particular body part.
  - Zoophilia involves sexual activity with animals (i.e. both actual sexual contact and sexual fantasies, higher in psychiatric patients).
  - Coprophilia is sexual activity involving feces.
  - Klismaphilia is sexual activity involving enemas.
  - Urophilia is sexual activity involving urine.
  - Masturbation is sexual self-gratification.
- Other paraphilias
  - Autogynephilia describes a man's propensity to be sexually aroused by thoughts or images of himself as a woman (with female attributes).
  - Asphyxiophilia or hypoxyphilia is when a patient uses hypoxia to achieve sexual excitement; this can be complicated by autoerotic asphyxiation.
  - Video voyeurs derive sexual gratification from videos, usually of women doing natural acts or women involved in sexual activity.
  - Infantophilia is a new subcategory of pedophilia in which the victims are younger than 5 years.
  - Zoophilia (Bestiality)

    Persistent and significant involvement in sexual activity with animals is rare.
  - Urophilia – Urine
  - Coprophila – Feces
  - Enemas – Klismaphilia
  - Necrophilia – Corpses

List of paraphilias

Abasiophilia: love of (or sexual attraction to) people who use leg braces or other orthopedic appliances

Acousticophilia: sexual arousal from certain sounds

Acrotomophilia: love of (or sexual attraction to) amputees

Agalmatophilia: sexual attraction to statues or mannequins or immobility

Algolagnia: sexual pleasure from pain

Amaurophilia: sexual arousal by a partner whom one is unable to see due to artificial means, such as being blindfolded or having sex in total darkness. (See: sensory deprivation)

Andromimetophilia: love of women dressed as men

Apodysophilia: desire to undress, see also nudism

Apotemnophilia: desire to have (or sexual arousal from having) a healthy appendage (limb, digit, or male genitals) amputated

Aquaphilia: arousal from water and/or in watery environments, including bathtubs or swimming pools

Aretifism: sexual attraction to people who are without footwear, in contrast to retifism

Asphyxiophilia: sexual attraction to asphyxia; also called breath control play; including autoerotic asphyxiation; see medical warnings

Autogynephilia: love of oneself as a woman (also see Blanchard, Bailey, and Lawrence theory for discussion on controversy)

Biastophilia: sexual pleasure from committing rape

Celebriphilia: pathological desire to have sex with a celebrity.

Coprophilia: sexual attraction to (or pleasure from) feces

Crush fetish: sexual arousal from seeing small creatures being crushed by members of the opposite sex, or being crushed oneself

Dacryphilia: sexual pleasure in eliciting tears from others or oneself

Dendrophilia: sexual attraction to trees and other large plants, popularized by the movie "Superstar" with Molly Shannon

Diaper fetishism: sexual arousal from diapers

Emetophilia (a.k.a. vomerophilia): sexual attraction to vomit

Ephebophilia (a.k.a. hebephilia): sexual attraction towards adolescents

Eproctophilia: sexual attraction to flatulence

Exhibitionism: sexual arousal through sexual behavior in view of third parties (also includes the recurrent urge or behavior to expose one's genitals to an unsuspecting person, known as indecent exposure)

Faunoiphilia: sexual arousal from watching animals mate

Fetishism: is the use of non-sexual or nonliving objects or part of a person's body to gain sexual excitement.

Examples include: Balloon fetishism — breast fetishism — foot fetishism (podophilia) — fur fetishism — leather fetishism — lipstick fetishism — medical fetishism — panty fetishism — robot fetishism — rubber fetishism — shoe fetishism — smoking fetishism — spandex fetishism — dental braces fetishism — transvestic fetishism (see below)

Contd...

Contd...

Frotteurism: sexual arousal from the recurrent urge or behavior of touching or rubbing against a nonconsenting person
Galactophilia: sexual attraction to human milk or lactating women (incorrect term)
Gerontophilia: sexual attraction towards the elderly
Hematophilia: sexual attraction involving blood (either on a sex partner/ attractive person or the liquid itself; not to be confused with hemophilia, a genetic disorder of the blood)
Harpaxophilia: sexual arousal from being the victim of a robbery or burglary
Hematolagnia: sexual attraction to blood
Hybristophilia: sexual arousal to people who have committed crimes, in particular cruel or outrageous crimes
Infantilism: sexual pleasure from dressing, acting, or being treated as a baby
Katoptronophilia: sexual arousal from having sex in front of mirrors.
Klismaphilia: sexual pleasure from enemas
Lust murder: sexual arousal through committing murder
Macrophilia: sexual attraction to larger people and large things (including larger body organs such as breasts and genitalia)
Maiesiophilia: sexual attraction to childbirth or pregnant women
Masochism: is the recurrent urge or behavior of wanting to be humiliated, beaten, bound, or otherwise made to suffer
Microphilia: sexual attraction to smaller people and things of smaller size
Mysophilia: sexual attraction to soiled, dirty, foul or decaying material
Necrophilia: sexual attraction to corpses
Necrozoophilia: sexual attraction to the corpses or killings of animals (also known as necrobestiality)
Nepiophilia: the same as infantophilia sexual attraction to children between the age of 0 - 3 yrs.
Pedophilia: sexual attraction to prepubescent children (British spelling: paedophilia)
Phalloorchoalgolagnia: sexual arousal by the experiencing of painful stimuli being administered to the male genitals.
Pictophilia: sexual attraction to pictorial pornography/erotic art
Plushophilia: sexual attraction to stuffed toys or people in animal costume, such as theme park characters
Pyrophilia: sexual arousal through watching, setting, hearing/talking/ fantasizing about fire
Retifism: sexual arousal from shoes
Sadism: sexual arousal from giving pain
Schediaphilia (aka Toonophilia): love (or sexual arousal) to cartoon characters/ situations
Sitophilia: sexual arousal from food
Somnophilia: sexual arousal from sleeping or unconscious people
Spectrophilia: sexual attraction to ghosts
Telephone scatologia: being sexually aroused by making obscene telephone calls

Contd...

Contd...

Teratophilia: sexual attraction to deformed or monstrous people

Transformation fetish: sexual arousal from depictions of transformations of people into objects or other beings

Transvestic fetishism: is a sexual attraction towards the clothing of the opposite gender (also known as transvestitism)

Trichophilia: love (or sexual arousal) from hair

Urolagnia: sexual attraction to urine

Vorarephilia: sexual attraction to being eaten by, and/or eating, another person or creature

Voyeurism: sexual arousal through watching others having sex (also includes the recurrent urge or behavior to observe an unsuspecting person who is naked, disrobing or engaging in sexual activities, see peeping tom)

Xenophilia: sexual attraction to foreigners (in science fiction, can also mean sexual attraction to aliens)

Zoophilia: emotional or sexual attraction to animals

Zoosadism: the sexual enjoyment of causing pain and suffering to animals

Note: Sadism and masochism are often grouped together, under sadomasochism, or (as a lifestyle interest) BDSM. See also " bondage and discipline" and algolagnia.

PHYSICAL EXAMINATION

Obtain a complete history and perform complete mental status, physical, and neurological examinations to assist with the evaluation and to rule out other disease processes. This particular patient population may be more difficult to interview because they may be more likely to have guilt associated with their disorder, therefore making them reluctant to openly share information with the interviewer. The interviewer must establish rapport with these patients and allow them to talk more freely about their disorder. By asking leading questions and then allowing the patient to reveal information on his or her own helps in the treatment and management of this disorder.

CAUSES

Rule out major medical or psychiatric illnesses. Look for both hard and soft neurological signs involving the striato-thalamo-cortical processing loop (theory). This theory states that a disruption of the striato-thalamo-cortical processing loop can cause abnormal filtering of information resulting in the brain's inability to block unimportant information, which is thought to cause a propensity to initiate or perpetuation paraphilias and other psychotic phenomena. It is important to point out that this is just a theory and much more research is needed to either confirm or disprove this concept as a cause of paraphilias.

TREATMENT

Medical Care

- Inpatient treatment indications
  - Patients are suicidal, homicidal, or gravely disabled (Suicide risk is high if they feel exposed or confronted.)
  - Patients are dangerous to themselves, others, or cannot take care of themselves
- Psychotherapy
  - *Cognitive-behavioral therapy:* This type of therapy involves applying behavioral therapy techniques to modify the patient's sexual deviations by altering distorted thinking patterns and making patients cognizant of the irrational justifications that lead to their sexual variations. This therapy also incorporates relapse prevention techniques, helping the patient to control the undesirable behaviors by avoiding situations that may generate initial desires. Many times, therapists apply the technique of "covert sensitization," in which patients' harmful sexual variation is paired with an unpleasant stimulus, such as that of a person with alcoholism who is administered Antabuse, in order to deter them from repeating the act. This approach has been proven effective in cases of pedophilia and sadism.
  - Another technique employed by therapists is that of orgasmic reconditioning. In this approach, a patient is reconditioned to a more appropriate stimulus by masturbating to his or her typical, less socially acceptable stimulus. Then, just before orgasm, the patient is told to concentrate on a more acceptable fantasy. This is repeated at earlier times before orgasm until, soon, the patient begins his masturbation fantasies with an appropriate stimulus.

- *Social skills training:* Because many believe that paraphilias develop in patients who lack the ability to develop relationships, many therapists and physicians use social skills training to treat patients with these types of disorders. They may work on such issues as developing intimacy, carrying on conversations with others, and assertive skills training. Many social skills training groups also teach basic sexual education, which is very helpful to this patient population.
- *Twelve-step programs:* Many physicians and therapists refer patients with paraphilias to 12-step programs designed for sexual addicts. Similar to alcoholics anonymous, these programs are designed to give control to group members, who lead most of the sessions. The program incorporates cognitive restructuring with social support to increase awareness of the problem. The group also focuses on the sense of a "higher power" and each individual's reliance upon his or her spirituality.
- *Group therapy:* This mode of therapy involves breaking through the denial so commonly found in people with paraphilias by surrounding them with other patients who share their illness. Once they begin to admit that they have a sexual divergence, the therapist begins to address individual issues such as past sexual abuse or other problems that may have led to the sexual disorder. When these issues have been identified, beginning Gestalt-type therapy (with the victim, if any) may be desirable to help patients get past the guilt and shame associated with their particular paraphilia. The goal of this type of therapy is to lead the patient to a "healthy remorse." These patients require lifetime therapy in order to reduce the likelihood of relapse.
- *Individual expressive-supportive psychotherapy:* This type of therapy requires a psychologically minded patient willing to focus on the paraphilia. The therapist should not set high goals but needs to break through the denial. Countertransfence and avoidance of the patient can be a

problem with this form of therapy. If the patients can break through the denial, then the patient can work on the unconscious meaning behind the paticular paraphila.

- Medications
  - Antidepressants
  - Long-acting gonadotropin-releasing hormones (GnRH, ie, medical castration)
  - Antiandrogens
  - Phenothiazine
  - Mood stabilizers
- Sex education and therapy
- Social skills and training

Surgical Care

Surgical castration

Consultations

- Neurologist, if neurological signs are present
- Attorney
- Pastor

Activity

Restrict activity if patients represent a danger to themselves, to others, or if they are gravely disabled.

Medication

The goals of pharmacotherapy are to reduce morbidity and prevent complications.

Antidepressants May be used to decrease aggression and treat underlying illness. **Fluoxetine (Prozac)** 10-80 mg PO qd antidepressant (SSRI) used to treat impulse control problems or underlying illness. Selectively inhibits presynaptic serotonin reuptake with minimal or no effect in the reuptake of norepinephrine or dopamine.

Lithium (Eskalith) Indicated for treating bipolar disorder. Influences reuptake of serotonin and/or norepinephrine at cell membrane. **Dosing: Adult** 300 PO tid/qid **Pediatric** <6 years: Not established 6-12 years: 15-60 mg/kg/d PO tid/qid; not to exceed usual adult dose >12 years: Administer as in adults **Antiandrogens** Used to reduce androgen serum levels. **Medroxyprogesterone (Depo-Provera)** Derivative of progesterone. Used for breast cancer, contraception, secondary amenorrhea, and abnormal uterine bleeding. May be used to reduce sex drive.

Adult :150 mg IM qd/qwk/qmo usually adjusted based on patient response, tolerance, and/or plasma testosterone

Pediatric Not recommended

Phenothiazines

Are effective in treating emesis possibly due to their effects in the dopaminergic mesolimbic system.

Fluphenazine (Prolixin)

Antipsychotic used to treat underlying illness or decrease aggression.

Adult :1-10 mg PO qd

Pediatric

Administer as in adults

Anxiolytics

These agents help induce impulse control. **Buspirone (BuSpar)** Unique anxiolytic that differs from benzodiazepines in that it does not exert anticonvulsant or muscle relaxer for GAD. A 5-HT1 agonist with serotonergic neurotransmission and some dopaminergic effects in CNS. Has anxiolytic effect but may take as long as 2-3 wk for full efficacy.

Adult

15 mg/d PO divided tid and increase by 5 mg/d q2-4d; titrate to 20-60 mg/d; not to exceed 60 mg/d

Pediatric

Not established

Long-acting gonadotropin-releasing hormones

These agents are used to reduce release of gonadotropin hormones. **Triptorelin (Trelstar)** Synthetic decapeptide agonist analog of GnRH also known as luteinizing hormone–releasing hormone (LHRH). Reduces LH, FSH, and testosterone, which may lead to reduced sex drive.

Adult

3.75 mg IM qmo

Pediatric

Not established

Mood stabilizer

These agents are used to treat bipolar disorders. **Divalproex sodium (Depakote)** Indicated for manic episodes associated with bipolar disorder. Recommended plasma concentration is 50-125 μg/mL.

Adult

750 mg PO qd in divided doses initially; 60 mg/kg/d maximum

Pediatric

10-15 mg/kg/d PO initially; 60 mg/kg/d maximum

Follow-up: Further Inpatient Care Patients may require further inpatient care if they represent a danger to themselves, to others, or if they are gravely disabled. **Further Outpatient Care** For the best results, patients require medication management and psychotherapy. **Inpatient and Outpatient Medications:** If the patient began medication therapy in the hospital, continue the same therapy and adjust as needed. If not, select medications and discuss the risks, benefits, adverse effects, and alternatives with the patient. Obtain informed consent before starting medication therapy. **Transfer:** If patients are charged with a crime or have been arrested, they may be incarcerated. **Deterrence/Prevention:** Education/ Legal ramifications. **Complications**

- Adverse medication effects
- Noncompliance with medications and therapy
- Pedophilia on the Internet

PROGNOSIS

- Patients with a good prognosis have the following characteristics:
  - Cooperative attitude
  - Normal sex life
  - Motivated outlook, with a desire to change
  - Voluntary approach to treatment
- Patients with a poor prognosis have the following characteristics:
  - Early onset of paraphilia
  - Legal charges pending
  - Unmotivated attitude
  - Uncooperative attitude
  - Paraphilia as the only sexual activity or outlet
  - Comorbidity
  - Lack of remorse over acts

Patient Education

- Sex education and social skills training
- Both the patient and the family should be educated regarding paraphilias. The family may need to be involved in a support group (e.g. church). If the patient is on medication the family needs to be informed of potential problems such as side effects and drug interations. If the patient is married, marital counceling needs to be part of the treatment plan. The family also needs to be aware of local laws in regard to paraphilas. If the patient is on probation, the family needs to be aware of court dates, if appicable, probation, and if the patient will need to be listed on the sexual offenders listing the community.
- Community notification of a sex offender may be required for some patients with paraphilas. It is important to point out that many patients with paraphilias have no legal charges and even health care workers are not required to report all paraphilias while others require mandatory reporting such as pedophilia. Some patients may find this notification as a

deterrent to the paraphila while others may not. Some experts suggest that, while required, it may hamper some patients who are tring to obtain help for there illness. This will continue to be a matter of community concern and debate for the unforseeable future. The patient should address these concerns with the treatment team.

Treatment

1. Psychoanalysis
2. behavior therapy
3. Drug therapy → Antipsychotics for severe/aggressive condition.
   → benperidol for severe/aggressive condition.
   → Antiandrogens (Cyproterone acetate or medoxy progesterone acetate) for excessive activity in paraphila
4. Other treatment:
   Castration and psychosurgery – Amygdalotomy

SEXUAL DYSFUNCTION

Definition

There are various mental disorders falling into the category of psychosexual. These include all mental impairments which cause the patient an inability to function as a normal member of society and deal with the opposite sex in a healthy manner. They have been of much controversy in recent years even though these disorders have been largely curable since before 1940. They however require aggressive and expensive treatment in order to bring about such cures so the diseases are often ignored.

Sexual dysfunction is a significant disturbance in the sexual response cycle, which is not due to an underlying organic cause.

Normal human sexual response cycle

1. Appetitive phase
2. Excitement phase
3. Plateau phase

4. Orgasmic phase
5. Resolution phase

Etiology

Most cases of sexual dysfunction arise from a combination of psychological and cultural relationship and organic factors. Together, they often give rise to performance anxiety and spectatoring (critical monitoring of one's own sexual responses), which are distracting and preclude sensual pleasure which is vital for enjoyable sexual experience.

A. Psychosocial and Cultural Factors

1. Ignorance and misinformation
   Many parents and schools fail to provide even basic sex education. Cultural beliefs may contribute to anxiety or guilt experienced by some people. Masturbation is believed by Chinese to lead to weakness and poor stamina or to make one stupid and mentally ill. Physical illness has been ascribed by traditional healers, to "loss of semen". A variety of sexual myths may also exist involving gender roles, age and appearance or performance expectations.
2. Conflict of values
   Normal recurring sexual feelings especially during adolescence may be in conflict with what is portrayed by parents, school or religion. A commonly held attitude is that sex is shameful, dirty or sinful.
3. Fears and trauma
   Fears of impregnation, pregnancy, sexually transmitted disease, e.g. AIDS, may exist. Sexual abuse, rape, premarital pregnancy or abortion could have occurred in the past.
4. Unconscious conflicts
   Parental sanctions against sexual enjoyment, dissociated memories of early sexual trauma or ingrained religious scruples may remain unconscious but give rise to conflicts.

B. Relationship Factors

Sexual problems should be understood in the context of the relationships in which they are manifest. Issues of trust, power and control or anger at the partner are common themes. Difficulties with communication, conflict and commitment are often present.

C. Organic Factors

A variety of drugs and medical illness may cause disturbances of the sexual response cycle (see Tables 20.1 and 20.2). Most frequently they affect male erectile function, but they may also affect arousal and orgasm in both sexes.

Table 20.1: Medical conditions associated with sexual dysfunction

Congenital	**Endocrine**
Hypospadias/phimosis	Diabetes mellitus
Spina bifida	Addison's disease
Inflammatory	Thyroid disorders
Prostatitis/urethritis/cystitis	Acromegaly
Peyronie's disease	**Vascular**
Mumps	Arteriosclerosis
Neurological	Leriche's syndrome
Pituitary tumor	Penile arteriovenous shunt
Parkinson's disease	**Traumatic or surgical**
Peripheral neuropathies	Penile urethral injury
CNS syphillis	Spinal cord injury
Metabolic	Pelvic fracture
Cirrhosis/liver failure	Radiation therapy
Chronic renal failure	Sympathectomy radical bladder/prostate surgery

The importance of organic factors in the aetiology of sexual dysfunction especially of erectile dysfunction has been greatly emphasized in recently years. This has stemmed from a better understanding of sexual physiology and from the discovery of effective pharmacological treatments. The role of psychological and relationship factors has tended to be ignored. The adaptation of a dichotomous paradigm of sexual dysfunction being either organic or psychogenic; or holding the assumption that organic factors necessarily take precedence over psychosocial factors, should be cautioned against.

Where an important physical factor is assessed to be the major contributing course, referral to a urological/medical clinic would be appropriate.

Table 20.2: Drugs associated with sexual dysfunction

Antihypertension drugs	**Psychotropic drugs**
Methyldopa	Antidepressants
Clonidine	Antipsychotics
Hydrochlorthiazide	Benzodiazepines
Propranolol	**Drugs of abuse**
Anticholinergic drugs	Alcohol
Antiparkinsanion agents	Amphetamines
Antihistamines	Opiates – heroin, morphine
Atropine	Cocaine
Other prescription drugs	
Cimetidine	
Digoxin	
Indomethacin	
Disulfiram	
Estrogens	

Clinical Assessment

Patients often feel embarrassed bringing up sexual problems directly and may complain initially of physical complaints instead, e.g. feeling tired and weak, having urinary symptoms, etc.

A careful and detailed sexual history should be elicited from both the patient and ideally from the partner as well. Areas covered should include:

i. The exact nature of dysfunction in relation to the phases of the sexual cycle and what conditions produce or reduce it.
ii. Duration of the problem. If brief and of recent onset, its relation to recent stress or adjustment.
iii. Variation with different settings, partners, erotic fantasies or masturbation.

iv. Past and current sexual experiences including masturbation and partner experiences.

The relationship with the partner/spouse is especially important. Consider:

i. Areas of conflict, difficulty or stress.
ii. The level of trust, understanding and love. Commitment to each other.
iii. Communication and ability to resolve conflicts.
iv. Individual attitudes to coital frequency, birth control, having children, etc.

The existence of a psychiatric disorder like depressive illness, anxiety phobic disorder, or psychosis may also adversely affect sexual function.

A concomitant medical disorder and consumption of drugs or alcohol can cause sexual dysfunction and should be carefully considered in every case.

I. DISORDERS OF APPETITIVE PHASE (SEXUAL DESIRE DISORDERS)

1. Hypoactive sexual desire disorder (Frigidity)
2. Sexual aversion disorder and lack of sexual enjoyment disorder.
3. Excessive sexual drive
   Men – Satyriasis
   Women – Nymphomania

1. Hypoactive Sexual Desire Disorder

- Is characterized by an absence of fantasies and desire for sexual activity.
- It is many times more common in females.
- Contributing factors are: fear of pregnancy, unsatisfactory past sexual experiences, marital disharmony or fatigue.

2. Sexual Aversion Disorder and Lack of Sexual Enjoyment Disorder

In sexual aversion disorder, there is an aversion to and avoidance of all sexual activity with a sexual partner.

In the lack of sexual enjoyment disorder (Sexual Anhedonia) the sexual response is usually is normal. However, there is a feeling of lack of subjective sexual pleasure. This disorder is more common in females.

II. DISORDERS OF EXCITEMENT AND PLATEAU PHASE

(Sexual arousal disorders or failure of genital response)
1. Male erectile disorder (impotence).
2. Female sexual arousal disorder.

1. Male Erectile Disorder

This disorder is characterized by an inability to have or sustain penile erection till the completion of satisfactory sexual activity.

Causes

Physical disorders, drugs and psychological factors like
1. Ignorance regarding the sexual act
2. Fear of failure
3. Interpersonal difficulties between sexual partners
4. Anxiety disorder
5. Mood disorder
6. Masturbation anxiety
7. Fatigue
8. Fear of pregnancy
9. Fear of damaging the sexual partner
10. Poor self-image

2. Female Sexual Arousal Disorder

It is characterized by subjective as well as objective lack of sexual arousal in the form of lack of lubrication or vaginal dryness.

III. DISORDERS OF ORGASMIC PHASE (ORGASMIC OR DYSFUNCTION DISORDERS)

1. Male orgasmic disorder (Male anorgasmia)
2. Female orgasmic disorder (Female anorgasmia)
3. Premature ejaculation

1. Male Orgasmic Disorder

Failure or marked difficulty to have orgasm, despite normal sexual excitement, during coitus. The causes can be biological – poor prostate surgery, drug-induced or psychological-marital conflicts.

2. Female Orgasmic Disorder

Failure or marked difficulty to have orgasm, despite normal sexual excitement during coitus – causes – can be biological – endocrinal disorders – psychological – marital conflicts.

3. Premature Ejaculation

Ejaculation before the completion of satisfactory sexual activity for both partners. In severe cases, it is characterized by ejaculation either before penile entry into vagina or soon after penetration. The causes – biological – psychological.

IV. SEXUAL PAIN DISORDERS

1. Non-organic vaginisms
2. Non-organic dyspareunia

1. Non-organic Vaginisms

This disorder is characterized by an involuntary spasm of lower 1/3rd of vagina, interfering with coitus. Penile entry is either painful or impossible.

2. Non-organic dyspareunia

This disorder is characterized by pain in the genital area of either male or female, during coitus.

V. SEXUAL DISORDERS DUE TO A GENERAL MEDICAL CONDITION

The disorders listed above may occur secondary to a general medical condition.

These sexual disorders are due to sexual stimulation being inadequate either in focus, intensity or duration.

Treatment of Sexual Dysfunctions

Most treatment programs for sexual dysfunction are based on principles of Behavior Therapy, although other psychological approaches are often incorporated at the same time, including marital therapy or psychodynamic approaches. Pharmacotherapy and surgery are appropriate for specific cases. Although drug treatment is effective, e.g. for erectile dysfunction, an exclusively biological approach is not satisfactory and increases the chance of treatment failure or relapse.

Treatment consists of one or more of the following methods:

a. Sexual Counseling and Therapy

The aim is to establish proper verbal and sexual communication between partners. Initial assessment helps to identify antecedents of the problem and evaluate the nature of the couples' relationship.

Many techniques are derived from the Masters and Johnson approach, especially sensate focus. Prescribed exercises between sessions ('homework') focus on verbal communication and on heightening sensory awareness to sight, touch and smell. Intercourse is prohibited and partners focus on mutual pleasuring by massage, caressing, etc. without stimulation of genitalia. Performance anxiety is reduced by removing the focus away from orgasm as a goal.

During subsequent sessions, encouragement is given for performing the exercises and resistance (e.g. excuses of having "no time") is dealt with. Concerns about performance (spectatoring) is common and can be countered by using fantasies to distract oneself.

Genital stimulation is prescribed only at a later stage, when expression of mutual needs is comfortably established. Finally, intromission and intercourse is permitted.

b. Specific Techniques and Exercises

Unique to each specific types of dysfunction, specific techniques are used in conjunction with sensate focus:

i. Premature ejaculation – The squeeze technique entails the female applying firm pressure to the coronal ridge of the glans when the male experiences the sensation of ejaculation. Ejaculation is stopped and erection is diminished before stimulation recommences again. The stop-start technique is similar, where stimulation is stopped with increasing excitement, before ejaculation occurs. Constant practice increases the amount of ejaculatory control. The female-on-top position is recommended.
ii. Vaginismus – graduated dilatation of the introitus with the fingers or prescribed dilators is taught to the woman and/or the partner.
iii. Impotence – Sensate focus exercises emphasize total body stimulation and pleasure rather than penetration performance. Having and enjoying the erection without sexual intercourse builds confidence and quells anxiety, paving the way for intercourse to orgasm eventually.

c. Pharmacotherapy

The introduction of sildenafil (Viagra) for the treatment of erectile dysfunction has been a recent revolution. As the first effective, acceptable and widely available treatment for erectile dysfunction, it has allowed for unprecedented interest and public awareness about sexual dysfunction.

Sildenafil is a phosphodiesterase inhibitor and enhances and maintains penile responses to sexual stimulation in men with erectile problems. It however does not work without sexual desire and stimulation; nor will it make normal erections harder or last longer.

Side effects include headaches, blurred vision, seeing objects in shades of blue or dizziness. Taking it together with nitrates may lead to fatal complications.

Oral medication with testosterone or yohimbine (an a_2-adrenoceptor antagonist) is of doubtful efficacy. Many men are increasingly being given androgen preparations for sexual complaints and 'male menopause'. This is useless in the absence of established androgen deficiency.

Intracavernosal injections of papaverine or prostaglandin (PGE_1) is of particular value to men with otherwise irreversible organic erectile dysfunction, e.g. diabetics. Even in men with largely psychogenic factors, it has a role in increasing confidence by demonstrating the erectile capability of the penis. Indeed, intracavernosal injections can be used as an evaluative tool to determine penile capacity for erection.

d. Mechanical Aids and Surgery

External vacuum devices are a viable option for some. Penile prosthetic implants or vascular surgery are indicated for specific cases of organic impotence.

Points of various therapy for sexual dysfunction

1. Treatment of the underlying physical or psychiatric disorder, if presence
2. Psychoanalysis
3. Hypnosis
4. Group psychotherapy
5. Behavior therapy
   a. Relaxation training
   b. Assertiveness training
   c. Systematic desensitization
   d. Biofeedback
6. Masters and Johnson's technique
   a. One of the successful methods of treatment for psychosexual dysfunctions.
   b. The patient is not treated alone but both the partners are treated together.
   c. This is called dual sex therapy.
   d. Treatment is symptom removal using simple behavioral technique.
   e. The techniques are
      i. Sensate focus technique: For important cases
      ii. Squeeze techniques or Semen's technique: for premature ejaculation.
7. Oral drug therapy
   a. Psychiatric treatment
   b. Benzodiazepine for anxiety
   c. Premature ejaculation
      i. Fluoxetine, trazodone
      ii. Tricyclic antidepressants

Contd...

Contd...

   d. Impotence: α-blockers, opiate antagonists, dopamine agonists.
   e. Sildenatil citrate (Viagra)
   f. Hormonal treatment-Androgens
8. Intracavernosal injection of vasoactive drugs (IIVD):
   Papaverine, an alkaloid and a vasoactive substance, has been used as an intracavernosal injection.
9. Physical devices:
   Various suction devices (for producing artificial penile tumescence) and penile prosthetic implants are available.
10. Vascular surgery:
   Rarely – needed for some patient with underlying vascular insufficiency for organic sexual disorder.

21 Alcoholism and Associated Disorders

INTRODUCTION

First used by Magnus Huss, a Swedish Public Health Authority, in 1849, the word "Alcoholism" was quickly adopted by many other languages, with only minor variation.

The DSM – IIIR describes two general diagnostic classes of symptoms and maladaptive behavioral changed associated with the regular use of psychoactive chemicals.

Nine classes of psychoactive drugs are associated with both abuse and dependence: Alcohol, stimulants (including cocaine and crack), cannabodies, hallucinogens, inhalants, opiates, phencyclidine (PCP), sedative-hypnotics and anxiolytics.

Alcohol is a natural substance formed by the reaction of fermenting sugar with yeast spores. Alcohol is classified as a food because it contains calories; however, it has no nutritional value.

Beers contain	:	3 to 6% alcohol
Wines average	:	10 to 20%
Distilled beverages	:	40 to 50%

PHASES OF ALCOHOLISM

Jellinek (1952) outlined 4 phases through which the alcoholic's pattern of drinking progresses.

Phase I: *The Prealcoholic Phase:*

This phase is characterized by the use of alcohol to relieve the everyday stress of tensions of life. One individual drinks because of social motivations, and finds that alcohol relieves stress.

Overtime, needs to increase the amount of alcohol needed for relief. This phase called as "non-addicted heavy drinker".

Phase II: *Early Alcoholic Phase*

This phase begins the black outs – brief periods of amnesia that occur during or immediately following a period of drinking. In this phase, person begins to drink alone and becomes preoccupation with the supply of drinks. Person wakes up in the morning and needs a drink to control tremors (the eye – opener). He may experience blackouts.

Phase III: *True Alcoholics (Crucial Phase)*

In this phase the individual has lost control and physiological dependence is clearly evident. In which, completely loses control over ability to choose whether or not to drink. The person experiences the following: isolation from other's aggression, loss of interest in any activity that once brought pleasure, impotence, nutritional impairment.

Phase IV: *Chronic (Chronic Alcoholic)*

This phase is characterized by emotional and physical disintegration. Emotional disintegration is evidenced by profound helplessness and self pity. Hallucinations, tremors, convulsions, severe agitation and panic are symptoms of alcoholism. Depression and ideas of suicide are common.

According to Jellinek, there are five "species" of alcohol dependence – on the basis of patterns of uses.

Patterns	*Characteristics*
A. Alpha (α) Alcoholism	• Drinking to relieve physical/ emotional pain. • No loss of control
B. Beta (β) Alcoholism	• Physical complications due to cultural drinking patterns • No dependence
C. Gamma (γ) Alcoholism	• Malignant alcoholism • Physical dependence • Inability to control drinking

Contd...

Contd...

Patterns	*Characteristics*
D. Delta (δ) Alcoholism	• Inability to abstain • Tolerance • Withdrawal symptoms • Social disruption
E. Epsilon (ε) Alcoholism	• Dipsomania • Spree – drinking

Etiological Factors

I. Biological Factors

(i) Genetic vulnerability – family history of substance with disorder.
(ii) Personality disorder
(iii) Reinforcing effects of drugs
(iv) Craving and withdrawal effects
(v) Biochemical factors (e.g. role of dopamine and norepinephrine in cocaine and opioid dependence)

II. Psychological Factors

(i) Curiosity
(ii) Early initiation of alcohol and tobacco
(iii) Poor impulse control
(iv) Low self-esteem
(v) Poor stress management skills
(vi) Childhood trauma/loss
(vii) Psychological distress

III. Social Factors

(i) Peer pressure
(ii) Modeling
(iii) Ease of availability of alcohol/drugs
(iv) Religious reasons
(v) Poor social/familial support
(vi) Rapid urbanization

Body Effects of Alcohol Dependence

I. Medical Complications

A. Gastrointestinal System:

1. Fatty liver, cirrhosis of liver, hepatitis, liver cell carcinoma, liver failure.
2. Gastritis, reflux esophasitis, peptic ulcer, carcinoma stomach and esophagus.
3. Malabsorption syndrome
4. Pancreatitis, acute, chronic and relapsing

B. Central Nervous System:

1. Delirium tremens
2. Rumfits
3. Alcoholic hallucinosis
4. Wernicke-Korsakoff psychosis
5. Alcoholic dementia
6. Suicide
7. Head injury and fractures

C. Miscellaneous:

1. Acne rosacea, palmar erythema, parotid enlargement, ascites
2. Fetal alcohol syndrome
3. Alcoholic hypoglycemia
4. Alcoholic myopathy
5. Anemia, thrombocytopenia, vitamin K factor deficiency
6. Hypothermia
7. Malnutrition, pellagra
8. Sexual dysfunction

II. Social Complications

1. Accidents
2. Marital disharmony
3. Divorce
4. Occupational problems
5. Criminality
6. Financial difficulties

COMPLICATIONS

A. Acute Intoxication

Symptoms of alcohol intoxication includes disinhibition of sexual or aggressive impulses, mood lability, impairment judgement, impaired social or occupational functioning, slurred speech, incoordination, unsteady gait, nystagmus and flushed face. Intoxications usually occurs at blood alcohol levels between 100 and 200 mg/dl.

B. Alcohol Withdrawal Syndrome

Within 4 to 12 hours of cessation of or reduction in heavy and prolonged alcohol use, the following symptoms may appear; coarse tremor of hands, tongue, or eyelids, nausea or vomiting, malaise or weakness, tachycardia, sweating, elevated blood pressure, anxiety, irritability, transient hallucinations or illusions, headache and insomnia.

Withdrawal syndrome characterized by one of the following 3 disturbances; delirium tremens, alcoholic seizures and alcoholic hallucinosis.

1. Delirium Tremens

It is the most severe alcohol withdrawal syndrome. It occurs usually within 2 – 4 days of complete or significant abstinence from heavy alcohol drinking in 5% of patients. This is an acute organic brain syndrome with the characteristic of clouding of consciousness, disorientation, poor attention span and distractibility, visual hallucinations and illusions, tachycardia, fever, sweating, hypertension, atoxia, insomnia, dehydration and electrolyte imbalance.

2. Alcoholic Seizures ("rum fits")

Generalized tomic clonic seizures occur in about 10% of alcohol dependence patients. Usually 12 – 48 hours after a heavy bout of drinking. Multiple seizures 2 – 6 at one time, are more common than single seizures.

3. Alcoholic Hallucinosis

This is characterized by the presence of hallucinations during abstinence, following regular alcohol intake. These hallucinations persist after the withdrawal syndrome is over, and classically occur in clear consciousness.

C. Neuropsychiatric Complications of Chronic Alcohol Use

1. Wernicke's Encephalopathy

This is an acute reaction to severe thiamin deficiency, the commonest cause being chronic alcohol use. Characteristically, the onset occurs after a period of persistent vomiting.

(a) Ocular signs – nystagmus, opthalmoplegia, papillary irregularities, retinal hemorrhages and impairment of vision.

(b) Higher mental function disturbance: Disorientation, confusion, recent memory disturbances, poor attention span and distractibility are common.

2. Korsakoff's Psychosis

Korsakoff's psychosis presents as an amnestic syndrome, characterized by gross memory disturbances with confabulation.

3. Marchiafava-Bignami Disease

It characterized by disorientation, epilepsy, ataxia, hallucinations and personality

4. Others

Alcoholic dementia, cerebellur degeneration and peripheral neuropathy.

Treatment

1. Detoxification

This is the treatment of alcohol withdrawal symptoms, i.e. symptoms produced by the removal of the "toxin" (alcohol). The usual duration of uncomplicated withdrawal syndrome is 7 – 14 days. The drugs of choice are benzodiazepines. These drugs are used in a standardized protocol with the dosage steadily decreasing every day before being stopped, usually on the tenth day.

2. Treatment of Alcohol Dependence

The important methods include:

(i) Behavior therapy:
The most commonly used behavior therapy is aversion therapy, using either a sub-threshold electric shock or an emetic like apomorphine.

(ii) Psychotherapy

(iii) Group therapy

(iv) Deterrent agents

(v) Anti-craving agents: e.g. acamprosate, naltrexone, fluoxetine, etc.

(vi) Psychosocial rehabilitation.

Substance – Abuse Epidemiology

Substance abuse ranks among the top three most serious public health problems. Estimate of prevalence of use is difficult because most users take more than one drug and take drugs in combination such as cocaine for stimulation and alcohol to come down more easily from the high.

The costs of substance abuse for two individual the family and society are evident in high rates of crime (often drug, and/or alcohol – related), medical costs, drug enforcement efforts. Absenteeism and accidents on the job resulting from effects of heavy alcohol and other drug use affect industry and business.

Theories of Addiction

Three prominent classes of theories of chemical dependence are:

1. The disease model
2. Sociopsychological models
3. Interactive models.

The Disease Model

Addiction meets the criteria for disease in as much as it (i) can be diagnosed, (ii) is primary and itself is the cause of other medical and psychiatric problems, (iii) is predictable and progressive in its course, (iv) is treatable.

The correspondence between addiction and other disease is evidenced in both physiologic and psychological aspects. The physical components include biologic factors such as genetic predisposition and chemically altered brain function. The psychologic components include an obsession with the use of the drug for its pleasurable qualities of a compulsive self-defeating drug-use pattern.

Theories on Addiction

Three prominent classes of theories of chemical dependence are:

1. The disease model
2. Socio psychological models
3. Interactive models.

The Disease Model

Addiction meets the criteria for disease in as much as it (i) can be diagnosed, (ii) is primary and itself is the cause of other medical and psychiatric problems, (iii) is predictable and progressive in its course, (iv) is treatable.

The correspondence between addiction and other diseases are evidenced in both physiologic and psychological aspects. The physical components include biologic factors such as general predisposition and chemically altered brain function. The psychologic components include an obsession with the use of the drug for its pleasurable qualities and a compulsive self-defeating drug-use pattern.

Jellinet (1960) is credited with articulating the disease model of alcoholism. The current disease model, revised from Jellinek's early work, incorporates the following:

1. There is unique entity that can be identified as alcoholism.
2. Alcoholics and pre alcoholic are essentially different from non-alcoholics.
3. Alcoholics may sometimes experience an irresistible physical craving for alcohol or a strong psychologic compulsion to drink.
4. Alcoholic gradually develop loss of control over drinking and possibly even an inability to stop drinking.
5. Alcoholism is a permanent and irreversible condition.
6. Alcoholism is a progressive disease that follows an inexorable development through a distinct series of phases as long as the person continues to ingest alcohol.

There are four phases of alcoholism:

1. Prealcoholism
2. Early alcoholism
3. Frank addiction
4. Chronic illness with identified behavior manifested in each.

Sociopsychologic Models

Socio psychologic theories include psychodynamics theories, family theories and learning and conditioning theories.

Early psychologic theories were psychoanalytic and derived from Freudian views on the individual's pursuit of euphoria as an escape from depression through use of a substitute for the gratification of oral and genital needs.

Further interpretation by Rado 1933, notes that the impulses to use the toxic agents, not the agent itself, makes individual an addict. Psycho analytic theory assets that drug addition is a symptom of underlying psychopathology that becomes embedded in lifestyle.

In adaptation model, addiction is an attempt is adapt to severe distress through the habitual use of drugs. This model suggest that adaptation may be directed nor toward relief of psychologic pain but toward escape from environmental stress and life crisis. **Stanton (1984)** describes the use of opiates by both parents and children as an attempt to relive intrafamilial stress.

Learning and conditioning theories are behaviorally based and assert that drug-use develops via learning and modeling and the positive reinforcement of mood alteration by the chemicals. Social learning theory stresses that people teach new behaviors, influence previously learned responses, and enhance the value of particular behaviors. Thus a behavior that is followed by reward or absence of negative consequences is likely to be modeled by an observer.

Psychologic addiction is a compelling from of addiction and is more prevalent than physiologic dependence.

Interactive Models

Interactive or multiple factor models acknowledge that it is difficult to predict the development of addiction. Interaction of variables result in illness, and these variables include individual and family dynamics and sociopsychologic and environmental factors.

Donoven's (1986) proposed risk factors for alcoholism also have applicability to other forms of drug dependence and include the following:

1. Heredity, as evidenced in family history, gender and neuropsychological deficits.
2. Deficits of psychologic structure, such as ego, weakness and antisocial personality.
3. Sociocultural factors.

Interactive models also allow for consideration of mediating factors that may serve to prevent addiction from emerging. These factors, include social class, adoption and age of placement, family dynamics and support systems.

In the interactive model, causality is dynamic, allowing for flexible interpretations of valid outcomes and changeability in understanding of the evolution of illness. In fact, specific individuals ad groups may manifest a variety of factors that cause the disease. Such a model provides for varying patterns of disease development and stresses the quantitative value of factors.

The Stuart Stress Adaptation Model Related to Substance Abuse

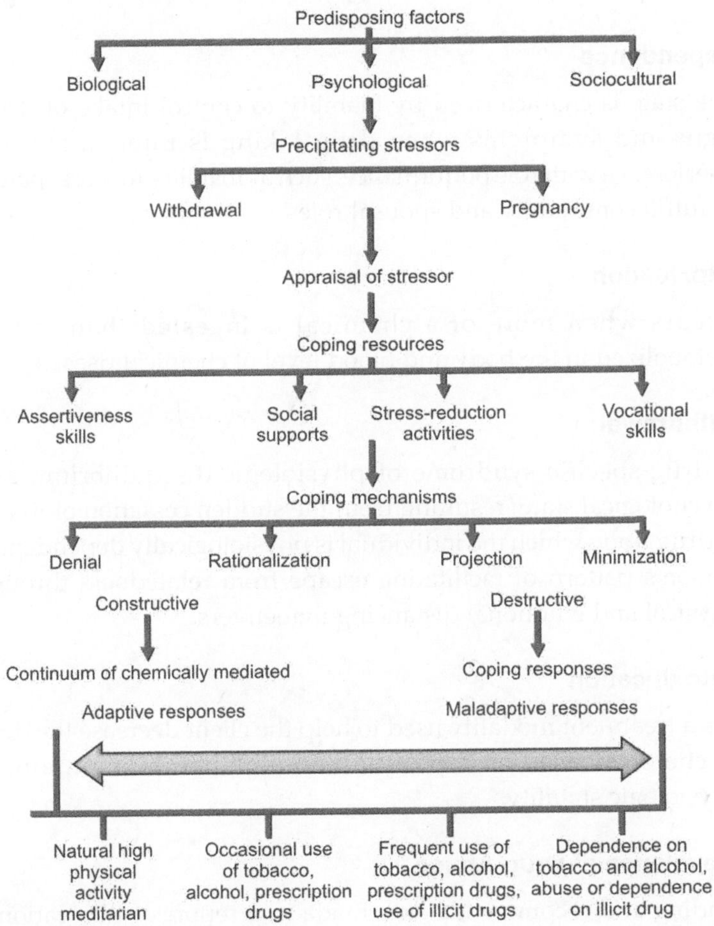

DRUG DEPENDENCE

Addiction

They defined as "a state of periodic or chronic intoxication produced by repeated consumption of a drug".

Habituation

Was defined as a "condition resulting from the repeated consumption of drug".

Dependence

The state is characterized by inability to control intake of drug, signs and symptoms when drug taking is interrupted and interference with role performance, such as inability to work, parent or fulfill community and spousal roles.

Intoxication

Occurs when more of a chemical is ingested than can be metabolized in the body and blood level of chemical rises.

Withdrawal

A drug-specific syndrome of physiologic disequilibrium and psychological state, resulting from the sudden cessation of intake of drug upon which the individual is physiologically dependent; a person's pattern of facilitating escape from relatedness through physical and emotional distancing maneuvers.

Detoxification

It is a treatment modality used to help the client decrease the dose of chemical used as rapidly as possible while maintaining physiologic stability.

Prevalence of Drug Abuse

Finding and recommendations made in a report of the National Committee on Drug Addiction (1977) focused on the following dependence-producing drug and other substances commonly misused in India.

1. Cannabis and its products (Bhang, Ganja)
2. Hallucinogen, e.g. LSD Lysergic acid diethylamide
3. Tranquillizers, hypotic and sedatives (Dizepam methaqalone and chloral hydrate)

4. Barbiturate (Phenobarbital and secubarbitol)
5. Amphetamines
6. Tobacco
7. Other narcotic drug (opium, pethidine, morphine, heroin)
8. Alcohol
   40 – 45% of prevalence substance abuse.

Etiology

There seems to (1982) be no unitary theory to explain drug dependence. Wilson and Kneisl have classified the theories of drug dependence as psychological, sociological and physiological.

Causative factors for narcotics and other substance abuse can be studied under the following heading:

1. Interpersonal and psychosocial
2. Socioeconomic
3. Cultural and ethnic
4. Youth culture
5. Pharmacological
6. Ecological.

I. Interpersonal and Psychosocial Factors

Psychoanalytically, they are described to be regressed and fixed at the oral stage of psychosexual development.

Wursmer (1972) has stated that families where the parents are self-centered and are preoccupied with success and prestige may lead their children in drug addiction. These children may feel personal insecurity, escape from a difficult situations due to self-doubt and absence of a strong ego.

II. Socioeconomic Factors

- Low socioeconomic status.
- Difficult life style, poverty and hopelessness lead to frustration and then to drug addiction.
- Broken families, unloving parents where there is no meaningful relationship are also contributory factors.
- Increasing in middle socioeconomic people.

III. Youth Culture

Adolescents try to follow the peer group. They also try to be a part of the group, use the drugs and get addicted.

IV. Pharmacological Factors

Some substances/drugs are likely to cause an addictive effect more than others. For instances, opium produces tolerance and physical dependence more in comparison to other drugs.

V. Ecological Factors

Freedman (1972) suggests that people and their drug environment are interwoven. To achieve a sense of belongingness some youth join the group of drug abusers. Social groups are another environmental pressure for drug addiction.

Diagnostic Criteria for Psychoactive Substance Abuse DSM – II R

At least three of the following:

1. Substance often taken in larger amounts or over a longer period than the person intended.
2. Persistent desire or one or more unsuccessful effort to cut down or control substance use.
3. A great deal of time spent in activities necessary to get the substance, taking substance or recovering from its effects.
4. Frequent intoxication or withdrawal symptoms when expected to fulfill a major role obligation at work school, home.
5. Important social, occupational or recreational activities given up or reduced because of substance use.
6. Continued substance use despite knowledge of having a persistent social, psychological, physical problem that is caused by use of substance.
7. Marked tolerance; need for markedly increased amount of substance in order to achieve intoxication or a desired effect.
8. Characteristic withdrawal symptoms.

Common Mood Altering Chemicals

Drug Names	*Effects*	*Site of Action*	*Length of Effect*
Hallucinogeng Mushroom (Psilocybin) LSD (Lysergic Acid Diethylamide) DOM (Dimethodymethylam phetamine)	Altered body image, Euphoria, Sharpened perceptions, somatic effects: dizziness, tremors, weakness, nausea, psychosis like symptoms emotional swings, suspiciousness, bizarre behaviour, increased blood pressure, increased temperature.Objective signs: Dilated pupils, flushing, tremors.	Central Nervous System (CNS) Brain	Onset 40 – 60 min duration 6 – 12 hr
Cannabinoids Marijuana Hashish	Failure in judgement and memory, mild intoxication, euphoria, relaxation, sexual arousal, panic states visual hallucinations.Objective Signs: Reddended eyes, dry mouth, in co-ordination. .Heart rate to 140/ min.	CNS Cardiovascular System Respiratory system	Administration and dose dependent Onset: 20 – 30 min Duration: 3 – 7 hr
Opiates: Opiates; semisynthetic and synthetic analgesics Codeine Morphine Heroin Dulaudid Methadone Designer drugs	Analgesia, Euphoria, Escape, Reduction in sexual and aggressive drives, Respiratory depression, sedation, sleepiness.Objective Signs: Hypertension, papillary constriction, constipation	Nervous tissue CNS (Opiate receptors) Respiratory system	Onset 20 – 30 min Duration 4 – 8 hr

Contd...

Contd...

Drug Names	*Effects*	*Site of Action*	*Length of Effect*
Sedative – hypnosis and anxiolytics: Barbiturates Secondal Nembutal Amytal Tuinol Benzodiazapines Buspirone	Drowsiness, sedation, euphoria, escape, loss of aggressive and sexual drives, emotional liability, poor judgement.	CNS Cardiovascular system Respiratory system	Onset 30 – 40 min Duration 4 – 5 hr
Stimulus Amphetamine Ritalin Preludin Cocaine Crack	Euphoria, gradiosity, stimulation, energy, anxiety, relief of fatigue, depression, paranoia.Objective Sign: Sweating dilated pupils, increased blood pressure, rapid HR.	CNS	Rapid onset 2 – 3 min upto 45 min. Duration: drug related
Inhalants Benzene (Paint thinner, cleaning fluid, glue) Nitrites Nitrous oxide	Euphoria, giddiness, headache, fatigue, drowsiness.Objective Signs: arrythorias, damage to kidney, liver abnormalities	Cardiac effect CNS	Onset: Immediate Duration: 20 – 45 min
Alcohol Beverage alcohol, beer, wine	Relaxation, sedation, release of inhibitions. Objective Signs: In co-ordination, nausea, vomiting, slurred speech	CNS Respiratory system	Onset: 20 min – 1 hr Duration: dose related

Contd...

Drug Names	*Effects*	*Site of Action*	*Length of Effect*
Xanthines Caffeine Nicotine Cigarettes Smokeless tobacco	Stimulation, restlessness, anxiety. Objective Signs: Decreased heart and respiratory rates, diarrhoea, gastric disorder, insomnia and tremors	CNS	Onset: 10 – 30 min Duration: 3 – 7 hr
	Stimulation Enhanced performance	CNS Respiratory system Cardiovascular system Endocrine system	Onset: Immediate Duration: 5 – 15 min

Management of Alcohol and Substance Abuse

Many psychological methods can use for management of management.

1. **Individual psychotherapy:**
   Individual psychotherapy used to give the alcohol person.
2. **Group psychotherapy:**
   Alcoholic anonymous and narcotic anonymous activities.
3. **Aversion therapy:**
   Pleasant event or substance make into unpleasant one, (e.g.) Alcohol is pleasant for a person. So, add chemical make unpleasant one.
4. **Anta Abuse:**
   Disulfaram drug used here. This drug affect aldehydate conversion. So it affects the general circulations system and produce the unwanted signs and symptoms.
5. **Behavioral therapy:**
   Reinforcement pattern used.
6. **Cognitive Therapy:**
   Helps to understand negative behavior.

Nursing Assessment

1. Nursing history
2. Observation for physical signs associated with alcohol abuse
   Telangiectasia – Vascular lesion formed by dilation of a group of small blood vessels, usually on the face.
   Palmer erythema – Red spots on the palms of hands.
   Peripheral neuropathy – Disease of nervous system in arms and legs.
   Acne rosacca – Skin disease of the nose, face and chin
   Poor hygiene
   Poor muscletone
3. Physical signs associated with other drugs use
   Poor hygiene
   Dental caries
   Very scarring
   Abscesses

Nursing Diagnosis

1. Alteration sensory perceptual related to confusion, disorient blackout, hallucinations.
2. High risk for injury related to ataxia, history of seizures.
3. Self-care deficit related to intolerance to activity, diminished self-esteem, discomfort.
4. High risk for infection related to homeless like style, practice of unsafe sex, severe withdrawal syndrome.
5. Alteration in nutrition less than body requirement related to report of inadequate dietary intake, change in appetite.
6. Sleep pattern disturbance related to sleep pattern reversal fleeting hystagmus.
7. Alteration in thought process related to mood swings, restlessness, impairment of recent memory, dementia.
8. Impaired communication related to inability to express feeling, slurring of speech, inappropriate speech patterns.
9. Alteration in self-concept.
10. Social isolation.
11. Dysfunctional family process.
12. Powerlessness.
13. Ineffective individual coping.

INTERVENTIONS

Intoxication

Intoxication occurs when more of a chemical is ingested than can be metabolized in the body and the blood level of the chemical rises.

During intoxication the client is unable to reason or make sound judgements. The main goal of nursing care is to maintain physiologic stability while the person's body metabolize the chemical.

Monitor vital signs every 15 minutes until fluctuations subside, then every 30 min for 2 hours than once an hour for the remainder of the 24 hours.

Take temperature every 2 hours through 24 hours.

Maintain open airway. Assist client with positioning for optimal ventilation.

Monitor I/O chart until vital signs are within normal limits for 24 hours.

Withdrawal Syndrome

Withdrawal is a chemical-specific syndrome that follows the cessation of or reduction in intake of mood altering chemical that the person used regularly.

Withdrawal may begin in 8 to 12 hours with short acting and may be delayed 1 to 3 days for long – acting drugs.

Detoxification is a treatment modality used to help the client decrease the dose of chemical used as rapidly as possible while maintaining physiologic stability.

Nursing care during withdrawal is supportive, acknowledging the client's experience with empathy.

Comfort measures such as hot tea, warm blankets and cuddling a pillow are usually appreciated by clients. They also need to know how long detoxification is expected to last.

Once acute withdrawal has subsided, the abstinence syndrome emerges. It may last for weeks and is thought to be a major factor in relapse. The abstinence syndrome is characterized by drug seeking, over concern with body discomfort, and decreased ability to tolerate stress.

Acute Health Problems

Besides the early cardio vascular dangers, other health problems are common. The nurse's role is three fold.

1. To help the client connect chemical use to physical consequences by means of formal and informal teaching.
2. To teach clients to manage chronic health problems that do not resolve after detoxification.
3. To implement protocols for medical treatment of problems while clients are treatment.

Management of Alcohol Withdrawal

The principles of alcohol detoxification according to evidence based practice guidelines are as follows:

- Long acting benzediazepines are the drugs of choice in treating alcohol withdrawal because they effectively reduce signs and symptoms of withdrawal, prevent seizures and have a better margin of safety than many other drugs.
- The use of a clinically valid and reliable withdrawal assessment tool such as CIWA – AR (Clinical Institute Withdrawal Assessment – Alcohol Revised) is recommended as basis for medication determinations.

Although neither magnesium nor thiamine reduces seizures administration of thiamine is recommended to prevent Wernicke's disease and Wernicke-Korsakoff syndrome.

Psychological Interventions

Motivational approaches

- Express empathy through reflective listening
- Avoid argument and direct confrontation
- Roll with resistance
- Support self-efficacy

Social Interventions

- Family counseling
- Group therapy
- Self-help groups: 12 step group: Alcoholic anonymous is model for 12-step support group. AA arms for total abstinence.
- Community treatment programs
- Employee Assistance programs.

Preventive Interventions

Primary Prevention:

Public speakers, school programs.

Secondary Prevention:

Early identification, presentation of assessment finding, education, advice regarding the need to reduce drinking with an emphasis on personal responsibility, self-help manuals and periodic follow-up.

Tertiary Prevention:

Involves decreasing the complications of addiction. Medical and psychiatric treatment setting still serve a major role here.

22 Psychiatry Emergency

INTRODUCTION

A psychiatric emergency is a disturbance in thought, mood and action which causes sudden distress to the individual and (or) sudden disability, thus requiring immediate management.

A psychiatric emergency is an acute disturbance of behavior, thought or mood of a patient which if untreated may lead to harm, either to the individual or to others in the environment. Thus the definition of a psychiatric emergency differs from other medical emergencies in that the danger of harm to the society is also taken into account.

Emergencies may be classified as major, where there is a danger to life either of the patient or to others in his environment or minor where there is no threat to life but causes severe incapacitation.

Emergency psychiatry is the clinical application of psychiatry in emergency settings. Conditions requiring psychiatric interventions may include attempted suicide, substance abuse, depression, psychosis, violence or other rapid changes in behavior. Psychiatric emergency services are rendered by professionals in the fields of medicine, nursing, psychology and social work. The demand for emergency psychiatric services has rapidly increased throughout the world since the 1960s, especially in urban areas. Care for patients in situations involving emergency psychiatry is complex. Professionals working in psychiatric emergency service settings are usually under a high risk of violence due to the mental state of their patients. Individuals may arrive in such a setting through their own voluntary request, a referral from another health professional, or through involuntary commitment

Psychiatric emergencies fall into 2 categories: Those without organic causes and those due to organic causes. A careful history and physical/mental state examination are vital in differentiating the two. Be sure to ask about past medical illness and hospitalizations: recent accidents, serious illness, use of alcohol or drugs, and personal crisis.

Types of Psychiatric Emergencies

Psychiatric emergencies are usually described as:

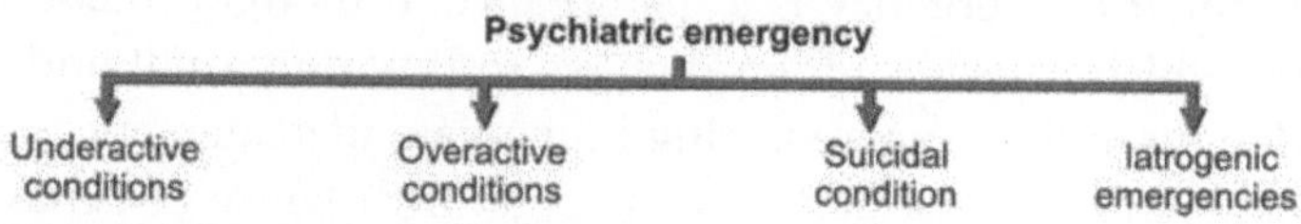

1. **Underactive Conditions:**

   The conditions in which underactive are:

   2. Depression
   3. Catatonia – stupor
   4. Grief and bereavement
   5. Insomnia

2. **Overactive Conditions:**

   These patients are increased psychomotor activity and they can be dangerous to themselves and to others. Overactive conditions are

   1. Excited behavior and violence
   2. Schizophrenia
   3. Mania
   4. Acute anxiety
   5. Organic disorder, delirium, dementia
   6. Drug reaction
   7. Acute psychosis
   8. Alcoholic disorders
   9. Drug withdrawal
   10. Panic disorder

3. **Suicide**
4. **Iatrogenic Emergencies:**
   1. Side-effects of psychotropic medication
   2. Over dose
   3. Withdrawal syndrome
   4. Other conditions: hyperventilation syndrome, insomnia, grief and bereavement, crisis, acute poisoning and epilepsy.

PSYCHIATRIC EMERGENCIES

Suicide

Suicide is the act of killing oneself. It is a type of Deliberate Self Harm (DSH).

Definition

1. Suicide defined as a human act of self-intentional and self-inflicted cessation (death).
2. Attempted suicide is an unsuccessful suicidal act with a non-fatal outcome.

Suicide rate in India was 11.2 per 100,000 in 2002. The rates vary across the country with states such as Kerala having the highest suicide rate of 30.8 per lakh in 2002. Suicide rates in Army, Air Force and Naval personnel were 0.04, 0.11 and 0.12 per thousand respectively. Rates are higher in urban than in rural settings. Studies of completed suicides show that 90-94% of the patients are mentally ill while committing the act. Depression accounts for nearly half the number of patients committing suicide followed by alcohol abuse (34%) and schizophrenia (13%) .

A meta-analysis of 249 studies on suicide during 1966-93 revealed that virtually all mental disorders carry an increased risk of suicide barring mental retardation and dementia. The suicide risk is highest for primary psychiatric disorder and least for organic disorders with substance use disorders falling in between . Indian studies show that most people attempting suicide are in the age group of 15-30 years and are predicted to increase further in the coming years . Suicide is common in the unmarried (in the married the loss of spouse increases the risk during the first year of the loss). Rates are also high in the unemployed and in those suffering from a concurrent medical illness. More men than women commit suicide though more women attempt it.

Psychosocial factors that predispose to suicide, include, for the person contemplating suicide to ventilate his problems and enable the counsellor to persuade the patient to seek professional help. However, a scientific validity of their usefulness is still lacking (Table 22.1).

Table 22.1: Psychiatric emergencies

Major emergencies
Suicidal patient grief reaction
Agitated and violent patient, Rape
Disaster
Medical emergencies in psychiatry
Panic attack
Deliriums due to life threatening conditions
Neuroleptic malignant syndrome
Serotonin syndrome
Overdosages of common psychiatric medications
Overdosages and withdrawal from addicting substances

Agitated and Violent Patients

Violence is a danger often faced in the emergency room setting. The risk of violence is especially high in those societies where there is easier access to firearms and alcohol/drug abuse. The use of alcohol also predisposes to violence. Specific psychiatric and medical disorders have also been associated with violent behavior (Tables 22.2 and 22.3).

Certain characteristics predict an assault in the emergency setting. Unemployed young (<40 years) men, with low socioeconomic status, past history of violence and who are usually non compliant with treatment. A threat to assault should always be taken seriously. Signs predicting an impending assault are anger, demanding immediate attention, loud voice, excitement, staring eyes, flared nostrils, flushed face, hands clenched or gripping,

Table 22.2: Psychiatric disorders associated with violent behavior

Schizophrenia especially paranoid
Mania
Paranoid psychosis
Personality disorder especially antisocial type
Alcohol intoxication or withdrawal
Substance intoxication with cocaine, amphetamines, anabolic steroids, phencyclidine
Substance withdrawal
Post traumatic stress disorder
Dementia
Learning disorder
Niacin
Pyridoxine
Vitamin B_{12}
Temperature distubrances
Hyperthermia
Hyhpothermia

Table 22.3: Medical disorders associated with violent behavior

Neurologic illnesses
Brain infections such as encephalitis, meningoencephalitis
Head injury with intracerebral, subarachnoid or subdural hematoma
Cerebral infarction
Seizure disorders (interictal, post ictal or temporal lobe epilepsy)
Hepatic encephalopathy
Huntington's disease
Parkinson's disease due to levodopa toxicity
Wilson's disease
Endocrinopathies
Thyrotoxicosis
Hypothyroidism
Cushing's syndrome
Hyper parathyroidism
Metabolic disorders
Hypoglycemia
Hypoxia
Electrolyte imbalance
Hypocholesterolemia
Infections
AIDS
Syphilis
Tuberculosis
Vitamin deficiencies
Folic acid

pacing about in the room, possessing weapons, pushing furniture, uncooperativeness and suspiciousness, slamming objects and sudden movements.

Protection against assault : Refer Table 22.4.

Table 22.4: Strategies to prevent assault

Verbal assault
Answer all questions softly, simply and honestly
Be empathic and calm
Keep hands visible
Keep the door open
Stay at least an arm's length away from the patient
Stay to the side of the patient
Use non threatening body language
Use reflective statements rather than judgmental ones
Physical assault
Call for help, if possible press the panic button to summon help
Deflect a kick with your legs
Deflect punches with your hands
Escape
Face the person sideways
If bitten do not pull away the bitten part, instead force the bitten part to the mouth and nose of the biter to block his respiration
If choked, tuck your chin to the chest to maintain the airway hands of the patient

Violent Behavior

Chaotic home environment, sudden loss (death, divorce, job, finances), recent humiliating life event, unfaithful partner, HIV and legal problems. In the young, suicides are common after declaration of the results of the board exams. The most common symptom in patients is hopelessness i.e. the belief that no action can save the patient from the trauma that he or she may be undergoing. A majority (56%) attempt suicide as an escape from an unbearable situation, 13% do so to produce a change in others or the environment and the rest have a combination of escape and manipulative motives. 50 to 80% of suicide attempters have communicated their intent to the family or to their treating psychiatrist.

Management : All psychiatric patients need to be asked about suicidal ideation as a part of routine assessment. Self destructive behaviors and previous attempts are the most powerful predictors of a future suicidal attempt. It needs to be clearly understood that asking about suicidal attempt does not provoke the patient to commit suicide or instil the idea of committing suicide.

Many patients feel relieved on being asked about suicidal ideation and being explained that their ideas are part of an illness.

In case the patient has arrived in the emergency department with history of an attempt, then, first the medical condition of the patient needs to be assessed for risk to life and admitted to the ICU under escort until the medical condition stabilizes. At the earliest opportunity he is referred for assessment by a psychiatrist.

Severely suicidal patients who are depressed need to be treated with electroconvulsive therapy (ECT). The procedure has an overall response rate of 75-85% . In schizophrenia, apart from ECT, atypical antipsychotics such as clozapine are reported to be having a specific antidepressant and anti-suicidal effect. Crisis intervention centres and help lines are available in most cities all over the world.

Drugs Used for Controlling Aggression

Nonspecific sedation may be required to first bring the patient under control before an assessment can be made. Emergency staff should be familiar with the administration of these drugs which should readily be available. If the patient is willing, drugs may be given orally, however, usually the parenteral route is necessary. The most commonly used drug is haloperidol 10 mg given as a single intramuscular dose and can be safely repeated at intervals of every half hour to a maximum of 60 mg. Lorazepam 2 mg up to a maximum of 10 mg is equally effective as haloperidol. It is especially useful where alcohol withdrawal is suspected.

Once the patient is under control, it is mandatory to carry out a careful physical examination and laboratory studies to exclude the common causes of violent behavior enumerated earlier. Often, if the patient is accompanied by relatives or friends, the diagnosis may be revealed by history.

Prevention of Assault on Health Workers

The casualty centre should have adequate security staff. Access to examination rooms and treatment areas should be limited. All consulting and examination rooms should have at least two exits. Similarly, all rooms should have a call button, which can be pressed in an emergency so that all available staff can rush to the aid of the medical person being assaulted. All suspicious patients should be watched and reported in detail for future risks.

Medical personnel should also be careful not to provoke an assault by being always polite and respectful,

Calm, avoiding prolonged eye contact with potentially violent patients, giving clear instructions, remaining at a safe distance unless unavoidable, keeping clear exits, removing all articles in their rooms which could be used for assault. All cases of assault must be investigated and discussed among the staff and the administration and lessons drawn for future .

Delirium is managed with environmental manipulation to help orient the patient (e.g. leaving a light on at night, frequent orientation to time, place, and person) and with drugs. Drugs should be prescribed only after the underlying disorder has been diagnosed or the process of determining the diagnosis has been initiated.

Haloperidol in low doses (0.5 to 2 mg) is frequently the drug of choice. Lorazepam 0.5 to 2 mg can reduce agitation and is preferable when substance withdrawal is the cause. Anticholinergic drugs (e.g, benztropine) should be used with caution in delirious patients, especially the elderly, because anticholinergic toxicity (atropine psychosis) can occur.

Substance intoxication and withdrawal : It may occur with a psychiatric disorder or as a primary presenting complaint. Alcohol, cocaine and phencyclidine are the substances that most commonly lead to violent behavior. Patients should be placed under observation in a secure room away from stimulation; attempting to talk the patient down is not recommended. Physical restraints or sedation may be necessary for violent patients. Lorazepam 2 to 4 mg stat or diazepam 10 to 20 mg stat is recommended to treat agitation.

Withdrawal from barbiturates, other sedatives and hypnotics (including benzodiazepines) and alcohol are similar clinically. When symptoms are severe, treatment in a hospital is safest and is mandatory if the patient is febrile (>38.3°C or 101°F), cannot hold down fluids to prevent dehydration, or has a severe underlying physical disorder. Alcohol withdrawal can be life threatening. Seizures can occur. Delirium tremens, a withdrawal syndrome that starts within 7 days of withdrawal (usually within 24 to 72 hr), is a medical emergency and should be treated in an ICU.

Management is usually with high doses of benzodiazepines, parenteral thiamine and maintenance of fluid and electrolyte balance.

Overdose of prescribed psychoactive drugs : It can also pose a threat to life apart from causing intoxication. Hence, the patient should be jointly managed by a physician and a psychiatrist. If the patient has taken a toxic dose and is awake, treatment consists of inducing emesis followed by administering activated charcoal. Overdose with tricyclic antidepressants or carbamazepine requires cardiac monitoring. Overdose with barbiturates or benzodiazepines and alcohol may cause respiratory arrest. Antipsychotic drugs, at therapeutic as well as toxic doses, can cause acute extrapyramidal adverse effects including dystonia, oculogyric crisis, torticollis, and akinesia. Akathisia is a common adverse effect of high-potency antipsychotics, when severe, it is accompanied by extreme anxiety or terror. Acute onset of oculogyric or orofacial dystonia in an otherwise healthy person may suggest purposeful or inadvertent ingestion of an antipsychotic. Immediate relief may be provided with a parenteral antihistaminic such as promethazine 25 mg IM.

Substance Dependence, Abuse and Intoxication

Another common cause of psychotic symptoms is substance intoxication. These acute symptoms may resolve after a period of observation or limited psychopharmacological treatment (Fig.22.1). However the underlying issues, such as substance dependence or abuse, is difficult to treat in the emergency room. Both acute alcohol intoxication as well as other forms of substance abuse can require psychiatric interventions. Acting as a depressant of the central nervous system, the early effects of alcohol are usually desired for and characterized by increased talkativeness, giddiness, and a loosening of social inhibitions. Besides considerations of impaired concentration, verbal and motor performance, insight, judgment and short-term memory loss which could result in behavioral change causing injury or death, levels of alcohol below 60 milligrams per deciliter of blood are usually considered non-lethal. However, individuals at 200 milligrams per deciliter of blood are considered grossly intoxicated and concentration levels at 400 milligrams per deciliter of blood are lethal, causing complete anesthesia of the respiratory system. Beyond the dangerous behavioral changes that occur after the consumption of certain amounts of alcohol, idioyncratic intoxication could occur in some individuals even after the consumption of relatively small amounts of alcohol. Episodes of this impairment usually consist of confusion, disorientation, delusions and visual hallucinations, increased

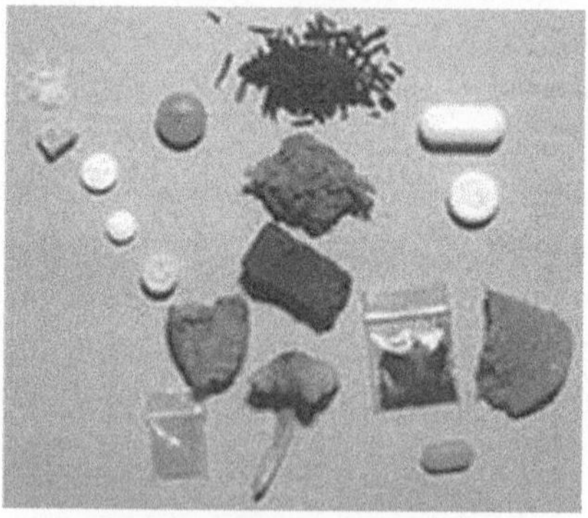

Fig. 22.1: Psychoactive drugs

aggressiveness, rage, agitation and violence. Chronic alcoholics may also suffer from alcoholic hallucinosis, wherein the cessation of prolonged drinking may trigger auditory hallucinations. Such episodes can last for a few hours or an entire week. Antipsychotics are often used to treat these symptoms.

Patients may also be treated for substance abuse following the administration of psychoactive substances containing amphetamine, caffeine, tetrahydrocannabinol, cocaine, phencyclidines, or other inhalants, opioids, sedatives, hypnotics, anxiolytics, psychedelics, dissociatives and deliriants. Clinicians assessing and treating substance abusers must establish therapeutic rapport to counter denial and other negative attitudes directed towards treatment. In addition, the clinician must determine substances used, the route of administration, dosage, and time of last use to determine the necessary short and long term treatments. An appropriate choice of treatment setting must also be determined. These settings may include outpatient facilities, partial hospitals, residential treatment centers, or hospitals. Both the immediate and long-term treatment and setting is determined by the severity of dependency and seriousness of physiological complications arising from the abuse.

Hazardous Drug Reactions and Interactions

Overdoses, drug interactions, and dangerous reactions from psychiatric medications, especially antipsychotics, are considered psychiatric emergencies. Neuroleptic malignant syndrome is a potentially lethal complication of first or second generation antipsychotics. If untreated, neuroleptic malignant syndrome can result in fever, muscle rigidity, confusion, unstable vital signs, or even death. Serotonin syndrome can result when selective serotonin reuptake inhibitors or monoamine oxidase inhibitors mix with buspirone. Severe symptoms of serotonin syndrome include hyperthermia, delirium, and tachycardia that may lead to shock. Often patients with severe general medical symptoms, such as unstable vital signs, will be transferred to a general medical emergency room or medicine service for increased monitoring.

Personality Disorders

Disorders manifesting dysfunction in areas related to cognition, affectivity, interpersonal functioning and impulse control can be considered personality disorders. Patients suffering from a personality disorder will usually not complain about symptoms resulting from their disorder. Patients suffering an emergency phase of a personality disorder may showcase combative or suspicious behavior, suffer from brief psychotic episodes, or be delusional. Compared with outpatient settings and the general population, the prevalence of individuals suffering from personality disorders in inpatient psychiatric settings is usually 7–25% higher. Clinicians working with such patients attempt to stabilize the individual to their baseline level of function.

Anxiety

Patients suffering from an extreme case of anxiety may seek treatment when all support systems have been exhausted and they are unable to bear the anxiety. Feelings of anxiety may present in different ways from an underlying medical illness or psychiatric disorder, a secondary functional disturbance from another psychiatric disorder, from a primary psychiatric disorder such as panic disorder or generalized anxiety disorder, or as a result of stress from such conditions as adjustment disorder or post-traumatic stress disorder. Clinicians usually attempt to first provide a "safe harbor" for the patient so that assessment processes and treatments can be adequately facilitated. The initiation of treatments for mood and anxiety disorders are important as patients suffering from anxiety disorders have a higher risk of premature death.

Disasters

Natural disasters and man-made hazards can cause severe psychological stress in victims surrounding the event. Emergency management often includes psychiatric emergency services designed to help victims cope with the situation. The impact of disasters can cause people to feel shocked, overwhelmed, immobilized, panic-stricken, or confused. Hours, days, months and even years after a disaster, individuals can experience tormenting memories, vivid nightmares, develop apathy, withdrawal, memory lapses, fatigue, loss of appetite, insomnia, depression, irritability, panic attacks, or dysphoria. Due to the typically disorganized and hazardous environment following a disaster, mental health professionals typically assess and treat patients as rapidly as possible. Unless a condition is threatening life of the patient, or others around the patient, other medical and basic survival considerations are managed first. Soon after a disaster clinicians may make themselves available to allow individuals to ventilate to relieve feelings of isolation, helplessness and vulnerability. Dependent upon the scale of the disaster, many victims may suffer from both chronic or acute post-traumatic stress disorder. Patients suffering severely from this disorder often are admitted to psychiatric hospitals to stabilize the individual.

Neuroleptic Malignant Syndrome

t is a hypermetabolic reaction to dopamine antagonists, primarily antipsychotic drugs, such as phenothiazines and butyrophenones. It usually occurs early in treatment and rarely during maintenance treatment. It develops in up to 3% of patients started on antipsychotics. Risk is increased in agitated male patients who have received large and rapidly increased doses. No genetic component is apparent. Its pathophysiologic basis is believed to be blockade of central dopamine receptors.

Characteristic signs are muscle rigidity, hyperpyrexia, tachycardia, hypertension, tachypnea, change in mental status and autonomic dysfunction. Laboratory abnormalities include respiratory and metabolic acidosis, myoglobinuria, elevated CK and leukocytosis. Mortality rates are between 10 to 20%.

Treatment includes cessation of antipsychotic drugs, supportive care, and aggressive treatment of myoglobinuria, fever, and acidosis. The dopamine agonist bromocriptine 2.5 to 20 mg tid or dantrolene up to 10 mg/kg IV q 4 h may be used as a muscle relaxant. Treatment is usually in an ICU. After recovery, reintroduction of the antipsychotic drug retriggers the syndrome in up to 1/3 of patients.

Serotonin Syndrome

It occurs when serotonergic agents are used in combination with MAOI inhibitors.

A sudden build up of serotonin systemically may lead to a life threatening condition manifesting in hyperthermia, diaphoresis, excitement or confusion, hyperreflexia, hypotension, tremor. The condition may progress to DIC, rhabdomyolysis and cardiovascular collapse. Urgent medical management is necessary. Drugs like dantrolene, a potent muscle relaxant and periactin, which is also a serotonin antagonist are useful.

Hospital Admission

The Emergency Care Process (Fig. 22.2)

The staff will need to determine if the patient needs to be admitted to a psychiatric inpatient facility or if they can be safety discharged to the community after a period of observation and/or brief treatment. Initial emergency psychiatric evaluations usually involve patients who are acutely agitated, paranoid, or who are suicidal. Initial evaluations to determine admission and interventions are designed to be as therapeutic as possible.

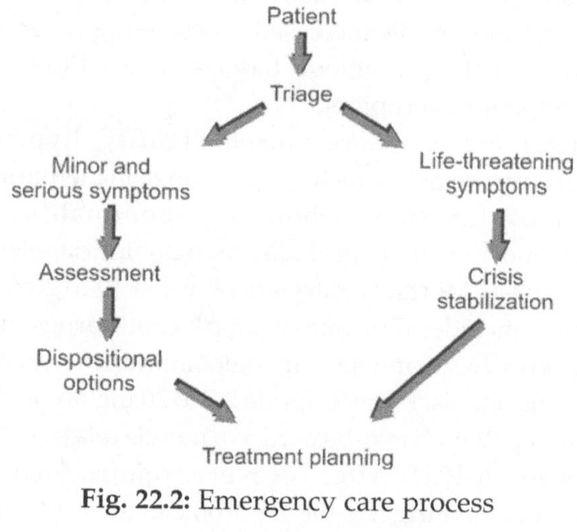

Fig. 22.2: Emergency care process

Delivery of Psychiatric Emergency Services

The place where emergency psychiatric services are delivered are commonly referred to as Psychiatric Emergency Services, Psychiatric Emergency Care Centres, or Comprehensive Psychiatric Emergency Programs. Mental health professionals from a wide area of disciplines, including medicine, nursing, psychology, and social work in these settings alongside psychiatrists and emergency physicians. The facilities, sometimes housed in a psychiatric hospital, psychiatric ward, or emergency room, provide immediate treatment to both voluntary and involuntary patients 24 hours a day. Within a protected environment, psychiatric emergency services exists to provide brief stay of two or three days to gain a diagnostic clarity, find appropriate alternatives to psychiatric hospitalization for the patient, and to treat those patients whose symptoms can be improved within that brief period of time. Even precise, psychiatric diagnoses are a secondary priority compared with interventions in a crisis setting. The functions of psychiatric emergency services are to assess patients' problems, implement a short-term treatment consisting of no more than ten meetings with the patient, procure a 24 hour holding area, mobilize teams to carry out interventions at patients' residences, utilize emergency management services to prevent further crises, be aware of inpatient and outpatient psychiatric resources, and provide 24/7 telephone counseling.

Treatment

Treatments in psychiatric emergency service settings are typically transitory in nature and only exist to provide dispositional solutions and/or to stabilize life-threatening conditions. Once stabilized, patients suffering chronic conditions may be transferred to a setting which can provide long-term psychiatric rehabilitation. Prescribed treatments within the emergency service setting vary dependent upon the patient's condition. Different forms of psychiatric medication, psychotherapy, or electroconvulsive therapy may be used in the emergency setting.

The introduction and efficacy of psychiatric medication as a treatment option in psychiatry has reduced the utilization of physical restraints in emergency settings, by reducing dangerous symptoms resulting from acute exacerbation of mental illness or substance intoxication.

Medications

With time as a critical aspect of emergency psychiatry, the rapidity of effect is an important consideration. Pharmacokinetics is the movement of drugs through the body with time and is at least partially reliant upon the route of administration, absorption, distribution and metabolism of the medication. A common route of administration is oral administration, however if this method is to work the drug must be able to get to the stomach and stay there. In cases of vomiting and nausea this method of administration is not an option. Suppositories can, in some situations, be administered instead. Medication can also be administered through intramuscular injection, or through intravenous injection (Fig. 22.3). The amount of time required for absorption varies dependent upon many factors including drug solubility, gastrointestinal motility and pH. If a medication is administered orally the amount of food in the stomach may also affect the rate of absorption. Once absorbed medications must be distributed throughout the body, or usually

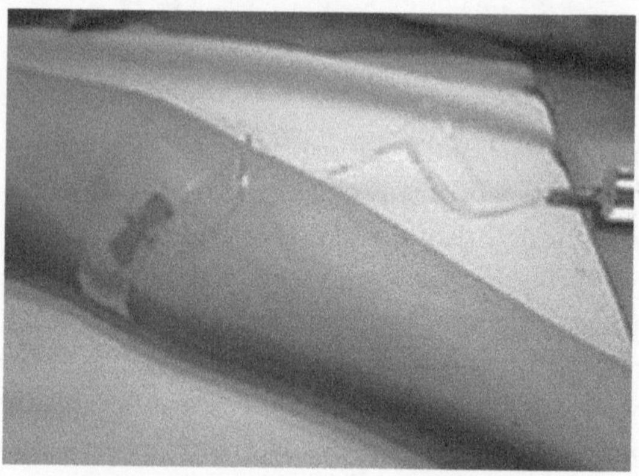

Fig. 22.3: A patient receiving an intravenous infusion

with the case of psychiatric medication, past the blood-brain barrier to the brain. With all of these factors affecting the rapidity of effect, the time until the effects are evident varies. Generally, though, the timing with medications is relatively fast and can occur within several minutes. As an example, physicians usually expect to see a remission of symptoms thirty minutes after haloperidol, an antipsychotic, is administered intramuscularly.

Psychotherapy

Other treatment methods may be used in psychiatric emergency service settings. Brief psychotherapy can be used to treat acute conditions or immediate problems as long as the patient understands his or her issues are psychological, the patient trusts the physician, the physician can encourage hope for change, the patient has motivation to change, the physician is aware of the psychopathological history of the patient, and the patient understands that their confidentiality will be respected. The process of brief therapy under emergency psychiatric conditions includes the establishment of a primary complaint from the patient, realizing psychosocial factors, formulating an accurate representation of the problem, coming up with ways to solve the problem, and setting specific goals. The information gathering aspect of brief psychotherapy is therapeutic because it helps the patient place his or her problem in the proper perspective. If the physician determines that deeper psychotherapy sessions are required, he or she can transition the patient out of the emergency setting and into an appropriate clinic or center.

ECT

Electroconvulsive therapy is a controversial form of treatment which is sometimes applied in psychiatric emergency service settings. Instances wherein a patient is depressed to such a severe degree that the patient cannot be stopped from hurting himself or herself or when a patient refuses to swallow, eat or drink medication, electroconvulsive therapy could be used as a therapeutic alternative. While preliminary research suggests that electroconvulsive therapy may be an effective treatment for depression, it usually requires a course of six to twelve sessions of convulsions lasting at least 20 seconds for those antidepressant effects to occur

CONCLUSION

The increasing incidence of alcohol and substance abuse in our country as well as the rise in levels of Unipolar depression, have led to an increased number of patients reporting to the emergency care unit. It is necessary for all clinicians to be familiar with common psychiatric emergencies especially suicide attempts and violent behavior and other psychiatric emergencies so as to improve the level of care offered to the patients.

BIBLIOGRAPHY

1. Crowe RR. Electroconvulsive therapy : a current perspective. N Engl J Med 1984; 311: 163-7.
2. Harris EC, Barraglough B. Suicide as an outcome for mental disorders, a meta-analysis. Br J Psychiatry 1997; 170: 205-28.
3. Jain V, Singh H, Gupta SC, Kumar S. A study of hopelessness, suicidal intent and depression in cases of attempted suicide. Ind J of Psychiatry 1999; 41: 2.
4. Murray CJ, Lopez AD. Alternative projections of mortality and disability by cause 1990-2020 : Global Burden of Disease Study. Lancet 1997; 349(9064) 1498-504.
5. Psychiatric Clinics of North America. Carol Bernstein, editor. WB Saunders Co 1999; 22(4): 789-803, 923-41.
6. Roy A. Suicide. In : Sadock BJ and Sadock VA, editors.Comprehensive Textbook of Psychiatry 7th ed. Lippincott Williams and Wilkins publishers. 2000; 2031-40.

23 Forensic Psychiatry

Forensic psychiatry deals with the legal aspects of psychiatry. Psychiatric nurse should be sufficiently aware of the legal aspects of psychiatry. This will help her to protect the patients right and avoid in giving poor advice or innocently involving herself in legal issues.

Legal aspect helps at many points in psychiatric care side through admission of a mentally ill person in a mental hospital, civil responsibility, criminal responsibility and standards of care.

The various legal aspects of psychiatry are briefly discussed below:

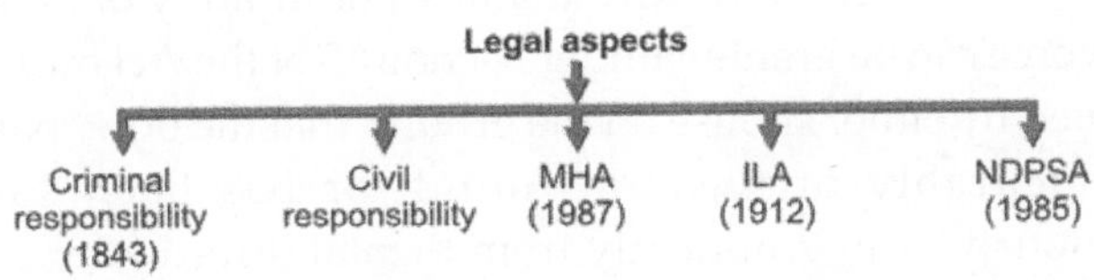

1. Criminal Responsibility

In January 1843, a young Scotsman, Daniel McNaughten shot dead Edward Drummond, the Secretary of British Prime Minister Sir Robert Peel. McNaughton wanted to kill British Prime Minister Robert Peel, under the influence of his delusions, but by mistake he shot his Secretary Edward Drummond on the back.

The Jury, after testification by 9 physicians, found McNaughten "not guilty by reasons of insanity". Queen Victoria, Sir Robert Peel and other prominent persons were outraged. Following this, 15 prominent judges were invited by the House of Lords.

They were asked to respond to a series of questions on criminal responsibility. The answers have now come to be known as McNaughton's Rule all over the world.

In India, Section 84, of Indian Penal Code (Act 45 of 1860) states that "nothing is an offense, which is done by a person, who at the time of doing it, by reason of unsoundness or mind, is incapable of knowing the nature of the act or that he is doing what is either wrong or contrary to low".

2. Civil Responsibility

1. Marriage

The Hindu Marriage Act (Act 25 of 1955) provides for conditions for a Hindu Marriage Act under section 5. One of the conditions, Section 5(ii) introduced by Act 68 of 1976, states that at the time of the marriage, neither party,

a) is incapable of giving a valid consent ... unsoundness of mind; or
b) though capable of giving consent, has been suffering from mental disorder of such a kind or to such an extent as to be unfit for marriage and the procreation of children; or
c) has been subject to recurrent attacks or insanity or epilepsy.

Divorce can be granted under Section 13 of the Act on a petition presented by either spouse on the ground that the other party "has been incurably of unsound mind, or has been suffering continuously or intermittently from mental disorder".

2. Adoption

A Hindu male "who is of sound mind" is not a minor, can adopt a child, with the consent of his wife unless" ... she has been declared by a court to be of unsound mind" (Act 78, 1965 Sec. 7).

A Hindu female "who is of sound mind" is not a minor, can adopt a child, with the consent of his wife unless" ... she has been declared by a court to be of unsound mind" (Act 78, 1965 Sec. 7).

3. Witness

Under the Indian Evidence Act, a lunatic is not incompetent to testify in the court as a witness unless he is prevented from understanding the questions put to him and giving rational answers to them.

4. Vote

Under Act 326 of Constitution of India, no person declared to be of unsound mind can vote.

5. Testamentary Capacity

A will is invalid under the following conditions (e.g.):

(i) Imbecility arising from advanced age or by excessive drinking.
(ii) Insane delusions making the testator incapable of rational views and judgement.

6. Transfer of Property

Under transfer of Property Act 1882, only persons competent to contract, are authorized to transfer property.

7. Contract

Under the Indian Contract Act 1872, every person to be competent to contract must be a major and of sound mind.

3. Indian Lunacy Act, 1912

Indian Lunacy Act based on British Acts. Indian Lunacy Act, Act 4 of 1912 was based largely on the earlier English Lunacy Act of 1890.

The Indian Lunacy Act had 8 chapters.

Chapter I: Defined a lunatic as "an idiot or person of unsound mind".

Chapter II: Reception of the lunatics

1. Voluntary Admission
2. Reception order

3. Patient admitted on petition
4. Transfer
5. Escape
6. Criminal lunatics
7. Reception after inquisition.

Chapter III: Care, Treatment and Discharge

Chapter IV: Proceeding in Lunacy in Presidency town

Chapter V: Proceeding in Lunacy outside presidency town

Chapter VI: Establishment of Asylums

Chapter VII: Expenses of Lunatics

Chapter VIII: Rules

4. The Mental Health Act, 1987

The Mental Health Bill became the Act 14 of 1987 on 22nd May 1987. The Act is divided into 10 chapters consisting of 98 sections.

Objectives:

It is considered necessary to

1. Regulate admission to psychiatric hospital or nursing home of mentally ill persons.
2. Protect society from the presence of mentally ill persons.
3. Protect human rights of such person.
4. Protect citizen from being detained in psychiatric hospitals without sufficient cause.
5. Regulate maintenance charges of mentally ill patient.
6. Provide facilities for establishing guardianship or custody of managing their own affairs.
7. Provide for establishment of central authority or state authority for mental health services.
8. Regulate the powers of government for establishing, licensing and controlling psychiatric hospitals for mentally ill persons.
9. Provide legal aid to mentally ill person.

Chapters

Chapter I: Deals with preliminary definitions.

The Act uses the term "mentally ill person" instead of "lunatic" and defines it as "a person who in need of treatment by reason of any mental disorder other than mental retardation".

The term "mentally ill prisoner" is used instead of "criminal lunatic". Psychiatric hospital and psychiatric nursing home instead of mental hospital.

Chapter II: Provides for establishment of mental health authorities at centre and state levels. These authorities will regulate and co-ordinate mental health services.

Chapter III: Deals with guidelines for establishment and maintenance of psychiatric hospitals and nursing home. There is a provision for a licensing authority and valid license which has to be renewed every 5 yr.

Chapter IV: Deals with the procedures of admission and detention in psychiatric hospitals or nursing homes.

Admission methods are:

1. **Voluntary admission:** Any person who considers himself to be mentally ill and wishes to be admitted to a psychiatric hospital may make a request to the medical officer and can be admitted as a voluntary patient. In case of minors the guardian may make such a request for that minor.

   The medical officer shall make enquiry within 24 hours and should admit the voluntary patient.

   Voluntary patient/minor patients with Guardian

   ↓

   Make request for admission

   Within 24 hours admission should made.

   (For Discharge, can do any time but within 30 days, if morethan 30 days , the medical officer shall call a board consisting of 2 medical officers within 72 hours of the 30 days and if the board is of the opinion that the individual needs further treatment the medical officer should keep him in the hospital for periods not exceeding 90 days at a time.)

2. **Admission under special circumstances:** Admission is made, if a relative or a friend of the mentally ill person, can make a request for admission and on examination, it found that it is in the best interest of the mentally ill for whom the request is being made, the Medical Officer may admit the patient. Such admissions have to be reviewed with 90 days and shall be kept in hospital only if found necessary on review.
3. **Reception order on application:** Application for reception order made by the Medical Officer incharge of the treatment of the magistrate within the local limits. If patient's danger for himself or to others, his parents or relative may make such application to the magistrate of the area in which the patient normally resides for such an order.
4. **Reception order without application on production of mentally ill person before magnitude:** A Police Officer may detain for protection of any person wandering, who in his opinion may be mentally ill and is liable to harm himself or others. If the parents/relative is available, inform the relative, but produce to the magistrate within 24 hours of taking the wanderer into protections. According to relative agrees the magistrate giving order to mental hospital for treatment.
5. **Admission as inpatient after inquisition:** If after the inquisition it is found that the individuals is to be detained in the mental hospital and it is in the best interest to the patient, the district court may do so, but the court should review his care from time to time.
6. **Admission as a mentally ill prisoner:**
   i. Detention of alleged mentally ill, pending report of the Medical Officer.
      The Magistrate may give order to keep the mentally ill on observation. It is not more than 10 days.
   ii. Detention of mentally ill, pending the removal to psychiatric facility.
      The Magistrate given in writing can direct to retain the individual for not more than 30 days. Pending the removal of the person to the psychiatric facility.

Chapter V: Deals with the inspection, discharge, leave of absence and removal of mentally ill persons.

Inspection: Three visitors appointed by the State Government or Central Government shall visit the institution at least once in every month for joint inspection.

Discharge: The Medical Officer incharge of hospital/ward on recommendation of 2 Medical Practitioner (one should be psychiatrist), may discharge a patient other than the voluntary patient. This discharge cannot be ordered by Medical Officer in case of prisoners.

An reception order may be discharged, following an application by the relative two originally applied for reception order. However, Medical Officer should certify that the person is not harmful for himself or others. Otherwise, his relative should be made responsible to see that the mentally ill does not harm himself or others.

If admitted the individual was alleged to be mentally ill and was admitted on a reception order finds himself to be of sound mind and has recovered from his illness, he make an application to the Magistrate for discharge but the application should be accompanied by a medical certificate. So, Magistrate feels satisfactory, provide the discharge order.

If individual had been detained under a reception order, was later found to be sound mind and capable of taking care or himself, the Medical Officer should give a discharge order with the findings duly certified by the District Court.

Leave of Absence: The applicant, under request the reception order was provided for admission of a mentally ill person, make an application for "Leave of Absence" to the Medical Officer. The Medical Officer may give permission for "Leave of absence". In case where the Medical Officer refuses to provide permission for "Leave of absence" an appeal can be made to the Magistrate who may after proper enquiry grant the "Leave of absence" on bond.

Chapter VI: Judicial inquisition regarding alleged mentally ill person possessing property, custody of his person and management of his property.

If the individual suffering mental illness the court feels that the alleged mentally ill person is incapable of looking after both himself and his property, an order can be issued for the appointment of a Guardian. For incapable of looking on property means manager can be appointed.

Chapter VII: Liability to meet the cost of maintenance of mentally ill persons detained in psychiatric hospitals or nursing homes.

Chapter VIII: Protection of human rights of mentally ill persons. It covered that

(i) No mentally ill person shall be subjected during treatment, to any indignity or cruelty.

(ii) No mentally ill person, under treatment shall be used for the purposes of research,

   a. such research is of direct benefit to him.
   b. A consent has been obtained in writing from the person (if a voluntary patient) or from the guardian/relative (if admitted in voluntarily).

(iii) No letters or communication sent by or to a mentally ill person shall be intercepted, detained or destroyed.

Chapter IX: Penalties and procedures.

Chapter X: Miscellaneous section.

5. **The Narcotic Drugs and Psychotropic Substances Act (NDPSA) 1985:** In India the Opium Act of 1857 was revised first in 1878 and then in 1950. On 16th September 1985, Act 61 of 1985 was enforced as NDPSA.

The act includes:

1. Narcotic Drugs (cannabis, cocaine, coca leaf, opium, poppy straw and all manufactured drugs).
2. Psychotropic substances (76 drugs and their derivatives).

Act: If any person produces, possesses, transports, imports, exports drugs or psychotropic substance except "ganja" he shall be punishable with:

1. Rigorous imprisonment for not less than ten years which may extend to 20 yr and

2. A fine of not less than one lakh rupees which may extend to 2 lakh rupees.
3. Punishment for repeat offence is rigorous imprisonment for not less than 15 yr which may extend to 30 yr. And a find of not less than 1.5 lakh rupees which may extend to 3 lakh rupees.

However, if a person is carrying small quantities e.g., 250 gm of heroin, 5 gm of charas, 5 gm of opium, 125 gm of cocaine then the punishment is simple imprisonment which may extend to one year or a fine or both. For less than 500 gm of ganja imprisonment is 5 yr.

If a person is found to be trafficking more than or equal to 1 kg of pure heroin punishment is death penalty.

Role of Nurse in Legal Psychiatry

1. Adequate knowledge regarding Indian Mental Health Act, Criminal and Civil responsibility and NDPSA.
2. She/he should aware about admission and discharge procedures.
3. Helps to qualified to work in psychiatric condition.
4. Should obtain informed consent for treatment and procedures such as:
   a. Explanation about the procedure to the patient.
   b. Advantages of therapy
   c. Clarify the doubts to relatives of patients
   d. Written consent
5. Maintain the standards of nursing care.
6. Maintenance of confidentiality of records.

24 Crisis and Grief

A crisis is defined by the mental health authorities as "A state of disequilibrium resulting from the interaction of an event with the individual's or family's coping mechanisms, which are inadequate to meet the demands of the situation, combined with the individual's or family's perception of the meaning of the event".

— **Taylor, 1982**

Crisis is an initial disturbance that results from a stressful event or a perceived threat to self.

A crisis may influence people's life in different ways. A crisis is an internal disturbance that an result from a stressful event or a perceived threat to self precipitators events of crisis include perceived losses, threats of losses or challenges.

In the Chinese language, two symbols communicate crisis: "danger" and "opportunity".

Characteristics of Crisis

- Crisis is a sudden event in one's life that disturbs homeostasis, during which usual coping mechanisms cannot resolve the problems.
- Crisis are precipitated by specific identifiable events.
- Crisis are personal by nature.
- Crisis are acute, not chronic and will be solved on one way or another within a brief period.
- Crisis is self-limiting acute and last one to six weeks.
- A crisis situation is dangerous to the person, he or she may harm self or others.

Types of Crisis

Crisis can be categorized as following:

1. **Maturational Crisis:**
   It is otherwise called as developmental crisis. Human beings go through different stages of development. The transition between these stages can be an emotionally disturbing period, e.g. Child's first real separation from home to attend school, a girl who attains puberty, attending college, staying away from home for the first time, getting married, etc.
2. **Situational Crisis:**
   Crisis are unanticipated or sudden events that threaten the individual's integrity such as the death of a loved one, loss of a job, and physical or emotional illness in the individual of family members.
3. **Adventitious Crisis:**
   Accidental uncommon or unexpected crisis, e.g. both the parents die and the child is left alone.

Signs and Symptoms of Crisis

The major feeding in a crisis is anxiety. The individual experiences a heavy burden of free-floating anxiety. The anxiety may be manifested through depression, anger and guilt feelings. Normally crisis will take about 4 to 6 weeks to resolve a crisis. The individual could be irrational. He may get angry and blame others for what happened to him. He may even neglect his responsibilities.

Stages of Crisis

Caplan (1964) outlined four specific phases through which individuals progress in response to a precipitating stressor.

Phase I: Threat to the individual resulting in anxiety: Anxiety increases when individual is exposed to a precipitating stressors.

Phase II: Increased tension and anxiety: When coping mechanisms failed in the Phase I, anxiety continuously increase and individual coping ability decrease. So, the individual begins to feel a great deal of discomfort at this point.

Phase III: Reorganization: When the individual experiences real anxiety and feels that he cannot go on any longer, its due to the flood of anxiety. The affected individual tries to reorganize his life inspite of the loss. He may make an attempt to escape the reality.

Phase IV: Resolution phase: At this phase the individual learns to adapt to new situation. The victims life is organized according to the loss in consideration and the new circumstances.

According to **Mary Verghese (1994)**, phase of crisis explained following ways:

1. Phase of denial
2. Phase of increased tension
3. Phase of disorganization
4. Attempt to reorganize
5. Phase of attempt to escape the problem
6. Phase of local reorganization
7. Phase of general reorganization

Resolution of Crisis

There are three ways:

1. **Pseudoresolution:** The individual uses repression and pushes out of consciousness the incident and the intense emotions associated it. But in future, if and when a crisis occurs, the repressed feeling may come to surface and influence the feelings aroused by the new crisis.
2. **Successful resolution:** The individual may go through the various stages of crisis but reaches the phase of general reorganization.
3. **Unsuccessful resolution:** The individual uses pathological adaptation at any phases of crisis resulting in a lower level of functioning.

Crisis Intervention

Crisis intervention is a technique used to help an individual or family to understand and cope with the intense feelings that are typical of a crisis.

Aims of Crisis Intervention

1. To provide a correct cognitive perception of the situation.
2. To assist the individual in managing the feelings.

Procedure for the crisis intervention:

I. **To provide a correct cognitive perceptions:**

1. **Assessment of the situation**
   - Purpose of identification of the problem.
   - To identify the support system available.
   - To identify the strength and limitation.
2. **Define the event/situation:**
   - To identify the event.
   - To bring the precipitating event to the awareness of the victim.
3. **Plan of action:**
   - Victim and people should have active involvement in developing the plan of action.
   - Guidance of the victim.
   - Instruction and supportive care to provide for victim by the therapist.

II. **To assist the individual in managing the feeling:**

1. Help the individual to be aware of the feelings.
2. Help the individual to attain mastery over the feelings.

Crisis Intervention: "Models"

1. **Crisis Roster Model**

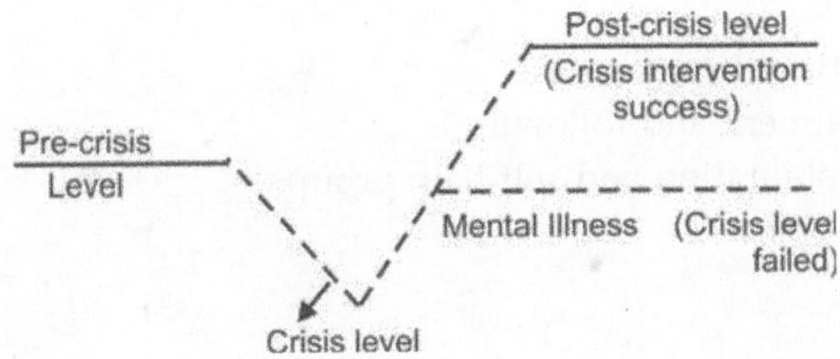

Pre-crisis level shows normal level of equilibrium between body and functions – crisis levels shows it is disturbed. If crisis intervention is adequate and successful the person come Normal activity and functioning. If it is failed, the person will develop mental illness.

Model (2): Stuart Model

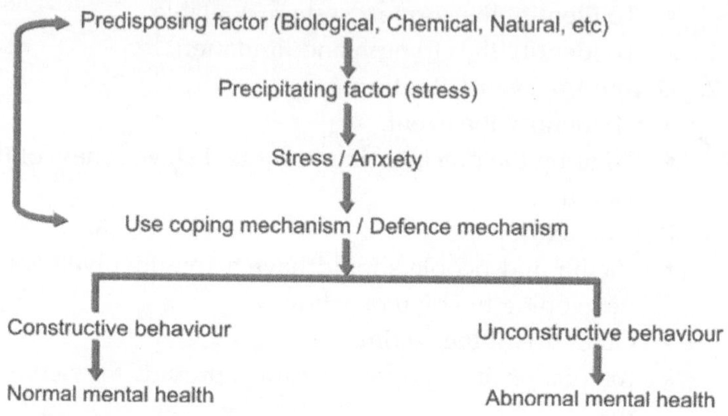

Crisis Intervention Methods

1. **Based on Caplan – three levels of crisis intervention.**
   i. **Primary Level:**
   Assess the crisis, define the crisis, assess the problem, and promote and support coping mechanism.
   ii. **Secondary Level:**
   Hot lines services link, walk-in-clinic, and counseling can use.
   iii. **Tertiary Level:**
   Treatment and following
   Rehabilitation and self-help groups

Model (3):

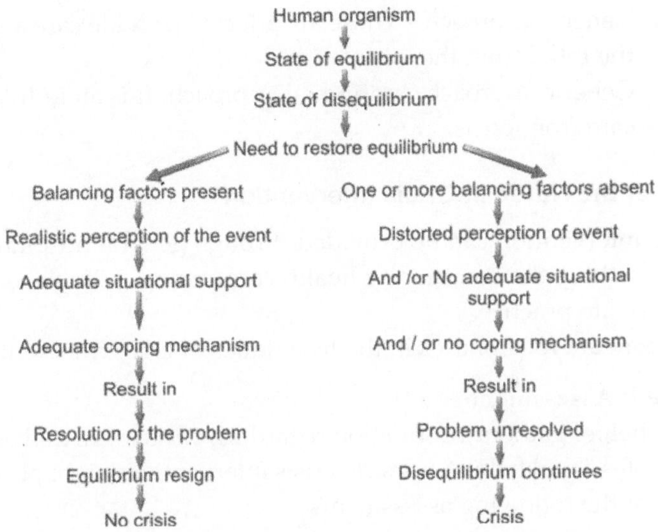

2. **Based on Stuart Model**

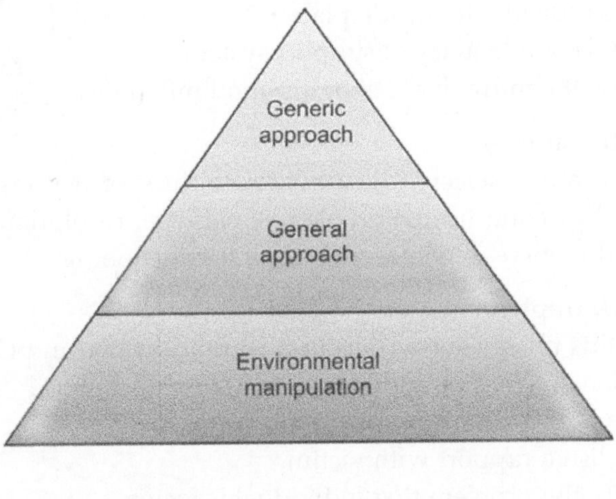

1. Environmental manipulation – Change the environment from the crisis situation.
2. General approach – Those are affected provide care and set the relief from the crisis.
3. Generic approach/Individual approach: It is an individual care from crisis.

Role of the Nurse in Crisis Intervention

Crisis intervention can be provided through general hospital, the home setting, the community health care setting, schools, offices and private practice.

There are four phases in the techniques of crisis intervention.

Phase I: Assessment

Here, helper gathers information regarding crisis event and assess the professional help. A nurse in crisis intervention might perform some of the following assessments:

4. To describe the even
5. Determine when it occurred.
6. Assess physical and mental status of the victim.
7. Assess coping mechanism skills.
8. Assess suicide/homicide plan.
9. Assess the adequacy of support system.
10. Assess the individual strengths and limitations.

Phase II: Planning

Here, the nurse selects the appropriate nursing actions for the identified nursing needs/problem. Goals are, resolution for the crisis and to increase in precrisis level of functioning.

Phase III: Implementation

During this phase, the actions that were identified in phase two are implemented. The implementation are,

- Use a reality oriented approach.
- Establish a rapport with victim.
- Clarify the problem that individual is facing.
- Guide the individual through a problem solving process.
- Identify external support system and new social networks.

Phase IV: Evaluation

To evaluate the outcome of crisis intervention, a reassessment is made to determine if the stated objective was achieved.

GRIEF

Introduction

A nurse works with many people who experience different types of loss. Coping mechanisms determine the person's ability to face and accept loss. Grief is a natural response to loss. The nurse assists patients/clients in understanding and accepting loss so that life can continue.

Grief

Grief is a form of sorrow that follows the perception or anticipation of a loss of one or more of valued or significant objects. These responses often include helplessness, loneliness, hopelessness, sadness, guilt and anger.

Grief involves thoughts, feelings and behaviours. Its purpose is to enable adjustment to a new way of life, which takes time.

The grieving person will try a variety of strategies in order to cope.

Worden (1991) describes the following tasks of grief that facilitate healthy adjustment to loss.

- Accepting the reality of the loss
- Experiencing the pain of grief
- Adjusting to an environment
- Re-investing emotional energy

Theories of the Grieving Process

Grief is a normal response to any loss. Behaviors and feelings associated with the grieving process occur in individuals suffering from losses such as a physical deformity or the death of a close friend.

There is a no right way to grieve. The concept and theories of grief are only tools that can be used to anticipate the emotional needs of individuals and families.

Theories

(1) Engel's Theory

Engel (1964) proposed that the grieving process has 3 phases that can be applied to grieving and dying people.

Phases:

1. Shock and disbelief
2. Developing awareness
3. Reorganization and restitution

1. **Shock and disbelief:**
   During the first phase, the individuals denies the reality of the loss and may withdraw, sit motionless or wander aimlessly. Physical reactions may include fainting, nausea, diarrhea, rapid heart rate, restlessness, insomnia and fatigue.
2. **Developing awareness:**
   In the second phase the individual begins to feel the loss acutely and may experience desperation. Suddenly anger, guilt, frustration, depression and emptiness occur.
3. **Reorganization and restitution:**
   During the third phase, inevitability of the loss is acknowledged. The loss is clear to the individual, who begins to reorganize life. New self awareness is also developed.

(2) Kubler-Ross Stages of Dying

The framework provided by Kubler-Ross (1969) is behavior oriented and includes 5 stages.

1. Denial 2. Anger 3. Bargaining 4. Depression and 5. Acceptance

1. **Denial:** The individual acts as though nothing has happened and may refuse to believe that a loss has occurred.
2. **Anger:** The individual resists the loss and may feel frustrated and angry or may experience a sense of helplessness and loss of control.
3. **Bargaining:** Postponement of the reality of the loss. The individual may attempt to make a deal in a subtle or overt way

to prevent the loss. The person frequently seeks the opinions of others during this stage.

4. **Depression:** Occurs when the loss is realized and the full impact of its significance is apparent. This stage may be accompanied by overwhelming loneliness and withdrawal.
5. **Acceptance:** Physiological reactions cease, and social interactions resume

(3) Martocchio's Phases (1985)

Martocchio (1985) describes 5 phases of grief that have overlapping boundaries and no expected order. Intense reactions of grief usually subside within 6 to 12 months and active mourning may continue for 3 to 5 yr. Phases are 1. Shock and disbelief, 2. Yearning and protest, 3. Anguish, disorganization and despair, 4. Identification in bereavement, and 5. Reorganization and restitution.

Complicated Grief

Some individuals find it more difficult to give than do others. A normal, healthy movement through their bereavement does not occur.

So indicators of unresolved or complicated grief includes:

- Over activity without a sense of loss.
- Alteration in relationships with friends and family.
- Hostilities against specific people.
- Agitated depression with tension, agitation, insomnia, feelings or worthlessness, extreme guilt and even suicidal tendencies.
- Inability to discuss the loss without crying.
- False euphoria.

Often, individuals with prolonged grief require long-term support, referral to psychiatric help or counselling.

Nursing Care and Grief

Goals for a person dealing with loss are to resolve grief, accept the reality of the loss, regain a sense to self-esteem, renew normal activities and relationships. Physiological needs must also be met.

During planning, the nurse has several resources, including family members, significant others, other team members and community support groups.

1. Promoting comfort:
   Personal hygiene – basic needs – pain control – sleep, appetite, mobility and psychological function.
2. Maintaining Independence
3. Preventing loneliness and isolation
4. Promoting spiritual comfort
5. Supporting the grieving family – supportive relationship with family

Grief Resolution

Although grief resolution of grief may require months or years, most individuals are under a nurse's care for only a short period of time. The nurse may become frustrates when, just as the person or family begins to express grief, the person leaves the health care unit or dies. Grieving is an individual process and resolution of loss does not follow a set schedule.

25 Suicide Prevention

SUICIDE

Commonest cause of death among psychiatric patients. Suicide is a type of Deliberate Self Harm (DSH) and is defined as a human act of self-intentioned and self-inflicted cessation.

An attempted suicide is an unsuccessful suicidal act with a non-fetal outcome.

Suicide Prevention (SUPRE)

Suicide (Latin *suicidium,* from *sui caedere,* to kill oneself) is the intentional taking of one's own life. Many dictionaries also note the metaphorical sense of "willful destruction of one's self-interest" (e.g., "political suicide"). Most common cause of death among psychiatric patients. Suicide is a type of Deliberate Self Harm (DSH) and is defined as a human act of self-intentioned and self-inflicted cessation. An attempted suicide is an unsuccessful suicidal act with a non-fetal outcome.

Views on suicide have been influenced by cultural views on existential themes such as religion, honor, and the meaning of life. The Abrahamic religions consider suicide an offense towards God due to religious belief in the sanctity of life. In the West it was often regarded as a serious crime. Japanese views on honor and religion led *to seppuku,* one of the most painful methods of suicide, to be respected as a means to atone for mistakes or failure, or as a form of protest during the Samurai era. In the 20th century, suicide in the form of self-immolation has been used as a form of protest, and in the form of kamikaze and suicide bombing as a military or terrorist tactic. *Sati* is a Hindu funeral practice in which the widow would immolate herself on her husband's funeral pyre, either willingly, or under pressure from the family and in-laws.

Medically assisted suicide (euthanasia, or the right to die) is currently a controversial ethical issue involving people who are terminally ill, in extreme pain, and/or have minimal quality of life through injury or illness. Self-sacrifice for others is not usually considered suicide, as the goal is not to kill one self but to save another.

Epidemiology of Suicide

Worldwide suicide rates have increased by 60% in the past 50 years, mainly in the developing countries. Most suicides in the world occur in Asia, which is estimated to account for up to 60% of all suicides. According to the World Health Organization, China, India and Japan may account for 40% of all world suicides.

The official suicide rate in India is 9.9/Lakh/Year. Highest suicide rate is in the age group of 18 – 30 yr. The ratio of attempted suicide to completed suicide is 10:1. The highest rates of suicide in India – Pondicherry, West Bengal, Kerala, Chennai and Bengalunu.

Gender and Suicide

In the Western world, males die much more often by means of suicide than do females, although females attempt suicide more often. This pattern has held for at least a century. Some medical professionals believe this stems from the fact that males are more likely to end their lives through effective violent means (guns, knives, hanging, etc.), while women primarily use more failure-prone methods such as overdosing on medications.

Age and Suicide

In the USA, males over the age of seventy die by suicide more often than younger males. There is no such trend for females. It is vary from developing countries like India. Adolescence and adulthood more common in suicide.

Season and Suicide

People die by suicide more often during spring and summer. The idea that suicide is more common during Christmas is a common misconception. There is also potential risk of suicide in some people experiencing *seasonal affective disorder*. Some studies have found that elderly people are more likely to commit suicide around their birthdays.

The Problem

In the year 2008, approximately one million people died from suicide: a "global" mortality rate of 16 per 100,000, or one death every 40 seconds. The World Health Organization noted that over one million people commit suicide every year, and that it is one of the leading causes of death among teenagers and adults under 35. There are an estimated 10 to 20 million non-fatal attempted suicides every year worldwide.

In the last 45 years suicide rates have increased by 60% worldwide. Suicide is now among the three leading causes of death among those aged 15-44 years (both sexes); these figures do not include suicide attempts up to 20 times more frequent than completed suicide. Suicide worldwide is estimated to represent 1.8% of the total global burden of disease in 1998, and 2.4% in countries with market and former socialist economies in 2020 (Fig. 25.1).

Suicide rate in India was 11.2 per 100,000 in 2002. The rates vary across the country with states such as Kerala having the highest suicide rate of 30.8 per lakh in 2002. Suicide rates in Army, Air Force and Naval personnel were 0.04, 0.11 and 0.12 per thousand respectively. Rates are higher in urban than in rural settings. Studies of completed suicides show that 90-94% of the patients are mentally ill while committing the act. Depression accounts for nearly half the number of patients committing suicide followed by alcohol abuse (34%) and schizophrenia (13%) .

Although traditionally suicide rates have been highest among the male elderly, rates among young people have been increasing to such an extent that they are now the group at highest risk in a third of countries, in both developed and developing countries.

Mental disorders (particularly depression and substance abuse) are associated with more than 90% of all cases of suicide; however, suicide results from many complex sociocultural factors and is more likely to occur particularly during periods of socioeconomic, family and individual crisis situations (e.g. loss of a loved one, employment, honour).

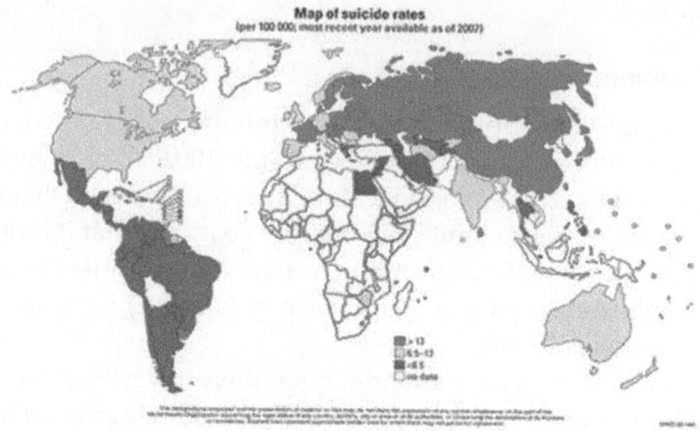

Fig. 25.1: Map of suicide rate

Causes

Suicide may occur for a number of reasons, including depression, shame, guilt, desperation, physical pain, emotional pressure, anxiety, financial difficulties, or other undesirable situations.

Neurotransmitter Theory

Diminished central serotonin plays a role in suicidal behavior Low concentrations of the serotonin metabolite 5-hydroxy-indoleacetic acid (5-HIAA) in the lumbar cerebrospinal fluid (CSF) were associated with suicidal behavior. This finding has been replicated many times and in different diagnostic groups. Postmortem neurochemical studies have reported modest decreases in serotonin itself, or 5-HIAA, in either the brainstem or frontal cortex of suicide victims.

Postmortem receptor studies have reported significant changes in presynaptic and postsynaptic serotonin binding sites in suicide victims. Taken together, these CSF, neurochemical, and receptor studies support the hypothesis that reduced central serotonin is associated with suicide.

Low Cholesterol

Excessively low cholesterol increases risk of suicide, perhaps by affecting serotonin levels, Genetic Factors Suicidal behavior, like other psychiatric disorders, tends to run in families.

In psychiatric patients a family history of suicide increases the risk both of attempted suicide and of completed suicide in most diagnostic groups.

Tryptophan hydroxylase (TPH) is an enzyme involved in the biosynthesis of serotonin. A polymorphism in the human TPH gene has been identified.

As low concentrations of 5-HIAA in CSF are associated with suicidal behavior, it was hypothesized that such individuals may have alterations in genes controlling serotonin synthesis and metabolism

Physical Disorder

Postmortem studies show that a physical illness is present in 25 to 75 percent of all suicide victims; a physical illness is estimated to be an important contributing factor in 11 to 51 percent of suicides. In each instance, the percentage increases with age.

Fifty percent of men with cancer who commit suicide do so within a year of receiving the diagnosis.

Cancer of the breast or genitals is found in 70 percent of women with cancer who commit suicide.

There are seven diseases of the central nervous system that increase the risk of suicide: epilepsy, multiple sclerosis, head injury, cardiovascular disease, Huntington's disease, dementia, and acquired immune deficiency syndrome (AIDS).

Four endocrine conditions are associated with increased suicide risk: Cushing's disease, anorexia nervosa, Klinefelter's syndrome, and porphyria. Mood disorders also attend these disorders.

The two gastrointestinal disorders with an increased suicide risk are peptic ulcer and cirrhosis, both physical disorders found among alcoholic persons.

The two urogenital problems with an increased suicide risk are prostatic hypertrophy and hemodialysis, both problems in which changes in mood occur.

Increased incidence of major depressive disorder in patients with cerebral disease, the association of suicide with cerebrovascular disorders and progressive organic deterioration leading to dementia.

Psychological Factors

Psychodynamic Theory

Freud

The first important psychological insight into suicide came from Sigmund Freud. Suicide is the extreme expression of anger at the love object who has abandoned the person.Mourning and Melancholia, Freud stated that suicide represented aggression turned inward against an introjected, ambivalently cathected love object.

Cognitive Theories

Aaron Beck stated that Hopelessness and dichotomous thinking increases risk for suicide

Sociocultural Factors

Durkheim's Theory

Durkheim's original theory is based on 26,000 suicides. Three patterns of suicide are described:

1. Egoistic
2. Anomic
3. Altruistic

1. Egoistic suicide is determined by a lack of meaningful family ties or social interactions.

2. Anomic suicide is committed by those who experience severe disorientation from society. Anomic suicide occurs when the relationship between an individual and society is broken by social or economic adversity.
3. Altruistic suicide results from excessive integration in society.

Marital Status

Married persons have the lowest suicide rates. The suicide rate for single persons is twice that of married persons and that of the divorced, separated, or widowed, four to five times higher.

Employment

The unemployed have higher suicide rates, probably owing to an interaction of socioeconomic circumstances, psychological vulnerability, and stressful life events.

During economic recessions and depressions and times of high unemployment, the suicide rate increases; during times of high employment and during war, the rate decreases.

Psychiatric Disorders

Depressive Disorders

- Depressive disorders (mood disorder) is the psychiatric diagnosis most commonly associated with suicide
- Male sex is a risk factor for suicide among depressed subjects.

Schizophrenia

- The suicide risk is high among schizophrenia patients: up to 10 percent die by committing suicide.
- Most persons with schizophrenia who commit suicide do so during the first few years of their illness, i.e. relatively young and about 75 percent are unmarried males.

Alcohol Use Disorders

- Alcoholic persons have an increased risk of suicide, with a lifetime suicide risk of 2.2 to 3.4 percent.

- More men than women are found among alcoholic suicide victims.
- Alcoholic persons usually commit suicide after years of alcohol abuse
- Comorbidity plays an important role

Other Substance Use Disorders Drug Dependence

- Suicide rate of heroin addicts is about 20 times greater than that of the general population.
- The availability of lethal amount of drugs, intravenous use, associated antisocial personality disorder, chaotic lifestyle, and impulsivity are some of the factors that predisposes drug-dependent persons to suicidal behavior, particularly when they are dysphoric, depressed, or intoxicated.

Personality Disorder

- Patients with borderline and antisocial personality disorders have an increased risk of suicide.

Panic Disorder

- 20 percent of individuals with panic disorder had made a suicide attempt at some time.
- Clinical assessment of suicide risk in panic and phobia patients should include determination of the presence or absence of major depressive disorder, substance abuse, and personality disorder.

Comorbidity

- Comorbidity is common among suicide victims; .
  1. Psychiatric disorders : Depression, alcoholism and drug dependence, schizophrenia
  2. Physical disorder : Cancer, AIDS and painful physical illness.
  3. Psychosocial factors : Failure in exam, failure in love, illegitimate pregnancy, loss of a loved one, occupation, etc.

Methods Used

Ingestion of poisons – 35%, hanging 23%, drowning 9%, jumping in front of train – 4% and burning 12%.

MLC

Sec. 309 of IPC, states that "whoever attempts to commit suicide and does any act towards the commission of such offense, shall be punishable with simple imprisonment for a term which may extend to one year and shall also be liable to fine".

Preventable

The management lies in preventing the act. This can be done at suicide prevention centres. Crisis intervention centers, psychiatric emergency services, medical emergency services, social welfare centers, even at home.

Important steps for preventing suicide are:

1. Take all suicidal threats; gestures or attempts seriously and notify a psychiatrist.
2. Inspect physical surrounding and remove all means of committing suicide, like sharp objects, ropes, drugs, etc.
3. Acute psychiatric emergency interview.
4. Counseling and guidance.
5. Treatment of psychiatric disorder with medication of ECT.
6. Follow up care – is very important to prevent future suicidal attempts or suicide.

Effective Interventions

Strategies involving restriction of access to common methods of suicide have proved to be effective in reducing suicide rates; however, there is a need to adopt multisectoral approaches involving other levels of intervention and activities, such as crisis centres.

There is compelling evidence indicating that adequate prevention and treatment of depression, alcohol and substance abuse can reduce suicide rates.

School-based interventions involving crisis management, self-esteem enhancement and the development of coping skills and healthy decision making have been demonstrated to reduce the risk of suicide among the youth.

Challenges and Obstacles

Worldwide, the prevention of suicide has not been adequately addressed due to basically a lack of awareness of suicide as a major problem and the taboo in many societies to discuss openly about it. In fact, only a few countries have included prevention of suicide among their priorities. Reliability of suicide certification and reporting is an issue in great need of improvement.

It is clear that suicide prevention requires intervention also from outside the health sector and calls for an innovative, comprehensive multi-sectoral approach, including both health and non-health sectors, e.g. education, labour, police, justice, religion, law, politics, the media.

World Suicide Prevention Day (10 September, 2007)

The focus of World Suicide Prevention Day this year is on suicide prevention from youth to old age. This theme has been adopted to emphasize that people of all ages commit suicide and that actions to prevent suicide included in national responses should meet the needs of different age groups.

World Suicide Prevention Day is an opportunity for people worldwide to unite in commitment and action to ensure that suicides are prevented, that people living with mental illness receive adequate treatment, that community-based care and close follow-up are available to people who attempt suicide, that access to common methods of suicides is restricted, and that media reports of suicides are more measured.

World Suicide Prevention Day (10 September, 2008)

Around one million people die each year by suicide. The focus of World Suicide Prevention Day this year is on suicide prevention by all, at all levels - personal, public and political. The 2008 theme, "Think Globally, Plan Nationally, and Act Locally" encourages people worldwide to unite in commitment and action to promote understanding about suicide and ensure that they are prevented. The impact of suicide can be devastating for all concerned.

On a personal level, friends and families require social support, on a national level governments need to recognize the causes of suicide and protect the most vulnerable groups in their communities. On a global scale, research and health organizations can identify global trends and encourage the sharing of information in effective prevention activities. About one million people commit suicide each year.

Every 40 seconds, the loss of a person who killed themselves shatters the lives of family and friends. For every person who completes a suicide, 20 or more may attempt suicide. For family and friends affected by suicide or attempted suicide, the emotional impact can last for many years.

World Suicide Prevention Day not only offers an opportunity to ensure that suicides are prevented, but also that people living with mental illness, in particular depression and alcohol use disorders, receive adequate treatment, that community-based care and close follow-up are available to people who attempt suicide, that access to common methods of suicides is restricted, and that media reports of suicides are more measured.

China, India and Japan - because of their large populations may account for up to 40% of all world suicides.

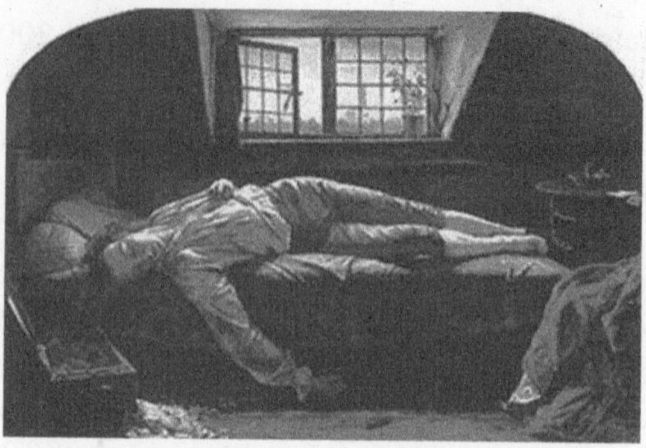

Fig. 25.2: A painting of the english romantic poet Thomas Chatterton, believed to have killed himself with arsenic in 1770

World Suicide Prevention Day (10 September, 2009)

Theme: "Suicide Prevention in Different Cultures" (Fig. 25.2)

Purpose:

- To improve education about suicide
- Disseminate information
- Decrease stigmatization and
- Most importantly, raise awareness that suicide is preventable.

26 Community Psychiatry

HISTORICAL DEVELOPMENT OF COMMUNITY MENTAL HEALTH NURSING

Born in 1963, the Community Psychiatry Movements has been hailed as the third psychiatric revolution.

The first revolution was the age of enlightment following the middle ages, when mental illness was viewed as a consequences of sin and witch craft. "Pinel Philippe" – made 1st revolution, by human care.

Second revolution was the development of psychoanalyis which offered hope for a causative explanation of psychiatric disorders. "Sigmund – Freud" made and developed psychoanalysis.

However, the community psychiatry movement was made possible by another revolution, the one ushered by the advent of psychopharmacology. Therefore, it may be more appropriate to refer to community psychiatry as the fourth psychiatric revolution.

Community mental health is defined to cover a variety of activities. It includes primary prevention activities that focus on promotion of mental health, prevention of occurrence of new cases of mental and emotional disorders. Secondary prevention activities that try to reduce the likelihood of mental and emotional illness from developing. In person at risk and tertiary preventive activities that address the care and management of individuals who experience serious and long-term psychiatric problems and then disabilities and who may need episodic or continuous hospitalization in a mental institution, psychiatric unit.

COMMUNITY MENTAL HEALTH NURSING

Definition

Community mental health nursing is the application of knowledge of psychiatric nursing in preventing, promoting, maintaining mental health of the people, to help in early diagnosis and care and to rehabilitate the clients after mental illness.

In community lining, the individual may to go through stressful situations. He/she may be able to cope with stress and adjustment take place. Sometimes this stress leads to mental illness.

The characteristics of community psychiatry are:

1. Provide mental health care in the community as opposed to institutional settings.
2. Focus services on a total community on population rather than on an individual patients.
3. Focus on preventive and promotive services as distinguished from therapeutic ones.
4. Provide continuity and comprehensiveness of services rather than the care based on illness episodes.
5. Provide indirect services such as consultation and mental health education rather than direct service to patients.
6. Plan community inducement to establish priorities for needed mental health services.
7. Develop and train new mental health workers who could provide basic mental health care.

   Generally and done by the core mental health discipline.

NATIONAL MENTAL HEALTH PROGRAMME

Mental health is an integral component of health, which is defined as a positive state of well-being (physical, mental, social) and not merely an absence of illness. Central Council of Health and Family Welfare (the highest policy making body for health in the country) on 18 – 20 August 1982, which recommended its implementation. The NMHP appeared almost simultaneously with the National Health Policy (1993).

Objectives of National Mental Health Programme (NMHP)

1. To ensure availability and accessibility of minimum mental health care for all in the foreseeable future, particularly to the most vulnerable and under privileged sections of populations.
2. To encourage applications of mental health knowledge in general health care and in social development.
3. To provide community participation in the mental health service development and to stimulate efforts towards self-help in the community.

Three aims are specified in the NMHP in planning mental health services for the country.

1. Prevention and treatment of mental and neurological disorders and then associated disabilities.
2. Use of mental health technology to improve general health services.
3. Application of mental health principles in total national development to improve quality of life.

Approaches to National Mental Health Programme

To achieve the objectives the following approaches were formed.

1. Diffusion of mental health skill.
2. Appropriate appointment to tasks in mental health care.
3. Equitable and balanced territorial distribution of resources.
4. Integration of basic mental health care into general health services.
5. Linkage to community development.
6. Mental health care

   It should include

   A) **Treatment:**
      1. Village and Sub Center Level
      2. Primary Health Center (PHC)
      3. District Hospital
      4. Mental hospital and teaching psychiatric units.

   B) **Rehabilitation of sub-program**

      It deals with treatment of epileptics and psychotics at the community level. Rehabilitation program established district level and higher level.

C) **Prevention sub-program**

It focus on prevention and control of alcohol related problems other prevention programs are juvenile delinquency and acute adjustment disorders, suicidal attempt and addictions.

7. Mental health training.
8. Mental retardation and drug dependence.

NATIONAL MENTAL HEALTH PROGRAM: BURDEN OF DISEASE

The World Bank report (1993) revealed that the Disability Adjusted Life Year (DALY) loss due to neuropsychiatric disorder is much higher than diarrhea, malaria, worm infestations and tuberculosis if taken individually. According to the estimates DALYs loss due to mental disorders are expected to represent 15% of the global burden of diseases by 2020.

During the last two decades, many epidemiological studies have been conducted in India, which show that the prevalence of major psychiatric disorder is about the same all over the world. The prevalence reported from these studies range from the population of 18 to 207 per 1000 with the median 65.4 per 1000 and at any given time, about 2 –3 % of the population, suffer from seriously, incapacitating mental disorders or epilepsy. Most of these patients live in rural areas remote from any modern mental health facilities. A large number of adult patients (10.4 – 53%) coming to the general OPD are diagnosed mentally ill. However, these patients are usually missed because either medical officer or general practitioner at the primary health care unit does not ask detailed mental health history. Due to the under-diagnosis of these patients, unnecessary investigations and treatments are offered which heavily cost to the health providers.

Program

The Government of India has launched the National Mental Health Program (NMHP) in 1982, keeping in view the heavy burden of mental illness in the community, and the absolute inadequacy of mental health care infrastructure in the country to deal with it.

National Mental Health Programme

(Rupees in thousands)

	Actual Expdr. 1996-97	*Budget Estimates 1997-98*	*Revised Estimates 1997-98*	*Budget Estimates 1998-99*
PLAN	89,90	3,00,00	3,00,00	4,00,00

During 1996-97 the District Mental Health Program has been started in 4 states with a budget grant of Rs. 22.5 lakh to each States as under:-

1. District Medak in Andhra Pradesh, Nogaon at Assam, Siker at Rajasthan and Trichy at Tamilnadu. The District Mental Health Program includes:
   (i) Training program of all the workers in the mental health team and at the identified Nodal Institute with in the states.
   (ii) Public education in mental health
   (iii) To increase awareness and reduce stigma.
   (iv) providing service both at OPD and indoor level for early detection and treatment of mental illness in the community itself and follow-up of discharge cases from mental Hospital.
   (v) Providing valuable-data and experience at the level of community in the state and center for future planning, Improvement in service and research.
2. During the year 1997-98 SFC was held and apart from continuing the ongoing projects DMH program has been extended in 7 States viz. Himachal Pradesh, Uttar Pradesh, Harayan, Panjab, Madhya Pradesh, Maharashtra and Arunchal Pradesh.
3. Training programs were conducted during the year by S.M.S. Medical College, Jaipur, Institute of Mental Health, Chennai; Institute of Mental Health, Hyderabad and Guwahati Medical College, Guwahati in addition to NIMHANS, Bengaluru.
4. During the year WHO Workshops were conducted under the National Mental Health Programme:

   (a) Workshop on district mental health Program at NIMHANS, Bengaluru.
   (b) Law, ethics and Psychiatry at IHBAS, Delhi.
   (c) Measurment of disability in relation to mental illness at NIMHANS, Bengaluru. (Proposed to be conducted)
5. Union Min. of Health with assistance of WHO helped procure basic essential equipment to three mansik arogyashalas at Ranchi, Gwalior and Agra.
6. "Spots on Television for public education in Mental health are proposed to be introduced by CHEB from this year.
7. Central Mental Health Authority also had its annual meeting in November, 1997 under the Chairmanship of Secy. Health. Implementation of the new Mental Health Act 1987 was reviewed in all the States and UTs.

Projected Targets for 1998-99

1. It is proposed to adopt more states in to the District mental health program in a phased manner (4-6 States every year).
2. Training programs to be undertaken through identified institutions.
3. To undertake co-ordination between Ministry of Health and Welfare Ministry and other Ministries/Agencies to achieve the broader objective of National Mental Health Program.
4. To involve NGOs in rehabilitation programs.

Aims

1. Prevention and treatment of mental and neurological disorders and their associated disabilities.
2. Use of mental health technology to improve general health services.
3. Application of mental health principles in total national development to improve quality of life.

Objectives

1. To ensure availability and accessibility of minimum mental health care for all in the foreseeable future, particularly to the most vulnerable and underprivileged sections of population.
2. To encourage application of mental health knowledge in general health care and in social development.
3. To promote community participation in the mental health services development and to stimulate efforts towards self-help in the community.
4. To prevent or treat psychiatric disorders.
5. To utilize appropriate mental health technology to improve general health services.
6. To apply mental health principles for improving quality of life for entire population.

Targets

- National co-coordinating group will be formed, comprises of representatives from all states, senior health administrators, professionals from relative fields like psychiatry, education, social welfare.
- Curriculam of mental health for the health workers.
- Non medical professionals, physicians at the PHC will have a 2 wk training program in mental health care.
- Creation of a post for psychiatrist at districts, he will be visiting PHC settings regularly, supervise and organize mental health training programs and continuing education programs.
- Appointment of a program officer for teaching and supervision.
- Provision of additional support for inclusion of community mental health components in teaching institutions.
- Psychotropic drugs will be included in the list of essential drugs in India.

Strategies or Approaches

1. Integration mental health with primary health care through the NMHP.

2. Provision of tertiary care institutions for treatment of mental disorders.
3. Eradicating stigmatization of mentally ill patients and protecting their rights through regulatory institutions like the Central Mental Health Authority, and State Mental health Authority.

Mental Health Care

1. The mental morbidity requires priority in mental health treatment
2. Primary health care at village and subcenter level
3. At Primary Health Center level
4. At the District Hospital level
5. Mental Hospital and teaching Psychiatric Units.

DISTRICT MENTAL HEALTH PROGRAM

Components

1. Training programs of all workers in the mental health team at the identified Nodal Institute in the State.
2. Public education in the mental health to increase awareness and reduce stigma.
3. For early detection and treatment, the OPD and indoor services are provided.
4. Providing valuable data and experience at the level of community to the state and Center for future planning, improvement in service and research.
   Agencies like World Bank and WHO have been contacted to support various components of the program. Funds are provided by the Govt. of India to the state governments and the nodal institutes to meet the expenditure on staff, equipments, vehicles, medicine, stationary, contingencies, training, etc. for initial
5. Years and thereafter they should manage themselves. Govt. of India has constituted central Mental Health Authority to oversee the implementation of the Mental Health Act, 1986. It provides

for creation of state Mental Health Authority also to carry out the said functions.

The National Human Rights Commission also monitors the conditions in the mental hospitals along with the government of India and the states are currently acting on the recommendation of the joint studies conducted to ensure quality in delivery of mental care.

Thrust Areas for 10th Five Year Plan

1. District Mental Health Programme in an enlarged and more effective form covering the entire country.
2. Streamlining/modernization of mental hospitals in order to modify their present custodial role.
3. Upgrading department of psychiatry in medical colleges and enhancing the psychiatry content of the medical curriculum at the undergraduate as well as postgraduate level.
4. Strengthening the Central and State Mental Health Authorities with a permanent secretariat. Appointment of medical officers at state headquarters in order to make their monitoring role more effective;
5. Research and training in the field of community mental health, substance abuse and child/adolescent psychiatric clinics.

Comments

1. For the first time in the last 40 years mental health has been chosen as the theme for the World Health Day 2001: "Mental Health: Stop Exclusion – Date to Care", Why? The recent evidence for the importance of mental health has been so striking that the WHO decided to give it a priority during year 2001, the beginning of 21st century.
2. There is no initiative from the mental health professional to take active part in this program. Most of them are not aware of the program.
3. There is shortage of professional manpower and training programs are not able to meet the demand in providing all medical private practitioners and medical officers.

4. Appropriate mental health can be provided at the subcenter and village level by minimum training of the health workers that will help in providing comprehensive health care at the most peripheral level.
5. The targets set for the program are not achieved till today after lapse of more than one decade. This indicates that there is a poor commitment of the government, psychiatrists, and community at large.
6. The program has given more emphasis on the curative services to the mental disorders and preventive measures are largely ignored. More public awareness programs are required.
7. The medical care in the hospitals is custodial in nature and this need to be changed to a therapeutic approach.

Eleventh Five Year Plan (2007 – 2012)

- DMHP will be extended to another 200 districts
- Reinforcement of upgrading psychiatry departments with adequate infrastructural facilities
- Construction of modern buildings with good infrastructure
- Provision of adequate man power for all psychiatry units
- Research, training programs have to be organized for qualitative and quantitative improvement
- ICE (information, education and communication) training programs has to be conducted.

Twelfth Five Year Plan (2012 – 2019)

- DMHP will be extended to remaining 193 districts
- 20 mental hospitals will be taken up for reconstruction
- Non – viable mental hospitals will be closed or merged with general hospitals (GHPU)
- Long-term community will be planned to cover all sections of population.

REVISED NATIONAL MENTAL HEALTH PROGRAMME (2003)

- Redesigning DMHP around a modal institution, a zonal medical college
- Strengthening medical colleges to improve psychiatric treatment facilities with adequate man power
- Stream lining and modernization of mental hospitals
- Research and development programs in the field of community mental health
- Promote intersectoral collaboration and linkages with other national programs
- Plan for cost effective intervention models
- Health and policy planning
- Focused IEC activities
- Provision of comprehensive community based mental health services will be cost effective and respects human rights
- Promotion of referral services
- Provision of essential psychotropic drugs; family support
- Home care support by provision of sufficient man power
- Crisis interventions, sheltered employment, provision of community care facilities
- Develops self help groups and provision of funds and space for their activities
- Human resource development — short-term training courses will be conducted for professionals and paraprofessionals
- Public mental health education: organizing awareness campaigns in community to enrich the knowledge related to all components of mental health; mass media will be used to enrich their knowledge
- Involvement of private sectors and voluntary organizations in provision of mental health care services at community. government has to support with funds to NGOs and voluntary organizations for provision of services
- Social skills training programs, life skill education programs has to be conducted to focus groups like school children.

- At district level, mental health teams has to be posted (one at district hospital level and another at District Medical Office), to render clinical care and the integration of mental health at peripheral institutions
- Services are focused to special sections of high risk population prone for stressful disorders

APPROACHES TO COMMUNITY MENTAL HEALTH CARE

Preventive Psychiatry

It is defined as preventing mental illness, promoting mental health, proper diagnosis and treatment of mental illness and rehabilitate of patient to avoid disable and reoccurrence of illness.
Concepts to preventive psychiatry.

1. Primary prevention
2. Secondary prevention
3. Tertiary prevention.

1. Primary Prevention

Primary prevention aims at promotion of mental health and prevention of mental disorders, i.e. reduction of occurrence of new cases of mental disorders. The community mental health nurse has a significant role in the primary prevention promotion of mental health can be done by nurse by educating the members of the community on principles of mental health and mental hygiene by providing them the healthy coping mechanism in handling day by day stresses in life, etc.

Role of Nurse in Primary Prevention

1. Advising the individuals in the community about importance of basic needs like good drinking water supply, housing with enough light, ventilation and adequate primary for healthy lining.
2. Educating the parents and other specific groups responsible for welfare of children about the importance of psychosocial development of the child need for love and affection importance

of play and recreation role modeling, caution against over protection, etc.

3. Education about the acquired lesions of the central nervous system, e.g. damage to train tissue resulting from trauma, infection, malnutrition, hypertension, encephalopathy, pollutants, nutritional deficiency and factors which are the major source of impairment leading to mental and neurological disorders.
4. Information on the prevention of peripheral nervous system damage caused due to inadequate or unbalanced diet, metabolic diseases, infections, traumas and toxins which in a long run leads to numerous social and psychiatric consequence.
5. Prevention of infection, trauma and chemical poisoning before, during and after birth.
   a. Preventive measures during antenatal period.
      i. Identify the pregnant women at risk. For example, primi para toxemia during pregnancy, abnormal presentations, pregnancy with associated physical disorders etc
      ii. Facilitate regular medical check up and appropriate intervention through trained professions.
      iii. Advice against the ill effects of drugs, X-rays, irradiation, smoking and alcoholism so that premature deliveries and fetal deformities can be prevented.
      iv. Help the women and family to develop competence in case of pregnant women who are at risk condition.
      v. Direct counseling of the pregnant women should be practiced to reduce the prevalence of developmental anomalies and low birth weight caused due to smoking and consumption of alcohol.
      vi. Give telarium toxoid to pregnant women in the first trimester in the areas where neonatal tetanus is prevalent and provide training to birth attendants in sterile technique for cutting the umbilical card.
      vii. Advice regarding the importance of timely immunization during pregnancy.

Measures during Pregnancy

1. Take appropriate care regarding the prevention of damage to brain during delivery, e.g. forcep delivery.
2. Guard against ill effects of ammonia due to prolonged labor.

Preventive Measures after Birth

1. Adequate balanced diet to the infant/child as a major component of prevention became malnutrition can impair cognitive and social development.
2. Protective measures against febrile convulsions and brain infection during infancy a childhood should be undertaken.
3. Encourage/advice the mother about the need for psychosocial development of the child importance of love and affection emotional security, caution against prolonged mother, child separation, adverse effects of over protection, problems related to child abuse etc.
4. Advice regarding the dietary correction in children suffering from phenylketoneuria and ceitiarism.

Other Preventive Measures

1. Education pertaining to the identification of high risk group in the community who are vulnerable for mental disorders during their life time. For example, growing children, pregnant women, old people, widowers, children's of broken homes, physically handicapped children, etc.
2. Undertake counseling services to the parents of physically and mentally handicapped children with particular reference to accept the handicapped and emotional support to the child and help them to be satisfied with limited goals in the field of achievement.
3. Organize child guidance and marital counseling centers with the help of mental health professionals in order to meet the requirement of such individuals in the community.
4. Educate the primary care workers like Anganwadi workers nursery teachers in the recognitions of sensory and motor handicaps in children.

5. Whenever possible undertaken schools health nursing. This will help in early identification of learning disabilities adjustment problems with peer group, school refusal and other anti social problems in school children.
6. Undertake brief genetic counseling sessions to the parents, families of mentally ill and in the community at large.

2. Secondary Prevention

Secondary prevention focus on early identification and effective treatment for those suffering with mental disorders.

1. **Early Detection of Mental Disorders in the Community**
   Nurses working in the hospitals or community can involve themselves in public mental health education. For example, education of the key persons in the community (like formal and informal leaders, school teachers, industrial workers, voluntary agencies about the early signs and symptoms of mental disorders will help in early identification of cases.
2. **Early Referral**
   Inform them about the available facilities for treatment of mental disorder like correct location of mental hospitals, emergency clinics, general hospital, psychiatric department private psychiatrists. So that appropriate referral could be made.
3. **Early Diagnosis and Effective and Prompt Treatment**
   Help the doctors by providing appropriate history and other necessary information for early diagnosis. Early and timely treatment like drugs and other social therapies should be facilitated appropriately depending upon the need of need patient.
4. **Consultation Service**
   Trained or specialized nurses in mental health can take up consultation services.
5. Training programs for para-professionals and non-professionals nurses can take up training programs in mental health for health workers to manage febrile convulsions, recognize, epilepsy convulsions, recognize epilepsy and how to reduce accidental injuries, etc.

3. Tertiary Prevention

Tertiary prevention aims to reduce the rate of disabilities due to longer duration of suffering from mental disorders. It aims to helps the patient in the readjustment with the family and community from where he comes through rehabilitation program.

Community based rehabilitation can be done through

a. Half way homes
b. Sheltered workshops
c. Day hospitals
d. Partial hospitalization
e. Day care center

Mental Health Services Available at

A. Local Levels

This can be divided into two levels.

a. Village and subcentre level and
b. Primary Health Center (PHC)

a. **Primary care at the village and subcenter level:**
   Multipurpose Workers (MPW) and Health Supervisors (HS) under the supervision of Medical Officer (MO) to be trained for:
   1. Management of psychiatric emergencies.
      - through simple crisis management skills.
   2. Administration and supervision of maintenance treatment for chronic psychiatric conditions.
   3. Recognition and management of grandmal epilepsy.
   4. Liaison with local school teachers and parents for the management of children with MR and behavior problems.
   5. Counselling in problems related to alcohol and drug abuse.

For each task, an appropriate difficulty or severity level will be specified, beyond which the problems would be automatically referred to next level of health care.

b. **Primary Health Center (PHC):**
   Medical Officer, aided by Health Supervisors to be trained for
   i. Supervision of MPW's performance of specified mental health tasks.

ii. Elementary diagnostic assessment of cases, and performing a standardized basic neurological examination.
iii. Treatment of functional psychosis.
iv. Treatment of uncomplicated cases of psychiatric disturbances associated with physical diseases like malaria, typhoid, mild to moderately severe depressive states, anxiety syndrome and initial stages of functional psychosis with appropriate drugs.
v. Management of uncomplicated psychosocial problems.
vi. Epidemiological surveillance of mental morbidity.
vii. Mental health training program.
viii. Outline of plan of action

It consists of set of targets and detailed activities.

Targets

i. Within one year each state of India will have adopted the present plan of action in the field of mental health.
ii. Within one year the Government of India will have appointed a focal point within the Ministry of Health specifically for mental health.
iii. Within one year, a national co-ordinating group will be formed comprising representatives of all states, senior health administration, and professionals from psychiatry, education, social welfare and related professions.
iv. Within one year, a task force will have worked out the outlines of a curriculum of mental health for the health workers identified in the different state as most suitable to apply basic mental health skills, and for Medical Officers working at PHC level.
v. Within five years, atleast 5000 of the target non-medical professionals will have undergone 2 week training on mental health care.
vi. On the recommendation of a task force, appropriate psychiatric drugs to be used PHC level will be included in the list of essential drugs in India.
vii. Psychiatric units with in-patients beds will be provided at all the Medical College Hospitals in the country within 5 years.

B. District Hospital

It was recognized that there should be atleast 1 psychiatrist attached to every district hospital as an integral parts of the district health services.

The District Hospital should have 30 to 50 psychiatric beds. The psychiatrist in a District Hospital was envisaged to devote only and part of his time in clinical care and greater part in training and supervision of non-specialist health workers.

C. Mental Hospitals and Teaching Psychiatric Units

The major activities of these higher centers of psychiatric care include:

1. Help in care of 'difficult' cases.
2. Teaching
3. Specialized facilities like occupational therapy, units, psychotherapy, counseling and behavior therapy.

D. International Agencies/Level

1. Day hospital/Centers
2. Half-way houses
3. Group homes
4. Foster homes
5. Sheltered workshop
6. Mental health emergency care
7. Self-help groups

The role of the nurses in hospital and community in psychiatric nursing.

I. Nurse's Role in Mental Hospitals

Nurse's role in dependent, interdependent and independent functions.

1. **Dependent functions:**

   The most familiar dependent nursing functions involve carrying out the physician's orders. The nurse is responsible for giving treatments and medications accurately and on time. The nurse assures that the patient receives all the prescribed laboratory tests, psychological tests and other appropriate consultations.

2. **Interdependent Functions:**
   It may range from sharing information with the health team to acting as co-therapist with members of other disciplines in family or group therapy.
3. **Independent Nursing Functions:**
   often gives rise to greatest sense of job satisfaction. These functions can range from taking vital signs to carrying out special types of nursing observations and supervision. Together the nurse and the patient develops goals and determine the course that seems most likely to lead to accomplishing these goals. Along the way the nurse must decide what teaching is necessary for the patient, his family and significant others. The nurse must judge how much can be learned from patient's milieu and what needs must be met within the patient's home environment, community or employment situation.

Nurse's Role in Multidisciplinary Team

The psychiatric team consists of psychiatrist, psychiatric nurse, psychologist, and psychiatric social worker. The purpose of this team is to provide a forum in which these members democratically share professional knowledge and together evolve a therapeutic plan of action. It implies that psychiatric nurse has an equal opportunity to share what she has learned about the patient, and her contributions and welcomes in developing a definite goal-directed plan of action.

The Nurse in a Psychiatric Institutional (Mental Hospital) Setting

The skills required are:

1. Basic nursing skills
2. Technical nursing skills
3. Occupational and recreational setting
4. Organizational skills
5. Interpersonal skills
6. Observational skills

7. Skills of communication with parents and co-workers.

In a psychiatric institutional setting the nurse may be called upon to work in the:

1. Outpatient department of the psychiatric hospital.
2. Day hospital
3. Acute emergency ward
4. Family care units
5. Special clinics like child guidance clinics, deaddiction wards, etc.
6. Rehabilitation units.

The nurse in a mental hospital has a role to play in:

1. The safe custody of patients.
2. Carrying out various treatment modalities (physical and psychological).
3. The administration of the ward.
4. Carrying out the therapeutic milieu.
5. Responsibility of health education to patients and their relatives.
6. Patient centered and research minded responsibilities.
7. Maintaining better adjustment and cordial relationships with her own professional colleagues.
8. Playing an active role in promoting mental health services. Day-to-day activities of a nurse in the mental hospital.

Nurse's functions and responsibilities can be categorized into:

1. Patient care
2. Education and supervision
3. Ward management
4. Interpersonal relationships and communication.

Roles of nurse in community psychiatric nursing:

Community mental health is best defined as "all activities undertaken in the community in the name of mental health".

Gerald Capla in 1967, described:

1. Responsibility to a population for mental health care delivery.
2. Treatment close to the patient in community-based centers.
3. Providing continuity of care.

4. Multidisciplinary team approach.
5. Providing of comprehensive services.
6. Emphasis on prevention as well as treatment.
7. Avoidance of unnecessary hospitalisation.
8. Role of nurse in community mental health care.

Introduction

The methods of treating mental illness have changed dramatically in the past century. The overall goal of community mental health as outlined by Mrs. Indira Gandhi in may 1981 while addressing the world health assembly is as follows. "In India, we would like to go homes instead of large numbers gravitating towards centralized hospitals. Services must begin where people are and where problems arise."

Definition

Community mental health- psychiatric nursing is the application of specialized knowledge to populations and communities to promote and maintain mental health, and to rehabilitate populations at risk that continue to have residual effects of mental illness.

Psychiatric nursing in the community setting differs markedly from its hospital counterpart. The community setting requires that the psychiatric nurse possess knowledge about a broad array of community resources and be flexible in approaching problems related to individual psychiatric symptoms, family and support systems and basic living needs such as housing and financial support.

Principles

General Principles

The home and community environment help clients sustain social, family, and self care functions. Keeping clients in their usual environments is preferred, as long as it is medically, socially and economically feasible to do so.

A health problem is a manifestation of several related problems and issues, residual or ongoing , in various aspects of life. A holistic approach is necessary.

Cost-effectiveness can be achieved only through well coordinated and integrated services. Close monitoring of the balance between the costs of providing services and adequate reimbursement is critical.

Home health care is delivered in a client's place of residence. When entering a client's home, the nurse is in that person's cultural surroundings and must respect them, as well as integrate cultural preferences and expectations into services.

High quality client care is an indisputable goal, regardless of changes in policy and regulation of home care services.

Specific Principles

Each person has a unique psychological makeup. Nurses must tailor an individualized care plan to the person's particular circumstances and consider his or her home and community surroundings. Goals for improving health status and developing personal resources must be realistic based on the client's condition.

A client's or family's reaction to an alteration in mental health status, mental disability or mental illness is often influenced by whether the condition is permanent, temporary, degenerative or unknown. Empathy for emotional reactions from clients and families to various mental illnesses can help establish a positive therapeutic relationship.

Nurses base client care on the therapeutic relationship. Therapeutic rapport is the foundation for providing appropriate psychiatric home care nursing services.

Roles in Each Levels of Prevention

The premise of the model of public health is based largely on the concepts set forth by Gerald Caplan (1964) during the initial community mental health movement. They include primary prevention, secondary prevention, and tertiary prevention. These concepts no longer have relevance only to mental health nursing, but also have been widely adapted as guiding principles in many clinical and community settings over a range of medical and nursing specialities.

(a) Primary Prevention

Services aimed at reducing the incidence of mental disorders within the population. Primary prevention targets both individuals and the environment. Emphasis is twofold:

1. Assisting the individuals to increase their ability to cope effectively with stress.
2. Targeting and diminishing harmful forces (stressors) within the environment.

Nursing in primary prevention is focused on the targeting of groups at risk and the provision of educational programs. Examples include:

1. Teaching parenting skills and child development to prospective new parents.
2. Teaching physical and psychosocial effects of alcohol/drugs to elementary school students.
3. Teaching techniques of stress management to virtually anyone who desires to learn.
4. Teaching groups of individuals' ways to cope with the changes associated with various maturational stages.
5. Teaching concepts of mental health to various groups within the community.
6. Providing education and support to unemployed or homeless individuals.
7. Providing education and support to other individuals to various transitional periods (e.g. Widows and widowers, new retirees, and women entering the work force in middle life.)
8. Antenatal care to the mother and educating her regarding the adverse effects of irradiation, certain drugs and prematurity.
9. Ensuring timely, efficient, obstetrical assistance to guard against the ill effects of anoxia and injury to newborn at birth.

10. Providing dietary corrections to those infants suffering from metabolic disorders.
11. Correction of endocrinal disorders.
12. Training programs for mentally and physically handicapped children like blind, deaf and mute.
13. Rendering crisis counselling to the parents to physically and mentally handicapped children.
14. Identifying the problems of scholastic performance and emotional disturbances among school going children and giving timely intervention. School teachers could be taught to recognize the beginning symptoms of problem.
15. Ensuring harmonious relationship among the members of the family, and teaching healthy adaptive techniques at the time of stress producing events.

These services can be offered in a variety of settings that are convenient for the public (e.g. churches, schools, colleges, community centres, YMCAs and YWCAs, work place of employee organizations, meetings of women's group, or civic or social organizations such as PTA's health fairs, and community shelters).

(b) Secondary Prevention

Services aimed at reducing the prevalence of psychiatric illness by shortening the course (duration) of the illness (Sadock and Sadock, 2003).

Secondary prevention is accomplished through early identification of problems and prompt initiation of effective treatment. Nursing in secondary prevention focuses on recognition of symptoms and provision of, or referral for, treatment.

Examples include:

1. Ongoing assessment of individuals at high risk for illness exacerbation (e.g. during home visits, at day care, in community health centers, or in any setting where screening of high-risk individuals might occur).
2. Provision of care for individuals in whom illness symptoms have been assessed (e.g. individual or group counseling,

medication administration, education and support during period of increased stress (crisis intervention), staffing rape crisis centres, suicide hotlines, homeless shelters, shelters for abused women, or mobile mental health units.

3. Referral for treatment of individuals in whom illness symptoms have been assessed. Referrals may come from support groups, community mental health centres, emergency services, psychiatrists or psychologists, and day or partial hospitalization. In patient therapy on a psychiatric unit of a general hospital or in a private psychiatric hospital may be necessary. Chemotherapy and various adjunct therapies may be initiated as part of the treatment.

The salient features of secondary prevention include:

1. Early diagnosis and case finding
2. Early referral
3. Screening programs
4. Early and effective treatment for patient and, if necessary, to relevant family members.
5. Mental health education
6. Crisis intervention
7. Consultation services.

(c) Tertiary Prevention

Services aimed at reducing the residual defects that are associated with severe or chronic mental illness.

Tertiary prevention is accomplished in two ways:

1. Preventing the complication of the illness.
2. Promoting rehabilitation that is directed toward achievement of each individual's maximum level of functioning.

Nursing in tertiary prevention focuses on helping clients learn or relearn socially appropriate behaviours so that they may achieve a satisfying role within the community.

Examples include:

1. Consideration of the rehabilitation process at the time of initial diagnosis and treatment planning.

2. Teaching the client daily living skills and encouraging independence to his or her maximum ability.
3. Referring clients for various aftercare services (e.g. support groups, day treatment programs, partial hospitalization programs, psychosocial rehabilitation programs, group home or other transitional housing).
4. Monitoring effectiveness of aftercare services (e.g. through home health visits or follow up appointments in community mental health centers).
5. Making referrals for support services when required (e.g. some communities have programs linking individuals with chronic mental disorders to volunteers who serve to develop friendships with the individuals and who may assist with household chores, shopping, and other activities of daily living with which the individual is having difficulty, in addition to participating in social activities with the individual).

   Nursing care at the tertiary level of prevention can be administered on an individual or group basis and in a variety of settings, such as inpatient hospitalization, day or partial hospitalization, group home or halfway house, shelters, home health care, nursing homes, and community mental health centers.

CONCLUSION

Nurses are unique in their ability to bridge the gap between the hospital and the community, between the psychiatrist and the community care given, and between the public and other health care providers. Therefore, nurse's role in community support service is primary.

General Hospital Psychiatric Units (GHPUs)

The next important phase of development of mental health services subsequent to mental hospital phase, was the setting up of General Hospital Psychiatric Units. This had been a slow and silent charge which brought about a qualitative change in the whole approach to psychiatric treatment in the last two decades. Though such units for mentally ill persons were started as early as 1933, major spurt came in the 1960s.

The GHPU provided a big push for the greater acceptance of psychiatric services by the public without fear of social stigma. These units have brought a change in the mental health training of professionals and research. In the last 3 decades more and more centres have come up all over the country. Most of them are 30 – 50 bed units. As of new there are about 3,000 beds under this facility in different parts of the country. It is estimated that 75% of the research work done comes from professionals working in these units. An extension of these units has been taken up systematically in at least 2 states, namely Kerala and Tamil Nadu and at present there is a psychiatrist in each district in these two states.

The first GHPU was established in 1933 at Calcutta (Kolkata). The establishment of GHPU had a number of advantages, namely: (i) They were situated right in the community and more accessible and approachable, (ii) Families could easily visit and relatives stayed with ill persons and leanrt to look after the ill persons, (iii) There was no stigma of the mental hospital and mental health care, (iv) There were no legal restrictions of admission and treatment and (v) Proximity of other medical departments assured high quality of care for the ill patients with associated physical problems. In the country, these centers also become the focus of research and post-graduate training in psychiatry.

BIBLIOGRAPHY

1. Lalitha K. Mental Health and Psychiatric Nursing. (1st edn). Gajanana book publishers and distributors. Bangalore; 2006.
2. Mohr WK. Psychiatric Mental Health Nursing. (6th edn). Lippincott Willliams and Wilkins. Philadelphia: 2003
3. Shives LR. Basic Concepts of Psychiatric Mental Health Nursing (7th edn). Lippincott Williams and Wilkins.

27 Assessment of Psychiatric Patients

MENTAL STATUS EXAMINATION

The **mental status examination** (or **mental state examination** in the UK and Australia) abbreviated **MSE**, is an important part of the clinical assessment process in psychiatric practice. It is a structured way of observing and describing a patient's current state of mind, under the domains of appearance, attitude, behavior, mood and affect, speech, thought process, thought content, perception, cognition, insight and judgement. There are some minor variations in the subdivision of the MSE and the sequence and names of MSE domains.

The purpose of the MSE is to obtain a comprehensive cross-sectional description of the patient's mental state, which when combined with the biographical and historical information of the psychiatric history, allows the clinician to make an accurate diagnosis and formulation, which are required for coherent treatment planning.

The data are collected through a combination of direct and indirect means: unstructured observation while obtaining the biographical and social information, focused questions about current symptoms, and formalized psychological tests. The MSE is not to be confused with the mini mental states examination (MMSE) which is a brief neuropsychological screening test for dementia.

History

The MSE derives from an approach to psychiatry known as descriptive psychopathology or descriptive phenomenology which developed from the work of the philosopher and psychiatrist Karl Jaspers. From Jaspers' perspective it was assumed that the only way to comprehend a patient's experience is through his or her own description (through an approach of empathic and non-theoretical enquiry), as distinct from an interpretive or psychoanalytic approach which assumes the analyst might understand experiences or processes of which the patient is unaware, such as defense mechanisms or unconscious drives.

In practice, the MSE is a blend of empathic descriptive phenomenology and empirical clinical observation. It has been argued that the term *phenomenology* has become corrupted in clinical psychiatry: current usage, as a set of supposedly objective descriptions of a psychiatric patient (a synonym for signs and symptoms), is incompatible with the original meaning which was concerned with comprehending a patient's subjective experience.

Purposes

The mental status examination is a core skill of psychiatrists and nurses and is a key part of the initial psychiatric assessment in and our patient or psychiatric hospital setting. It is a systematic collection of data based on observation of the patient's behavior while the patient is in the clinician's view during the interview. The purpose is to obtain evidence of symptoms and signs of mental disorders, including danger to self and others, that are present at the time of the interview. Further, information on the patient's insight, judgment, and capacity for abstract reasoning is used to inform decisions about treatment strategy and the choice of an appropriate treatment setting. It is carried out in the manner of an informal enquiry, using a combination of open and closed questions, supplemented by structured tests to assess cognition. The MSE can also be considered part of the comprehensive physical examination performed by physicians and nurses although it may be performed in a cursory and abbreviated way in non-mental-health settings. Information is usually recorded as free-form text using the standard headings, but brief MSE checklists are available for use in emergency situations, for example by paramedics or emergency department staff. The information obtained in the MSE is used, together with the biographical and social information of the psychiatric history, to generate a diagnosis, a psychiatric formulation and a treatment plan.

Once the history and MSE are complete, documenting this event accurately and efficiently is important

MENTAL STATUS EXAMINATION

Appearance

Record the patient's sex, age, race, and ethnic background. Document the patient's nutritional status by observing the patient's current body weight and appearance. Remember recording the exact time and date of this interview is important, especially since the mental status can change over time such as in delirium.

Recall how the patient first appeared upon entering the office for the interview. Note whether this posture has changed. Note whether the patient appears more relaxed. Record the patient's posture and motor activity. If nervousness was evident earlier, note whether the patient still seems nervous. Record notes on grooming and hygiene. Most of these documentations on appearance should be a mere transfer from mind to paper because mental notes of the actual observations were made when the patient was first encountered. Record whether the patient has maintained eye contact throughout the interview or if he or she has avoided eye contact as much as possible, scanning the room or staring at the floor or the ceiling.

Attitude toward the Examiner

Next, record the patient's facial expressions and attitude toward the examiner. Note whether the patient appeared interested during the interview or, perhaps, if the patient appeared bored. Record whether the patient is hostile and defensive or friendly and cooperative. Note whether the patient seems guarded and whether the patient seems relaxed with the interview process or seems uncomfortable. This part of the examination is based solely on observations made by the health care professional.

Mood

The mood of the patient is defined as "sustained emotion that the patient is experiencing." Ask questions such as "How do you feel most days?" to trigger a response. Helpful answers include those that specifically describe the patient's mood, such as "depressed," "anxious," "good," and "tired." Elicited responses that are less helpful in determining a patient's mood adequately include "OK," "rough," and "don't know." These responses require further questioning for clarification.

Establishing accurate information pertaining to the length of a particular mood, if the mood has been reactive or not, and if the mood has been stable or unstable also is helpful.

Affect

A patient's affect is defined in the following terms: Expansive (contagious), euthymic (normal), constricted (limited variation), blunted (minimal variation), and flat (no variation). A patient whose mood could be defined as expansive may be so cheerful and full of laughter that it is difficult to refrain from smiling while conducting the interview. A patient's affect is determined by the observations made by the interviewer during the course of the interview.

Speech

Document information on all aspects of the patient's speech, including quality, quantity, rate, and volume of speech during the interview. Paying attention to patients' responses to determine how to rate their speech is important. Some things to keep in mind during the interview are whether patients raise their voice when responding, whether the replies to questions are one-word answers or elaborative, and how fast or slow they are speaking.

Thought Process

Record the patient's thought process information. The process of thoughts can be described with the following terms: Looseness of association (irrelevance), flight of ideas (change topics), racing (rapid thoughts), tangential (departure from topic with no return), circumstantial (being vague, i.e., "beating around the bush"), word salad (nonsensical responses, i.e., jabberwocky), derailment (extreme irrelevance), neologism (creating new words), clanging (rhyming words), punning (talking in riddles), thought blocking (speech is halted), and poverty (limited content).

Throughout the interview, very specific questions will be asked regarding the patient's history. Note whether the patient responds directly to the questions. For example, when asking for a date, note whether the response given is about the patient's favorite color. Document whether the patient deviates from the subject at hand and has to be guided back to the topic more than once. Take all of these things in to account when documenting the patient's thought process.

Thought Content

To determine whether or not a patient is experiencing hallucinations, ask some of the following questions. "Do you hear voices when no one else is around?" "Can you see things that no one else can see?" "Do you have other unexplained sensations such as smells, sounds, or feelings?"

Importantly, always ask about command-type hallucinations and inquire what the patient will do in response to these commanding hallucinations. For example, ask "When the voices tell you do something, do you obey their instructions or ignore them?" Types of hallucinations include auditory (hearing things), visual (seeing things), gustatory (tasting things), tactile (feeling sensations), and olfactory (smelling things).

To determine if a patient is having delusions, ask some of the following questions. "Do you have any thoughts that other people think are strange?" "Do you have any special powers or abilities?"

"Does the television or radio give you special messages?" Types of delusions include grandiose (delusions of grandeur), religious (delusions of special status with God), persecution (belief that someone wants to cause them harm), erotomanic (belief that someone famous is in love with them), jealousy (belief that everyone wants what they have), thought insertion (belief that someone is putting ideas or thoughts into their mind), and ideas of reference (belief that everything refers to them).

Aspects of thought content are as follows:

- *Obsession and compulsions:* Ask the following questions to determine if a patient has any obsessions or compulsions. "Are you afraid of dirt?" "Do you wash your hands often or count things over and over?" "Do you perform specific acts to reduce certain thoughts?" Signs of ritualistic type behaviors should be explored further to determine the severity of the obsession or compulsion.
- *Phobias:* Determine if patients have any fears that cause them to avoid certain situations. The following are some possible questions to ask. "Do you have any fears, including fear of animals, needles, heights, snakes, public speaking, or crowds?"
- *Suicidal ideation or intent:* Inquiring about suicidal ideation at each visit is always important. In addition, the interviewer should inquire about past acts of self-harm or violence. Ask the following types of questions when determining suicidal ideation or intent. "Do you have any thoughts of wanting to harm or kill yourself?" "Do you have any thoughts that you would be better off dead?" If the reply is positive for these thoughts, inquire about specific plans, suicide notes, family history (anniversary reaction), and impulse control. Also, ask how the patient views suicide to determine if a suicidal gesture or act is ego-syntonic or ego-dystonic. Next, determine if the patient will contract for safety. For homicidal ideation, make similar inquiries.
- *Homicidal ideation or intent:* Inquiring about homicidal ideation or intent during each patient interview also is important. Ask the following types of questions to help determine homicidal

ideation or intent. "Do you have any thoughts of wanting to hurt anyone?" "Do you have any feelings or thoughts that you wish someone were dead?" If the reply to one of these questions is positive, ask the patient if he or she has any specific plans to injure someone and how he or she plans to control these feelings if they occur again.

- *Sensorium and cognition:* Perform the Folstein Mini-Mental State Examination.
- *Consciousness:* Levels of consciousness are determined by the interviewer and are rated as (i) coma, characterized by unresponsiveness; (ii) stuporous, characterized by response to pain; (iii) lethargic, characterized by drowsiness; and (iv) alert, characterized by full awareness.
- *Orientation:* To elicit responses concerning orientation, ask the patient questions, as follows: "What is your full name?" (i.e. person). "Do you know where you are?" (i.e. place). "What is the month, date, year, day of the week, and time?" (i.e. time). "Do you know why you are here?" (i.e. situation).
- *Concentration and attention:* Ask the patient to subtract 7 from 100, then to repeat the task from that response. This is known as "serial 7s." Next, ask the patient to spell the word "world" forward and backward.
- *Reading and writing:* Ask the patient to write a simple sentence (noun/verb). Then, ask patient to read a sentence (e.g. "Close your eyes"). This part of the MSE evaluates the patient's ability to sequence.
- *Visuospatial ability:* Have the patient draw interlocking pentagons in order to determine constructional apraxia.
- *Memory:* To evaluate a patient's memory, have them respond to the following prompts. "What was the name of your first grade teacher?" (i.e. for remote memory). "What did you eat for dinner last night?" (i.e. for recent memory). "Repeat these 3 words: 'pen,' 'chair,' 'flag.' "(i.e. for immediate memory). Tell the patient to remember these words. Then, after 5 minutes, have the patient repeat the words.

- *Abstract thought:* Assess the patient's ability to determine similarities. Ask the patient how 2 items are alike. For example, an apple and an orange (good response is "fruit"; poor response is "round"), a fly and a tree (good response is "alive"; poor response is "nothing"), or a train and a car (good response is "modes of transportation"). Assess the patient's ability to understand proverbs. Ask the patient the meaning of certain proverbial phrases. Examples include the following. "A bird in the hand is worth 2 in the bush" (good response is "be grateful for what you already have"; poor response is "one bird in the hand"). "Don't cry over spilled milk" (good response is "don't get upset over the little things"; poor response is "spilling milk is bad").
- *General fund of knowledge:* Test the patient's knowledge by asking a question such as, asking the patient to list the last 5 presidents of the India or to list 5 major India cities. Obviously, a higher number of correct answers are better; however, the interviewer always should take into consideration the patient's educational background and other training in evaluating answers and assigning scores.
- *Intelligence:* Based on the information provided by the patient throughout the interview, estimate the patient's intelligence quotient (i.e. below average, average, above average).

Insight

Assess the patients' understanding of the illness. To assess patients' insight to their illness, the interviewer may ask patients if they need help or if they believe their feelings or conditions are normal. Impaired insight is characteristic of psychosis and dementia, and is an important consideration in treatment planning and in assessing the capacity to consent to treatment.

Judgment

Estimate the patient's judgment based on the history or on an imaginary scenario. To elicit responses that evaluate a patient's judgment adequately, ask the following question. "What would you do if you smelled smoke in a crowded theater?" (Good response is "call 911" or "get help"; poor response is "do nothing" or "light a cigarette"). Impaired judgment is not specific to any diagnosis but may be a prominent feature of disorders affecting the frontal lobe of the brain. If a person's judgment is impaired due to mental illness, there might be implications for the person's safety or the safety of others

Impulsivity

Estimate the degree of the patient's impulse control. Ask the patient about doing things without thinking or planning. Ask about hobbies such as coin collecting, golf, skydiving, or rock climbing.

Reliability

Estimate the patient's reliability. Determine if the patient seems reliable, unreliable, or if it is difficult to determine. This determination requires collateral information of an accurate assessment, diagnosis, and treatment.

OTHER DIAGNOSTIC EVALUATIONS

Perform a complete physical examination, including a neurological examination. Obtaining collateral information from family members, friends, and colleagues is important. These individuals all can help in formulating an accurate account of the events that led to the patient's visit to the psychiatrist.

- *Psychological evaluation:* Some evaluations require a battery of psychological tests, including neuropsychological testing when deemed appropriate. This series of tests can help determine what types of deficits the patient might have, can help identify any Axis II diagnoses, and can help identify other factors, such as factitious disorders or malingering.
- *Laboratory testing*
- *Diagnosis:* Use the *Diagnostic and Statistical Manual of Mental Disorders, Fourth Edition, and Text Revision* (*DSM-IV-TR*) Axis I-V.

- *Differential diagnosis:* Determine the patient's differential diagnosis, for both medical and psychiatric illnesses, based on all information gathered from the patient interview, MSE, psychological testing, review of medical history, and current laboratory reports.
- *Formulation:* Use the biopsychosocial model. The formulation is for the current situation and identifies the specific event, state of mind, topics of concern and defense mechanism(s) used, relationships, and the strengths that the patient brings to the treatment setting.
- *Treatment:* The treatment approach that is best suited as a starting point should be noted, including psychotherapeutic, psychopharmacologic, behavioral, and social interventions. This also is an excellent place to document further consultations that are deemed necessary. A statement regarding the patient's agreement (or lack thereof) with participating in the various portions of the recommended treatment also is wise to add.
- *Prognosis:* Patients' prognoses are dependent on the specific illness with which they are diagnosed. However, patients should be encouraged to pursue treatment regardless of their prognosis and should be encouraged to be compliant with the treatment plans formulated for them. Make them understand that their prognosis is always better when they are compliant with medications and follow-up appointments and instructions.

TREATMENT PLAN

Physical

- *Causes:* Multiple etiologies based on findings from history, MSE, physical examination, lab studies, and other required diagnostic tests
- *Differential diagnosis:* Multiple etiologies
  - Differentials -*DSM-IV-TR* Axis I-V
  - Other problems to consider — Medical and neurological illnesses

Work-up

- Lab studies
  - Routine — Sequential multiple analysis, CBC count with differential, urinalysis, urine drug screen, thyroid-stimulating hormone and thyroid function test, urine pregnancy test, rapid plasma reagent, and HIV test if indicated
  - Other laboratory tests based on interview and other examinations - Vitamin B_{12}/folate levels; medication levels, including lithium, imipramine, and digoxin; prothrombin time, activated partial thromboplastin time, and International Normalized Ratio; amylase, lipase, sedimentation rate, luteinizing hormone, follicle-stimulating hormone, hepatitis panel, and copper level
- Imaging studies — CT scan, MRI, other imaging studies based on interview (e.g. positron emission tomography scan, ultrasound)
- Other tests — Electroencephalogram, ECG
- Procedures — Dexamethasone-suppression test, catecholamine level, lumbar puncture, Amytal interview, hyperventilation, sodium lactate infusion
- Histologic findings — Based on final diagnosis (e.g. Alzheimer disease amyloid plagues)
- Staging — Based on final diagnosis.

Treatment

- Medical care: Based on final diagnosis
- Surgical care: Based on final diagnosis
- Consultations: Neurologist, internal medicine specialist, psychologist, social services personnel, others
- Diet: Based on final diagnosis
- Activity: Based on final diagnosis, restrict if patient represents a danger to self or others or is gravely disabled
- Medications: Based on final diagnosis

Follow-up

- Further inpatient care — If patients are suicidal, homicidal, or incapable of taking care of themselves
- Further outpatient care — Based on final diagnosis
- In/out patient medications — Based on final diagnosis
- Transfer — Hospital, nursing home, jail, long-term care facility, or other (based on final diagnosis)
- Deterrence/prevention — Education, early intervention, medication compliance
- Complications — Based on final diagnosis
- Prognosis — Based on final diagnosis
- Education — Medication, disease process, social skills training, vocational rehabilitation, coping, problem-solving skills.

SPECIAL CONCERNS

Medical/Legal Pitfalls

Become familiar with local, state, and national laws regarding specific situations. Cases of domestic violence are reportable in certain states; therefore, be aware of the physician's responsibility to the patient and to the law.

Special Concerns

- *Confidentiality:* Health care professionals should discuss with the patient what can and cannot be kept confidential based on both legal and ethical considerations. In most cases, patients must give permission to release information and their medical records. The exception to confidentiality is cases of suicidal and homicidal ideations.
  - Child abuse, abuse of elderly people: Clinicians are mandatory reporters of abuse and must do so if abuse is suspected.
  - Tarasoff I (1976): This case resulted in the "Duty to Warn," as established by the case of Tarasoff versus the Regents of the University of California.

- Tarasoff II (1982): This case was the second ruling, expanding Tarasoff I and resulting in the "Duty to Protect."

- *Admission types*
  - Informal voluntary: These are patients admitted to the hospital but who are free to leave at any time, even against medical advice.
  - Formal voluntary: These are patients admitted to the hospital who can leave the hospital only when discharged by the physician. Requests to leave the hospital may be made by the patient, but they must be made in writing. During a specific period of time, the person is evaluated by the physician and is either released or committed (i.e. changed to involuntary type of admission for further evaluation and treatment).
  - Involuntary: Patients not recognizing their need for hospitalization may be placed in the hospital to ensure the safety of themselves or others or because they are considered gravely disabled. Before patients are admitted under this type of admission, they are evaluated by a physician and, if deemed necessary, admitted for safety reasons. Patients are then evaluated by a second physician. Both physicians must agree to keep a patient in the hospital. The judicial system may place someone in the hospital for treatment, but generally, patients are kept in the hospital under the least restrictive measure to receive treatment. Patients do have the right to file a "writ of habeas corpus," a legal procedure to allow the courts to decide if a patient has been hospitalized without due process of law.
- *Seclusion (empty room for safety) and restraint (device to restrict patient s movement for safety) procedures:* The American Psychiatric Association task force on seclusion and restraint provides guidelines for these procedures. Become familiar with local laws and hospital rules regarding the use of these procedures.
- *Informed consent procedures:* Written or at least verbal confirmation, with documentation in the medical record, of

informed consent must be obtained before performing a procedure or administering a medication. The patient must be competent to discuss the risks, benefits, alternatives, and adverse effects of a procedure or medication. A competent adult may refuse treatment. If a patient is not competent to give informed consent, a guardian may give consent or the court may rule about administering a procedure or medication to ensure the safety of the patient or others.

MINI-MENTAL STATE EXAMINATION

The **mini-mental state examination** (**MMSE**) or **Folstein test** is a brief 30-point questionnaire test that is used to screen for cognitive impairment. It is commonly used in medicine to screen for dementia. It is also used to estimate the severity of cognitive impairment at a given point in time and to follow the course of cognitive changes in an individual over time, thus making it an effective way to document an individual's response to treatment.

In the time span of about 10 minutes it samples various functions including arithmetic, memory and orientation. It was introduced by Folstein *et al.* in 1975. The standard MMSE form which is currently published by Psychological Assessment Resources is based on its original 1975 conceptualization, with minor subsequent modifications by the authors.

The MMSE test includes simple questions and problems in a number of areas: the time and place of the test, repeating lists of words, arithmetic, language use and comprehension, and basic motor skills.

The Mini Mental State Exam is generally a reliable, valid measure of cognitive impairment. However, highly educated people tend to score higher on the MMSE even when they do have Alzheimer's disease.

The MMSE takes only 5 to 10 minutes to complete. Although it might seem like a simple procedure, only trained clinicians — such as physicians, nurses, and psychologists — should give and score the MMSE. The MMSE asks questions that assess five areas:

The MMSE is far more sensitive in detecting cognitive impairment than the use of informal questioning or overall impression of a patient's orientation.

- The test takes only about 10 minutes, but is limited because it will not detect subtle memory losses, particularly in well educated patients.
- People from different cultural groups, or low intelligence, or education may score poorly on this examination in the absence of cognitive impairment and well educated people may score well despite having cognitive impairment.
- The MMSE provides measures of orientation, registration (immediate memory), short-term memory (but not long-term memory) as well as language functioning.
- The examination has been validated in a number of populations. Scores of 25-30 out of 30 are considered normal; 18-24 indicate mild to moderate impairment; scores of 17 or less indicate severe impairment.

Before administering the MMSE it is important to make the patient comfortable and to establish a rapport with the patient. Praising success may help to maintain the rapport and is acceptable, but persisting on items the patient finds difficult should be avoided.

Recording the MMSE

The score achieved by the patient should be clearly recorded. The score is recorded using a denominator of 30 unless the patient was unable to complete the test due to a physical handicap (e.g. blindness), in which case the value of the questions not able to be completed is subtracted from 30 and the resulting number used as the denominator for the test score.

- If a denominator of less than 30 is used, the nature of the physical handicap should be indicated on the MMSE form.
- The appropriate description of the patient's level of consciousness should also be indicated: Alert = remains awake easily; Drowsy = finds it difficult to stay awake; Stupor = difficult to rouse; Coma = unable to rouse (if a person is unconscious, the MMSE score is 0/30).

Orientation

- What is the year, season, date, day and month (1 point for each; maximum total 5 points).
- Where are we: town, county, country, which hospital, surgery or house, and which floor (1 point for each; maximum total 5 points).

Registration

- Ask the patient if you may test their memory.
- Say the names of three unrelated objects (e.g. apple, table, penny) clearly and slowly, taking about one second for each.
- After you have said all three, ask the patient to repeat them.
- The first repetition is considered the test of registration and determines the patient's score out of 3, but keep saying the words until the patient can repeat all three (up to six trials).
- If the patient does not eventually learn all three, it is unlikely that recall can be meaningfully tested but it should still be attempted (see below).

Attention and Calculation

- Ask the patient to begin with 100 and count backward by 7. Stop after 5 subtractions (93,86,79,72,65).
- Score the total number of correct answers (maximum total 5 points).
- If the patient cannot or will not perform this task, ask them to spell the word "world" backwards. The score is the number of letters in correct order, e.g. dlrow = 5; dlorw =3.

Recall

- Ask for the 3 objects repeated above (e.g. apple, table, and penny). Give 1 point for each correct object (maximum total 3 points).

Language

- **Naming**: Show the patient a wrist-watch and ask them what it is. Repeat for pencil. Score one for each correct answer (maximum total 2 points).
- **Repetition**: Ask the patient to repeat the sentence "No ifs, ands or buts" after you. Allow only one trial. Score 1 if the repetition is completely correct and 0 if it is not.
- **3-stage command**: Give the person a piece of blank white paper and ask them to follow a 3-stage command: "Take a paper in your right hand, fold it in half and put it on the floor" (1 point for each part that is correctly followed) (maximum total 3 points).
- **Reading**: Write "CLOSE YOUR EYES" in capital letters and show it to the patient. Ask him or her to read the message and do what it says (give 1 point if they actually close their eyes).
- **Writing**: Give the patient a blank piece of paper and ask them to write a sentence of their choice (do not dictate a sentence); the sentence must contain a subject and verb and must make sense. Spelling, punctuation and grammar are not important (1 point).
- **Copying**: Show the person a drawing of 2 pentagons which intersect to form a quadrangle. Each side should be about 1.5 cm. Ask them to copy the design exactly as it is. All 10 angles need to be present and the two shapes must intersect to score 1 point. Tremor and rotation are ignored.

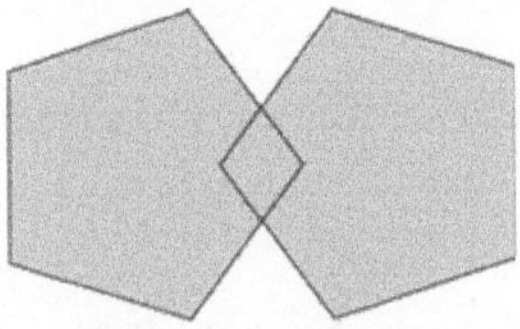

Close your eyes

SAMPLES OF THE FOLSTEIN MMSE

Name: ____________ Age: ____________ DOB____________
Place Seen: ____________ Date: ____________
Time: ____________
Ask Client his/her:
Name: ____________ DOB ____________
Completed by: ____________
Total: ____________

Orientation

Maximum Correct — Client's Score

1) 5 ( ) what is the – date ______, day of week ______, month ______, Season ______, year ______?
2) 5 ( ) Where are we – name of country ______, province ______ City ______, place ______, floor______?

Registration

3) 3 ( ) Name 3 objects (HOUSE, TREE, CAR). Take 1 second to say each. Then ask the Client all 3 after you have said them. Give 1 point for each correct answer.
Then repeat them until he learns all 3. Count trials and record.

TRIALS

____

Attention and Calculation

4) 5 ( ) Serial 7's
100 – 7 = ( ), 93 = ( ), 86 = ( ), 79 = ( ), 72 = ( ), 65.
One point for each correct answer. (Alternatively spell "WORLD" backwards).

Recall

5) 3 ( ) Ask for 3 objects – HOUSE ( ), TREE ( ), CAR ( )

Language

6) 9 ( ) Name a pencil, and watch ( ) 2 points
   Repeat the following – "NO IFS, ANDS OR BUTS" ( ) 1 point
   Follow a 3 – stage command:
   "Take the paper in your right hand, fold it in half, and put it on the floor." ( ) 3 points
   Read and obey the following: CLOSE YOUR EYES ( ) 1 point
   Write a sentence (1 point)
   Copy design (1 point)

Comments:

____

____

____

____

____

____

____

____

____

NEUROLOGICAL EXAMINATION

A **neurological examination** is the assessment of sensory neuron and motor responses, especially reflexes, to determine whether the nervous system is impaired. It can be used both as a screening tool and as an investigative tool, the former of which when examining the patient when there is no expected neurological deficit and the latter of which when examining a patient where you do expect to find abnormalities. If a problem is found either in an investigative or screening process then further tests can be carried out to focus on a particular aspect of the nervous system (such as lumbar punctures and blood tests).

Generally a neurological examination is focused toward finding out if there are lesions in the central nervous system and peripheral nervous systems or whether there is another diffuse process which is troubling the patient. Once the patient has been thoroughly tested, it is then the role of the physician to determine whether or not these findings combine to form a recognizable medical syndrome such as Parkinson's disease or motor neuron disease. Finally, it is the role of the physician to find the etiological reasons for why such a problem has occurred, for example finding if the problem was due to inflammation or congenital

Neurologic Examination

Equipment Needed

- Reflex Hammer
- 128 and 512 (or 1024) Hz Tuning Forks
- A Snellen Eye Chart or Pocket Vision Card
- Pen Light or Otoscope
- Wooden Handled Cotton Swabs
- Paper Clips

General Considerations

- Always consider left to right symmetry
- Consider central vs. peripheral deficits
- Organize your thinking into seven categories:
  1. Mental Status
  2. Cranial Nerves
  3. Motor
  4. Coordination and Gait
  5. Reflexes
  6. Sensory
  7. Special Tests

Mental Status

The Mini Mental State Examination is a useful screening tool.

Cranial Nerves

Observation

- Ptosis (III)
- Facial Droop or Asymmetry (VII)
- Hoarse Voice (X)
- Articulation of Words (V, VII, X, XII)
- Abnormal Eye Position (III, IV, VI)
- Abnormal or Asymmetrical Pupils (II, III)

I. Olfactory

Not Normally Tested

II. Optic

- Examine the Optic Fundi
- Test Visual Acuity
  1. Allow the patient to use their glasses or contact lens if available. You are interested in the patient's best **corrected** vision.
  2. Position the patient 20 feet in front of the Snellen eye chart (or hold a Rosenbaum pocket card at a 14 inch "reading" distance).
  3. Have the patient cover one eye at a time with a card.
  4. Ask the patient to read progressively smaller letters until they can go no further.
  5. Record the smallest line the patient read successfully (20/20, 20/30, etc).
  6. Repeat with the other eye.

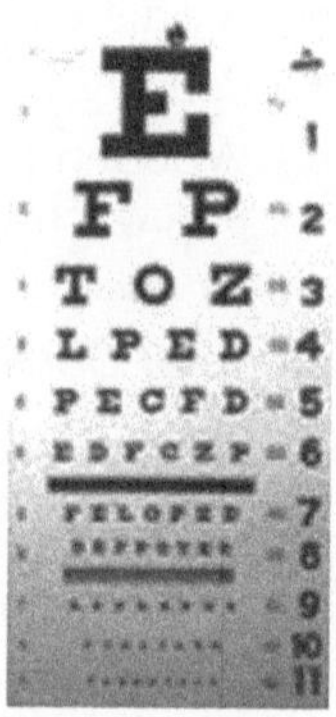

Screen Visual Fields by Confrontation

0. Stand two feet in front of the patient and have them look into your eyes.
1. Hold your hands about one foot away from the patient's ears, and wiggle a finger on one hand.
2. Ask the patient to indicate which side they see the finger move.

3. Repeat two or three times to test both temporal fields.
4. If an abnormality is suspected, test the four quadrants of each eye while asking the patient to cover the opposite eye with a card.

Test Pupillary Reactions to Light

0. Dim the room lights as necessary.
1. Ask the patient to look into the distance.
2. Shine a bright light obliquely into each pupil in turn.
3. Look for both the direct (same eye) and consensual (other eye) reactions.
4. Record pupil size in mm and any asymmetry or irregularity.
5. If abnormal, proceed with the test for accommodation.

Test Pupillary Reactions to Accommodation

0. Hold your finger about 10cm from the patient's nose.
1. Ask them to alternate looking into the distance and at your finger.
2. Observe the pupillary response in each eye.

III. Oculomotor

- Observe for Ptosis
- Test Extraocular Movements
  1. Stand or sit 3 to 6 feet in front of the patient.
  2. Ask the patient to follow your finger with their eyes without moving their head.
  3. Check gaze in the six cardinal directions using a cross or "H" pattern.
  4. Pause during upward and lateral gaze to check for nystagmus.
  5. Check convergence by moving your finger toward the bridge of the patient's nose.

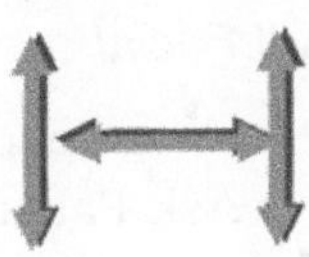

- Test Pupillary Reactions to Light

IV. Trochlear

Test Extraocular Movements (Inward and Down Movement).

V. Trigeminal

- Test Temporal and Masseter Muscle Strength
  1. Ask patient to both open their mouth and clench their teeth.
  2. Palpate the temporal and massetter muscles as they do this.
- Test the Three Divisions for Pain Sensation
  1. Explain what you intend to do.
  2. Use a suitable sharp object to test the forehead, cheeks, and jaw on both sides.
  3. Substitute a blunt object occasionally and ask the patient to report "sharp" or "dull."

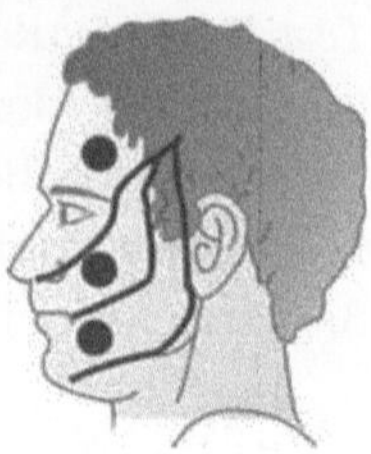

- If you find and abnormality then:
  1. Test the three divisions for temperature sensation with a tuning fork heated or cooled by water.
  2. Test the three divisions for sensation to light touch using a wisp of cotton.
- Test the Corneal Reflex.

1. Ask the patient to look up and away.
2. From the other side, touch the cornea lightly with a fine wisp of cotton.
3. Look for the normal blink reaction of **both** eyes.
4. Repeat on the other side.
5. Use of contact lens may decrease this response.

VI. Abducens

Test Extraocular Movements (Lateral Movement).

VII. Facial

- Observe for Any Facial Droop or Asymmetry
- Ask Patient to do the following, note any lag, weakness, or assymetry:
  1. Raise eyebrows
  2. Close both eyes to resistance
  3. Smile
  4. Frown

5. Show teeth
6. Puff out cheeks

- Test the Corneal Reflex.

VIII. Acoustic

- Screen Hearing
  1. Face the patient and hold out your arms with your fingers near each ear.
  2. Rub your fingers together on one side while moving the fingers noiselessly on the other.
  3. Ask the patient to tell you when and on which side they hear the rubbing.
  4. Increase intensity as needed and note any asymmetry.
  5. If abnormal, proceed with the Weber and Rinne tests.
- Test for Lateralization (Weber)
  1. Use a 512 Hz or 1024 Hz tuning fork.
  2. Start the fork vibrating by tapping it on your opposite hand.
  3. Place the base of the tuning fork firmly on top of the patient's head.
  4. Ask the patient where the sound appears to be coming from (normally in the midline).
- Compare Air and Bone Conduction (Rinne)
  1. Use a 512 Hz or 1024 Hz tuning fork.
  2. Start the fork vibrating by tapping it on your opposite hand.
  3. Place the base of the tuning fork against the mastoid bone behind the ear.
  4. When the patient no longer hears the sound, hold the end of the fork near the patient's ear (air conduction is normally greater than bone conduction).
- Vestibular Function is Not Normally Tested.

IX .Glossopharyngeal

X. Vagus

- Listen to the patient's voice, is it hoarse or nasal?
- Ask Patient to Swallow

- Ask Patient to Say "Ah"
  - Watch the movements of the soft palate and the pharynx.
- Test Gag Reflex (Unconscious/Uncooperative Patient)
  1. Stimulate the back of the throat on each side.
  2. It is normal to gag after each stimulus.

XI. Accessory

- From behind, look for atrophy or assymetry of the trapezius muscles.
- Ask patient to shrug shoulders against resistance.
- Ask patient to turn their head against resistance. Watch and palpate the sternomastoid muscle on the opposite side.

XII. Hypoglossal

- Listen to the articulation of the patient's words.
- Observe the tongue as it lies in the mouth
- Ask patient to:
  1. Protrude tongue
  2. Move tongue from side to side.

MOTOR

Observation

- Involuntary Movements
- Muscle Symmetry
  - Left to Right
  - Proximal vs. Distal
- Atrophy
  - Pay particular attention to the hands, shoulders, and thighs.
- Gait

Muscle Tone

1. Ask the patient to relax.
2. Flex and extend the patient's fingers, wrist, and elbow.
3. Flex and extend patient's ankle and knee.

4. There is normally a small, continuous resistance to passive movement.
5. Observe for decreased (flaccid) or increased (rigid/spastic) tone.

Muscle Strength

- Test strength by having the patient move against your resistance.
- Always compare one side to the other.
- Grade strength on a scale from 0 to 5 "out of five":

Grading Motor Strength

Grades	*Descriptions*
0/5	No muscle movement
1/5	Visible muscle movement, but no movement at the joint
2/5	Movement at the joint, but not against gravity
3/5	Movement against gravity, but not against added resistance
4/5	Movement against resistance, but less than normal
5/5	Normal strength

- Test the following:
  1. Flexion at the elbow (C5, C6, biceps)
  2. Extension at the elbow (C6, C7, C8, triceps)
  3. Extension at the wrist (C6, C7, C8, radial nerve)
  4. Squeeze two of your fingers as hard as possible ("grip," C7, C8, T1)
  5. Finger abduction (C8, T1, ulnar nerve)
  6. Oppostion of the thumb (C8, T1, median nerve)
  7. Flexion at the hip (L2, L3, L4, iliopsoas)
  8. Adduction at the hips (L2, L3, L4, adductors)
  9. Abduction at the hips (L4, L5, S1, gluteus medius and minimus)
  10. Extension at the hips (S1, gluteus maximus)
  11. Extension at the knee (L2, L3, L4, quadriceps)
  12. Flexion at the knee (L4, L5, S1, S2, hamstrings)
  13. Dorsiflexion at the ankle (L4, L5)
  14. Plantar flexion (S1)

Pronator Drift

1. Ask the patient to stand for 20-30 seconds with both arms straight forward, palms up, and eyes closed.
2. Instruct the patient to keep the arms still while you tap them briskly downward.
3. The patient will not be able to maintain extension and supination (and "drift into pronation) with upper motor neuron disease.

Coordination and Gait

Rapid Alternating Movements

1. Ask the patient to strike one hand on the thigh, raise the hand, turn it over, and then strike it back down as fast as possible.
2. Ask the patient to tap the distal thumb with the tip of the index finger as fast as possible.
3. Ask the patient to tap your hand with the ball of each foot as fast as possible.

Point-to-Point Movements

1. Ask the patient to touch your index finger and their nose alternately several times. Move your finger about as the patient performs this task.
2. Hold your finger still so that the patient can touch it with one arm and finger outstretched. Ask the patient to move their arm and return to your finger with their eyes closed.
3. Ask the patient to place one heel on the opposite knee and run it down the shin to the big toe. Repeat with the patient's eyes closed.

Romberg

1. Be prepared to catch the patient if they are unstable.
2. Ask the patient to stand with the feet together and eyes closed for 5-10 seconds without support.
3. The test is said to be positive if the patient becomes unstable (indicating a vestibular or proprioceptive problem).

Gait

Ask the patient to:

1. Walk across the room, turn and come back
2. Walk heel-to-toe in a straight line
3. Walk on their toes in a straight line
4. Walk on their heels in a straight line
5. Hop in place on each foot
6. Do a shallow knee bend
7. Rise from a sitting position

Reflexes

Deep Tendon Reflexes

- The patient must be relaxed and positioned properly before starting.
- Reflex response depends on the force of your stimulus. Use no more force than you need to provoke a definite response.
- Reflexes can be reinforced by having the patient perform isometric contraction of other muscles (clenched teeth).
- Reflexes should be graded on a 0 to 4 "plus" scale:

Tendon Reflex Grading Scale

Grades	*Descriptions*
0	Absent
1+ or +	Hypoactive
2+ or ++	"Normal"
3+ or +++	Hyperactive without clonus
4+ or ++++	Hyperactive with clonus

- Biceps (C5, C6)
  1. The patient's arm should be partially flexed at the elbow with the palm down.
  2. Place your thumb or finger firmly on the biceps tendon.
  3. Strike your finger with the reflex hammer.
  4. You should feel the response even if you can't see it.

- Triceps (C6, C7)
  1. Support the upper arm and let the patient's forearm hang free.
  2. Strike the triceps tendon above the elbow with the broad side of the hammer.
  3. If the patient is sitting or lying down, flex the patient's arm at the elbow and hold it close to the chest.
- Brachioradialis (C5, C6)
  1. Have the patient rest the forearm on the abdomen or lap.
  2. Strike the radius about 1-2 inches above the wrist.
  3. Watch for flexion and supination of the forearm.
- Abdominal (T8, T9, T10, T11, T12)
  1. Use a blunt object such as a key or tongue blade.
  2. Stroke the abdomen lightly on each side in an inward and downward direction above (T8, T9, T10) and below the umbilicus (T10, T11, T12).
  3. Note the contraction of the abdominal muscles and deviation of the umbilicus towards the stimulus.
- Knee (L2, L3, L4)
  1. Have the patient sit or lie down with the knee flexed.
  2. Strike the patellar tendon just below the patella.
  3. Note contraction of the quadraceps and extension of the knee.
- Ankle (S1, S2)
  1. Dorsiflex the foot at the ankle.
  2. Strike the Achilles tendon.
  3. Watch and feel for plantar flexion at the ankle.

Clonus

If the reflexes seem hyperactive, test for ankle clonus: ++

1. Support the knee in a partly flexed position.
2. With the patient relaxed, quickly dorsiflex the foot.
3. Observe for rhythmic oscillations.

Plantar Response (Babinski)

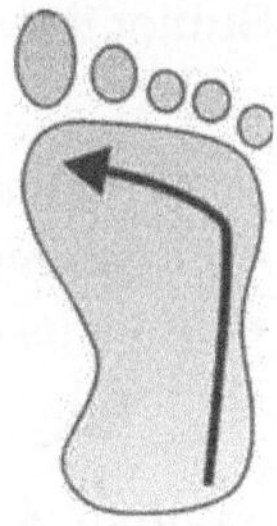

1. Stroke the lateral aspect of the sole of each foot with the end of a reflex hammer or key.
2. Note movement of the toes, normally flexion (withdrawal).
3. Extension of the big toe with fanning of the other toes is abnormal. This is referred to as a positive Babinski.

Sensory

General

- Explain each test before you do it.
- Unless otherwise specified, the patient's eyes should be closed during the actual testing.
- Compare symmetrical areas on the two sides of the body.
- Also compare distal and proximal areas of the extremities.
- When you detect an area of sensory loss map out its boundaries in detail.

Vibration

- Use a low pitched tuning fork (128 Hz).
  1. Test with a **non-vibrating** tuning fork first to ensure that the patient is responding to the correct stimulus.
  2. Place the stem of the fork over the distal interphalangeal joint of the patient's index fingers and big toes.
  3. Ask the patient to tell you if they feel the vibration.
- If vibration sense is impaired proceed proximally:
  1. Wrists
  2. Elbows
  3. Medial malleoli
  4. Patellas
  5. Anterior superior iliac spines
  6. Spinous processes
  7. Clavicles

Subjective Light Touch

- Use your fingers to touch the skin lightly on both sides simultaneously.
- Test several areas on both the upper and lower extremities.
- Ask the patient to tell you if there is difference from side to side or other "strange" sensations.

Position Sense

1. Grasp the patient's big toe and hold it away from the other toes to avoid friction.
2. Show the patient "up" and "down."
3. With the patient's eyes closed ask the patient to identify the direction you move the toe.
4. If position sense is impaired move proximally to test the ankle joint.
5. Test the fingers in a similar fashion.
6. If indicated move proximally to the metacarpophalangeal joints, wrists, and elbows.

Dermatomal Testing

If vibration, position sense, and subjective light touch are normal in the fingers and toes you may assume the rest of this exam will be normal.

Pain

- Use a suitable sharp object to test "sharp" or "dull" sensation.
- Test the following areas:
  1. Shoulders (C4)
  2. Inner and outer aspects of the forearms (C6 and T1)
  3. Thumbs and little fingers (C6 and C8)
  4. Front of both thighs (L2)
  5. Medial and lateral aspect of both calves (L4 and L5)
  6. Little toes (S1)

Temperature

- Often omitted if pain sensation is normal.
- Use a tuning fork heated or cooled by water and ask the patient to identify "hot" or "cold."
- Test the following areas:

1. Shoulders (C4)
2. Inner and outer aspects of the forearms (C6 and T1)
3. Thumbs and little fingers (C6 and C8)
4. Front of both thighs (L2)
5. Medial and lateral aspect of both calves (L4 and L5)
6. Little toes (S1)

Light Touch

- Use a fine whisp of cotton or your fingers to touch the skin lightly.
- Ask the patient to respond whenever a touch is felt.
- Test the following areas:
    1. Shoulders (C4)
    2. Inner and outer aspects of the forearms (C6 and T1)
    3. Thumbs and little fingers (C6 and C8)
    4. Front of both thighs (L2)
    5. Medial and lateral aspect of both calves (L4 and L5)
    6. Little toes (S1)

Discrimination

Since these tests are dependent on touch and position sense, they cannot be performed when the tests above are clearly abnormal.

- Graphesthesia
    1. With the blunt end of a pen or pencil, draw a large number in the patient's palm.
    2. Ask the patient to identify the number.
- Stereognosis
    1. Use as an alternative to graphesthesia.
    2. Place a familiar object in the patient's hand (coin, paper clip, pencil, etc).

3. Ask the patient to tell you what it is.

- Two Point Discrimination
  1. Use in situations where more quantitative data are needed, such as following the progression of a cortical lesion.
  2. Use an opened paper clip to touch the patient's finger pads in two places simultaneously.
  3. Alternate irregularly with one point touch.
  4. Ask the patient to identify "one" or "two."
  5. Find the minimal distance at which the patient can discriminate.

PROCESS RECORDING

Introduction

Process recording is a tool used by professionals in the field of psychiatry, clinical psychology, nursing, social work and in teaching. It helps and guides in the acquisition of the skills, self reflection. It focuses on one's thoughts, beliefs actions and reactions in relation to practice. A good process recording will capture the various facets of a practice moment and allow for identification of what one performed and where improvement is needed. The process recording addresses and examines the content and the process of the interaction with the client/client system.

The art of effective communication is a dynamic process. Nurses are continuously attempting to cope up with the wide range of human experiences. Nurses effectively uses the interpersonal techniques based on their intellectual level, maturity of judgment and capacity for adaptability.

Many of the students' response are superficial and stereotyped rather than being of a meaningful therapeutic nature. Thus, the nursing student needs to develop more perceptiveness so that she can affect constructive intervention through verbal exchange. Ruesch proposes that the closer that the understanding, the acknowledgement and the reply of the therapist matches the empirical experience of the patient, the more effective therapy becomes.

Definition

"A verbatim account of a visit for purposes of bringing out the interplay between the nurse and the patient in relation to the objectives of the visit"

— **Walker**

"Process recording as an exact written report of the conversation between the nurse and the patient during the time, they were together in psychiatric set-up".

— **Hudson**

"Process recording is a written reports or verbatim recording of all that transpired immediately before, during and immediately following nurse patient interaction. It may be written during the interaction or immediately after the one-one interaction".

"Process recording is a record of the nurse's feeling about what was going at the time and as far as possible, how patient said what he did".

Aims of Process Recording

The aim of process recording is to improve the quality of the interaction of better effect to the patient and as a learning experience for the nurse to continuously improve her clinical interaction pattern.

Purposes/Objectives/Goals

Process recording will be used as a:

1. Teaching tool
2. Communicative tool
3. Self evaluation tool
4. Diagnostic tool
5. Therapeutic tool
6. A prerequisite for nursing process.

a. For the Client

- Plays a vital role in establishing and maintaining therapeutic nurse-patient relationship.

- Gains competence in maintaining good interpersonal relationship.
- Clients can be helped more efficaciously by the nurse, who has the knowledge and dynamic of human behavior and skills in using their own behavior as a therapeutic tool.
- Helps in identification and understanding of client's total needs and the methods of assisting clients to workout solution to their health and related problems are being recognized.
- Workout solutions for clients' health problems and related other problems.

b. For the Student Nurse

- Serve as a basic instrument in guiding the student nurses' learning by addressing areas.
- Structures thinking related to professional practice.
- Helps the student nurses to clarify thinking about the purpose of an interview and their role in it.
- Conceptualizes thinking and develops abilities in organizing ongoing activities and transactions with client systems.
- Applies nursing theories into practice.
- It is a basic tool which stimulates communication and self awareness.
- Assist in planning, structuring and evaluating the interaction at a conscious level rather than in an intrusive level
- Heightens awareness of onset in action and as a part of transaction.
- Distinguishes facts from judgments and impressions.
- Aids in identification of strengths and weakness, areas where the student-nurse needs improvement, without feeling of threatened or exposed.
- Gains competence in communication, interaction and related skills.
- Becomes as a base of assimilation of new knowledge and skills associated with it.
- Provide an opportunity to gain ease and freedom in written expression that are important for professional development.
- Gains deeper insight and feedback in his/her practice.

- Offers a base for developing summarized and other educational institutions.
- Helps in rethink each interview with the conscious that the experiences and interactions with client must come through clearly to the field instructor who reads the recordings.
- To gain competency in interpreting and synthesizing raw data under supervision.
- Aids to learn and identify the thoughts and feelings in relation to others.
- Increases the ability to identify problems and gain skills in solving them.

C. For Field Instructors

- Provide an opportunity to individualize both student nurse and client with the students are working.
- Assess quickly the students' ability to respond to the feeling content of interviews or activities with the client.
- Reflects extend to which student nurses are able to integrate theory gained from previous experiences, classroom courses and outside readings.
- Provides direction and a structural framework for the supervisory conferences and evaluation.

Elements of Communication Studies through Process Recording/Skills Developed through Process Recording

1. Conversational skills
2. Skills in interviewing for a specific purpose.
3. Verbal and non- verbal cues to the patient's needs
4. Skill in meeting the patient's needs
5. Awareness of behavior in relation to the patient.
6. Control of behavior as a result of awareness.
7. Recurrent themes in the nurse-patient interaction
8. Skills in verbal intervention
9. Interaction patterns.

Phases in Process Recording

1. Preparing the student for process recording
2. Recording nurse-patient interactions
3. Evaluating the interactions by the instructor and the student

Preparing the Student for Process Recording

- The teacher must help the student to define clearly the appropriate objectives to be accomplished regarding nurse-patient interaction
- Then the process record should be discussed with the student in the light of these objectives and also to determine how it can be used best to accomplish the desired goals.
- Teacher should help the student to learn how to go about writing a process record. The teacher should not expect the student to be detailed process recording unless this relationship of means to an end is clearly seen and understood by both the teacher and the student.

Recording Nurse-Patient Interactions

There are four important parts in process recording;

1. The exact report of the patient-nurse conversation (verbatim).
2. The student's conscious feeling and her interpretation of the patient's feelings
3. Analyses for meanings and cues to patient's need
4. The instructor's and the student's evaluations of the total process recording experience.

A number of conditions need to be met if process recording is to be an effective teaching and learning instrument. These are:

- A minimum of two people
- Reassurance of the patient regarding the confidentiality of the interview. The student also must be impressed with the importance of keeping the interview material confidential.
- Recording of all the verbal interaction
- Notations on thoughts, feelings, and actions that the student experiences during the interaction

- Notations on the non-verbal communication of the patient.
- Notation of the interaction done as soon as possible after the interaction occurs, noting the time lapse between interaction and actual recording.

Evaluating the Interactions by the Instructor and the Student

1. After the interaction, data have been collected by the student, the teacher, and student has to analyses the recordings based on objectives.
2. Self-evaluation by the student to develop a deeper understanding of her own behavior and the effect of her behavior on others.
3. Develop keener insight into the behavior of the patient.

Prerequisites

- Psychiatric clinical setting
- Getting consent of the patient for the possibility of cassette recording
- Confidentiality — client to obtain co-operation for process recording.

Suggested Outlines for Process Recording

1. **Introductory material:**
   Client's identification data/client background information
   - Name
   - Age
   - Gender
   - Race
   - Educational status
   - Occupation
   - Religion
   - Caste
   - Monthly family income
   - Ward No.

- Bed No.
- ORD No.
- H/o any health problems
- Date of admission
- Length of stay in hospital
- Date, time and place of interaction
- Number of visits made by nurse in what capacity and context.
  - I. Personal history
    - Past medical history
    - Past psychiatric history
    - Present medical history
  - II. Family history
  - III. Socioeconomic history
  - IV. Provisional diagnosis (if any)
  - V. Presentation of complaints
    1. According to the patient
    2. According to the relatives

2. **Aims and objectives:**
   - Patient point of view
   - Student-nurse point of view
   - Short -term goal (in the beginning) may be more appropriate.
   - Long-term goal — second stage (working phase) the objectives can be more long term in nature. Focusing on;
     - Corrective psychodynamics
     - Preparing the family for future plans
     - Follow-up
     - Rehabilitation

3. **Record of interaction between nurse and the patient:**
   This should include truthful recording of:
   - What the nurse said and did
   - What the client said and did
   - Nonverbal behaviors of patient such as changing the position, looking at various things, eye contact, biting the

nails, nurse's thoughts and feelings also be recorded so that a self evaluation can be made as to how these influence her behavior.

- First interview: date.......... Time......... Duration.........
  - Specific objectives
  - Participants
  - Conversation
  - Inference
  - Interview technique used
  - Introspective observation

4. **Analysis of interaction:**

   It should include:

   - Interpretation of verbal and nonverbal behavior of the patient.
   - How the student-nurse understands the client system's situation and behavior.
   - Clients' thoughts and feelings.
   - Communication technique used, briefly characterize the transaction.
   - Evaluation based on objectives, effect of techniques used.
   - What interaction skills were useful and were not useful.
   - Plans made for further interaction.
   - Did you achieve your purpose/goals? If not why?.
   - Recording time; it can be 30 minutes. The active time can be 20 minutes, with 10 minutes for conclusion and recording. While interacting with the client, nurse makes short note of it andafter interaction, immediately written, conclusion are made.
   - Turning in; what you think the client is expecting from the interaction? What are you expecting or anticipating (describe your thoughts and feelings prior to interaction).
   - Even though video or cassette recording gives accurate information, the impact of these instruments will make an unnatural influence.

Verbatim

Participants	*Conversations*		*Inference*
	Verbatim (Conversation)	*Nonverbal Communication*	

-Staff signature/ student nurse.

CONCLUSION

Overall impression of the interview, follow-up visit (fixing the time and place for the next interview).

SUMMARY

1. Phases of one - one relationship.
2. Clients' behavior – physical, psychological, emotional, and social.
3. Evaluation – whether the objectives achieved or not.
4. Interview tactics used with illustrations and outcome.
5. Areas need improvement.
6. Evaluation clients' condition at the time of termination of relationship.
7. Clients' response to various therapies intervened.
8. Plan/contract for future interventions – how you and your client decided to work on; indicate next steps.

— Signature of student nurse

9. Comments of instructor on students' performance.
10. Over all assessment: how effective the student nurses' interaction pattern and performance.
11. Points/comment where improvement is needed.

— Signature with date and time.

Final Pointers for Student-Nurses who are Maintaining Process Recording

1. Remember the focus is on you, i.e. the student nurse, not the client. It is important to remember what is communicated (verbal and nonverbal)

2. Ability to recall will improve overtime.
3. Remember that you are writing honestly about the interaction for professional development.
4. Be sure to leave room throughout (e.g. wide margins) for comment from field instructor as they have to review and provide feedback before you submit the process recording to the field liaison.
5. Editing to be done before submitting to the instructor.

Approaches

a. **Purpose of client contact:**
The student-nurse should be directed toward formulating a statement of purpose in concise, clear, and specific in relation to the proposed interview or encounter . it shows the relatedness between this meeting and the previous contact and should reflect the student-nurses' awareness of the particular function of the agency and of the clients capacity and motivation.

b. **Observation:**
This section of the recording will vary in length and content in accordance with the stage of the nurse-client relationship. The student record general impressions of the physical and emotional climate at the outset of meeting and its impact on the client. Significant chances in the client's appearance and/or surroundings are also important.

c. **Content:**
The actual description of the interactions during the planned contact. Although each student develop their own style of writing
This section should include,
- A description of how the interview/activity began.
- Pertinent factual information and responses of both the client and the student in relation to it.
- A descriptive of the interaction between the client and student in dealing with the purpose and concerns identified in the client contact. This includes fact and feelings revealed by both client and the nurse.

- A description of the client's preparation for the next interview/activity and a statement of how the contact ended.

d. **Impressions:**

As early as the student's first contact with the client. They have to make a statement of impressions based on the facts. This process gradually develops into analytical thinking as the student begins to integrate course content and gains understanding of the interaction between self and the client.

e. **Workers role:**

Highlight the student's activity with the client and reflect use of the professional skills and techniques. The student should include and evaluate of their effectiveness as a helping person in each interview or encounter with the client.

f. **Plan:**

The student should make a brief statement of the next contact and record some of their thoughts about the long-range goals for the client.

Professional Skills Sets

1. **Self understanding:**
   - Self esteem
   - Acceptance of others
   - Responsible assertiveness
   - Self control
2. **Talking and listening:**
   - Voice, speech and language
   - Body language
   - Active listening
3. **Ethical decision making:**
   - Understanding the legal duties of professional helpers.
   - Understanding the fundamental values and ethics of social work
   - Identifying ethical and legal implications.
   - Ethical decision making

Merits

- Improves skills of communication and techniques of interpersonal relationship.
- Improves the more specific therapeutic conversation than talking other ways.
- Improves the abilities to face stressful situations.
- Helps to understand the psychopathology of various illnesses.
- Understand the use of mental mechanisms.
- Awareness of emotional maturity.
- Patient learns to listen to other talks.
- As a self evaluation.

Demerits

- Time consuming.
- Interpretation may go wrong.
- Cannot record tone of voice, mannerisms and other nonverbal behavior.
- Relationship may change from therapeutic to social relationships.

28 Nursing Standards

"Standards are professionally developed expressions of the range of acceptable variations from a norm or criterion"

—Avedis Donabedian.

Standards may be defined as "Benchmark of achievement which is based on a desired level of excellence."

Criteria are predetermined elements against which aspects of the quality of medical service may be compared.

WHY ARE STANDARDS IMPORTANT?

- Outlines what the profession expects of its members.
- Promotes guides and directs professional nursing practice – important for self-assessment and evaluation of practice by employers, clients and other stakeholders.
- Provides nurses with a framework for developing competencies
- Aids in developing a better understanding and respect for the various complementary roles that nurses have (Registered Nurses Association of BC (2003) and the College of Nurses of Ontario (2002).

WHAT IS A PROFESSION?

Characteristics of a Profession according to Houle (1980)

1. Concept of mission open to change.
2. Mastery of theoretical knowledge.
3. Capacity to solve problems.
4. Use of theoretical knowledge.
5. Continued seeking of self-enhancement by its members.

6. Formal training.
7. Credentialing system to certify competence.
8. Creation of subculture.
9. Legal reinforcement of professional standards.
10. Ethical practice.
11. Penalties against incompetent or unethical practice.
12. Public acceptance.
13. Role distinctions that differentiate professional work from that of other vocations and permit autonomous practice.
14. Service to society.

PROFESSIONALIZATION OF NURSING

Professionalization is the process by which an occupation achieves professional status. The status of nursing as a profession is important because it reflects the value society places on the work of nurses and the centrality of this work to the good of society.

Professional nursing practice involves "specialized skills essential to the performance of a unique, professional role" the two main concepts that are in the forefront of professional nursing and its services ideal are *accountability and autonomy*.

Accountability is the state of being responsible and answerable for one's own behavior. The sphere of a nurse's accountability is to self, the client, the employing agency, and the profession. The standards of clinical nursing practice by ANA and standards of the various specialty nursing practices document the professional nurse's scope and limits of accountability. By virtue of these *standards*, society holds nurses and those under their supervision accountable for their actions.

Autonomy in nursing is the freedom and the authority to act independently. It implies control over one's practice, and it applies to both decisions and actions.

An accountability based governance system is a predominant feature of professional practice models. Responsibility and authority are established in specified processes rather than in particular individuals who, in turn, determine the placement of accountability. The nurse is central to the organization and is supported by major service components such as standards, quality assurance, continuing education, and peer process.

Professional Standards and Nursing Process

Professional standards ensure that the highest level of quality nursing care is promoted. Excellent nursing practice is a reflection of sound ethical standards. Client care requires more than just the application of scientific knowledge. A nurse must be able to think critically, solve problems, and find the best solution for client's needs to assist clients in maintaining, regaining, or improving their health. Critical thinking requires the use of scientifically based and practice-based criteria for making clinical judgments. These criteria may be scientifically based on research findings or practice based on standards developed by clinical experts and quality improvement initiatives.

Standards of Professional Performance

The ANA Standards of Professional Performance describes a competent level of behavior in the professional role, including activities related to quality of care, performance appraisal, education, collegiality, ethics, collaboration, research, and resource utilization, this document serves as objective guidelines for nurses to be accountable foe their actions, their patients, and their peers . the standards provide a method to assure clients that they are receiving high-quality care, that the nurses know exactly what is necessary to provide nursing care, and that measure are I n place to determine whether the care meets the standards.

ANA Standards of Professional Performance

Standards	*Definition*	*Measurement criteria*
I. Quality of practice	The registered nurse systematically enhances the quality	1. Demonstrates quality by documenting the application of the nursing process in a and effectiveness of responsible, accountable and nursing practice ethical manner.

Contd...

Contd...

Standards	*Definition*	*Measurement criteria*
		2. Uses quality improvement activities to initiate changes in nursing practice and health care delivery system 3. Uses creativity and innovation to improve nursing care delivery 4. Incorporates new knowledge to initiate changes in nursing practice if desired outcomes are not achieved. 5. Participates in quality improvement activities.
II. Education	The nurse attains knowledge and competency that reflects current nursing practice	1. Participates in ongoing educational activities related to clinical knowledge and professional issues 2. Demonstrates commitment to life long learning 3. Seeks experiences to maintain clinical skills 4. Seeks knowledge and skills appropriate to the practice setting 5. Maintains professional records that provide evidence of competency and lifelong learning.
III. Professional practice evaluation	The nurse evaluates one's own nursing practice in relation to professional practice standards and guide line, relevant statutes, rules and regulations.	1. Engage in self evaluation on a regular basis 2. Seeks constructive feedback regarding ones own practice 3. Takes action to achieve goals identified during the evaluation process 4. Participates in systematic peer review as appropriate 5. Practice reflects knowledge of current practice standards, laws and regulations 6. Provides age appropriate care in culturally and ethnically sensitive manner

Contd...

Contd...

Standards	*Definition*	*Measurement criteria*
IV. Collegiality	The nurse interacts with and contribute to the professional development of peers and other health care providers as colleagues	1. Shares knowledge and skills with peers and colleagues 2. Provides peers with feedback regarding their practice 3. Interacts with peers and colleagues 4. To enhance ones own professional nursing practice 5. Maintains compassionate and caring relationships with peers and colleagues 6. Contributes to an environment that is conductive to clinical education nursing students as appropriate 7. Contributes to a supportive and healthy work environment
V. Collaboration	The nurse collaborates with patient, family, and others in the conduct of nursing practice	1. Communicates with the patient, significant others, and health care providers regarding patient care and nursing's role in the provision of care 2. Collaborates with patient, family and others health care providers in the formulation of overall goals and the plan of care and in the decisions related to care and delivery of services 3. Partners with others to effect change and generate positive outcomes 4. Document referrals, including provisions for continuity of care, as needed
VI. Ethics	The nurse integrates ethical provisions in all areas of practice	1. Practice is guided by *code of ethics for nurses with interpretive statement* 2. Maintains therapeutic and professional patient-nurse relationship 3. Delivers care in the manner of that preserves patient

Contd...

Contd...

Standards	*Definition*	*Measurement criteria*
		autonomy, dignity, and rights. 4. Seeks available resourced in formulating ethical decisions 5. Reports illegal, incompetent or impaired practice 6. Maintain patient confidentiality within legal and regulatory parameters.
VII. Research	The nurse integrates research findings in practice	1. Utilize best available evidence including research findings to guide practice decisions 2. Participates in research activities as appropriate to the nurse's education and position such as the following: 3. Identifying clinical problems suitable for nursing research a. Participating in data collection b. Participating in a unit, organization, or community research committee c. Sharing research activities with others conducting research d. Critiquing research for application to practice e. Uses research findings in the development of policies, procedures, and practice guidelines for patient care f. Incorporates research as a basis for learning
VIII. Resource utilization	The nurse considers factors related to safety effectiveness, cost, and impact on practice in the planning and delivery of nursing services.	1. Evaluates factors related to safety, effectiveness, availability and cost when practice options would result in the same expected patient outcome 2. Assists the patient and family in identifying and securing appropriate and available services to address health related needs

Contd...

Contd...

Standards	*Definition*	*Measurement criteria*
		3. Assigns or delegates tasks as defined by the state nurse practice acts and according to the knowledge and skills of the designated care giver 4. Assigns or delegate tasks based on the needs and condition of the patient, the potential for harm, the stability of the patients condition, the complexity of the task, and the predictability of the outcome 5. Assists the patient and family in becoming informed consumers about the cost, risks, and benefits of treatment and care
IX. leadership	The nurse provides leadership in the professional practice setting and the profession	1. Engages on team work. 2. Works to create and maintain healthy work environments. 3. Teach others to succeed through mentoring. 4. Exhibits creativity and flexibility during change. 5. Directs coordination of care across settings and care givers. 6. Serves in key roles in the work settings by participating on committees, councils, and administrative. 7. Promotes advancement of the profession. 8. Display the ability to define a clear vision, the associated goals, and a plan to implement and measure progress. 9. Demonstrates energy, excitement and a passion for quality work. 10. Willingly accepts mistakes by self and others, thereby creating a culture in which risk-taking is not only safe, but expected.

Standards of Care

The standards of care in the ANA nursing: Scopes and standards of practice (2004) describe a competent level of nursing care. The levels of care are demonstrated through the nursing process. The nursing process is the foundation of clinical decision making and includes all significant actions taken by nurses in providing care to clients. Within these are the nursing responsibilities for diversity, safety, education, health promotion, treatment, self care, and planning for the continuity of care. Standards of care are important if a legal dispute arises over whether a nurse practiced appropriately in a particular case.

ANA Standards of Practice

Standards	*Measurement criteria*
1. *Assessment* The nurse collects comprehensive data pertinent to the patients health or situation	1. Collects data in a systematic and ongoing process. 2. Data collection involves the patient, significant others, and health care providers, when appropriate 3. Prioritise data collection activities based on the patients immediate condition or needs determine the priority of data collection 4. Collects pertinent data using appropriate assessment techniques 5. Document relevant data in a retrievable form
2. *Diagnosis:* The nurse analyzes the assessment data to determine the diagnoses or issues	1. Derives diagnoses from the assessment data 2. Validates the diagnoses with patient, significant others, and health care providers, when possible. 3. Documents diagnoses in a manner that facilitates the determination of expected outcomes and plan of care
3. *Outcomes identification:* The nurse identifies expected outcomes for a plan individualize to the patient or the situation	1. Derieves outcomes from the diagnoses 2. Formulates outcomes mutually with the patient and the health care providers, when possible. 3. Outcomes are culturally appropriate and realistic in relation to the patients present and potential capabilities 4. Defines expected outcomes in terms of the patient, patient values, ethical considerations, environment, or situation with such

Contd...

Contd...

Standards	*Measurement criteria*
	consideration as associated risks, benefits, costs, current scientific evidence, and clinical expertise when formulating expecting outcomes. 5. Outcomes are attainable in relation to resources available to the person 6. Outcomes include a time estimate for attainment for expected outcome. 7. Outcomes provide direction for continuity of care 8. Modifies expected outcomes based on changes in the status of the patient or evaluation of the situation. 9. Documents outcomes as measurable goals.
4. *Planning:* The nurse develops a plan that prescribes strategies and alternatives to attain expected out comes	1. The plan is individualized to the patient and patients condition or needs 2. Develops the plan with the patient, significant others, and health care providers, when appropriate. 3. Includes strategies within the plan that address each of the identified diagnosis or issues, which may include strategies for promotion and restoration of health and prevention of illness, injury, and disease. 4. Provides for continuity within the plan. 5. Incorporates an implementation pathway or timeline within the plan. 6. Utilizes the plan to provide direction to other members of the health care team. 7. Defines the plan to reflect current status , rules, and regulations and standards. 8. Integrates current trends and research affecting care in the planning process. 9. Considers the economic impact of the plan. 10. Uses standardized language or recognized terminology to document the plan.
5. *Implementation* The nurse implements the identified plan of care	1. Interventions are consistent with the established plan of care 2. Implements interventions in a safe and appropriate manner, documents interventions 3. Utilizes evidence-based interventions and treatments specific to the diagnosis or problem. 4. Collaborates with nurse colleagues to implement the plan 5. Utilizes community resources and systems to implement the plan

Contd...

Contd...

Standards	*Measurement criteria*
5A. *Coordination of care.* The registered nurse coordinates care delivery.	1. Coordinates implementation of the plan. 2. Documentation of the care.
5B. *Health teaching and health promotion*	1. Provides health teaching that address such topics as healthy lifestyles , risk reducing behaviors, developmental needs, activities of daily living, and preventive self-care. 2. Uses health promotion and health teaching methods appropriate to the situation and the patient's developmental level, learning needs, readiness, ability to learn , language preference, and culture. 3. Seeks opportunities for feedback and evaluation of the effectiveness of the strategies used.
5C. *Consultation:* The advanced practice registered nurse and the nursing role specialist provide consultation to influence the identified plan, enhance the abilities of others and effect change.	1. Synthesizes clinical data, theoretical rmeworks, and evidence when providing consultation. 2. Facilitates the effectiveness of a consultation by involving the patient in decision-making and negotiating role responsibilities. 3. Communicates consultation recommendations that facilitates change.
5D. *Prescriptive authority and treatment:* The advanced practice registered nurse uses prescriptive authority, procedures, referrals, treatments, and therapies in accordance with state and federal laws and regulations.	1. Prescribes evidenced-based treatments, therapies, and procedures considering the patient's comprehensive health care needs. 2. Presribes pharmacological agents based on a current knowledge of pharmacology and physiology and based on clinical indicators, the patient's status needs, and the results of diagnostic and laboratory tests. 3. Evaluates therapeutic and potential adverse effects and potential adverse effects of pharmacological and non pharmacological treatment. 4. Provides patients with information about intended effects and potential adverse effects of proposed prescriptive therapies. 5. Provides information about costs, alternative treatments and procedures, as appropriate.
6. *Evaluation!* The nurse evaluates progress towards attainment of outcomes	1. Evaluation is systematic, ongoing and criterion-based 2. Involves the patient, significant others, and the health care providers in the evaluation process, when appropriate

Contd...

Contd...

Standards	*Measurement criteria*
	3. Uses ongoing assessment data to revise diagnoses, outcomesand plan of care as needed
	4. Documents revisions in diagnoses, outcomes, and the plan of care
	5. Evaluates the effectiveness of interventions in relation to outcomes.
	6. Documents the patients response to interventions

Code of ethics: Nursing has a code of ethics that defines the principles by which nurse provide care to their clients. In addition, nurses incorporate their own values and ethics into practice. The code of ethics for nurses with interpretive statements provides a guide for carrying out nursing responsibilities that provide quality nursing care and provides for the ethical obligations of the profession.

Standard of Nursing Care

In order to ensure quality care the nursing care needs some standards. Standards are degree of excellence. The aim of standard nursing care is to support and contribute to excellent practices. The role of nurse is constantly changing to meet the growing needs of health services.

Objectives

- Plan
- Holistic approach
- Appropriate diagnosis
- Realistic goal
- Selecting appropriate media
- Quality care rather than quantity
- Economize time, material, energy

Types of standard care

- Structure — Things we use
- Process — Things we do
- Outcome — The result

Characteristics of standard care

- Dynamic
- Reflects changes
- Not static

Brief description of methods and procedure

S - Successful termination of helping relationship for client.

T - To have clear idea or conception of the distinct goal, nursing the patient and health needs of society.

A - Assertive planning.

N - Nature of client nurse interaction.

D - Directing others.

A - Analytical thinking.

R - Respect status and policies.

D - Data collection in accordance with goal.

Standard: Nursing practice requires that a conceptual model for nursing be the basis for the independent part of that practice.

Elements: Nurses are required to have clear idea or conception of the distinct goal nursing, the patient, the health needs of the society, the source of client difficulty, the focus, and modes of nursing intervention and the expected consequences of nursing activities.

Standard: Nursing practice requires the effective use of the nursing process.

Elements: Nurses are required to collect data in accordance with their conception of the goal of nursing, client, the source of client difficulty, the four and modes of intervention conceptual models for nursing.

Standard: Nursing practice requires that the helping relationship be the nature of client-nurse interaction.

Elements: Nurses are required to increase the likelihood that the client will perceive the health service experience as understandable, manageable and meaningful at the outset.

Nurses are required to ensure a successful termination of the helping relationship.

Standard: Nursing practice requires nurses to fulfil professional responsibilities.

Elements: Nurses are required to respect status and policies relevant to the profession and the practice setting. Nurses are required to comply with the code of ethics of their profession. Nurses are required to function as members of a health team.

Standard in Nursing Practice

Professional responsibilities

- Health team member
- Ethics
- Policies

Conceptual

- Health needs of society
- Nursing intervention

Effective use of nursing process

- Data collection
- Diagnosis
- Goal
- Intervention
- Evaluation

Unity

- Setting standards
- Planning individual patient care
- Monitoring and evaluating patient and environment
- Coordinating services to the patient.

NATIONAL HEALTH POLICY — INDIA

Objectives

The main objective of this policy is to achieve an acceptable standard of good health amongst the general population of the country.

Goals to be Achieved by 2000-2015

1. Eradicate polio and yaws by 2005.
2. Eliminate leprosy.
3. Eliminate kala azar.
4. Eliminate lymphatic filariasis.
5. Achieve zero level growth of HIV/AIDS by 2007.
6. Reduce mortality by 50 % on account of TB, malaria, and other vector and water borne diseases by 2010.
7. Reduce prevalence of blindness by 0.5% by 2010
8. Reduce IMR to 30/1000 and MMR to 100/lakh by 2010.
9. Improve mental health care services

POLICIES UNDER NHP-2002 AND THE PROBLEMS TACKLED

Financial Resources

The public health investment in the country over the years has been comparatively low, and as a percentage of GDP has declined from 1.3 percent in 1990 to 0.9 percent in 1999. In this frame work, it has been the expectation that the principal contribution for the funding of public health services will be from the resources of the States, with some supplementary input from central resources.

Delivery of National Public Health Programs

It is self-evident that in a country as large as India, which has a wide variety of socioeconomic settings, national health programs have to be designed with enough flexibility to permit the State public health administrations to craft their own program package according to their needs. Since, for various reasons, the responsibility of the Central Government in funding additional public health services will continue over a period of time. Over the last decade or so, the Government has relied upon a 'vertical' implementation structure for the major disease control programs. Through this, the system has been able to make a substantial dent in reducing the burden of specific diseases. However, such an organizational structure, which requires independent manpower for each disease program, is extremely expensive and difficult to sustain.

The State of Public Health Infrastructure

For the out door medical facilities in existence, funding is generally insufficient; the presence of medical and para-medical personnel is often much less than that required by prescribed norms; the availability of consumables is frequently negligible; the equipment in many public hospitals is often obsolescent and unusable; and, the buildings are in a dilapidated state. In the indoor treatment facilities, again, the equipment is often obsolescent; the availability of essential drugs is minimal; the capacity of the facilities is grossly inadequate, which leads to over-crowding, and consequentially to a steep deterioration in the quality of the services. As a result of such inadequate public health facilities, it has been estimated that less than 20 percent of the population, which seek OPD services, and less than 45 percent of that which seek indoor treatment, avail of such services in public hospitals. This is despite the fact that most of these patients do not have the means to make out-of-pocket payments for private health services except at the cost of other essential expenditure for items such as basic nutrition.

Extending Public Health Services

While there is a general shortage for medical personnel in the country, this shortfall is disproportionately impacted on the less developed and rural areas. No incentive system attempted so far, has induced private medical personnel to go to such areas and even in the public health sector, effort to deploy medical personnel in such underserved areas, has usually been a losing battle.

Role of Local Self- Government Institutions

Some states have adopted a policy of devolving programs and funds in the health sector through different levels of the Panchayati Raj Institutions. Generally, the experience has been an encouraging one. The adoption of such an organizational structure has enabled need- based allocation of resources and closer supervision through the elected representatives. The policy examines the need for a wider adoption of the mode of delivery of health services, in rural as well as urban areas, in other parts of the country.

Norms for Health Care Personnel

It is observed that the deployment of doctors and nurses in both public and private institutions will follow a policy of specific recommendation.

Education of Helath Care Professionals

Medical and dental colleges are not evenly spread across the country. Apathy from the uneven geographical distribution of medical institutions, the quality of education is highly uneven and in several instances even sub-standard. Syllabus is excessively theoretical, making it difficult for the fresh graduate to effectively meet even the primary health care needs of the population. There is a general reluctance on the part of graduate doctors to serve in areas distant from their native place.

Need for Specialists in Public Health and Family Medicine

In any developing country with inadequate availability of health services, the requirement of expertise in the areas of public health and family medicine is markedly more than the expertise required for other clinical specialties. Also, the current curriculum in the graduate and postgraduate courses is outdated and unrelated to contemporary community need. The more talented medical graduates generally seek education in clinical disciplines, while the remaining go into general practice. While the availability of postgraduate educational facilities is 50 percent of the total number of qualifying graduates each year, and case considered adequate, the distribution of the disciplines in the postgraduate training facilities is overwhelmingly in favor of clinical specializations.

Nursing Personnel

The ratio of nursing personnel in the country, e.g. a doctor is very low according to professionally accepted norms. There is also an acute shortage of nurses trained in superspecialty disciplines for deployment in tertiary care facilities.

Urban Health

In most of the urban areas public health services are very meager. To the extent that such services exist, there is no uniform organizational structure. The urban population in the country is presently as high as 30 percent and is likely to go up to around 33 percent by 2010. The bulk of the increase is likely to take place through migration, resulting in slums which are available do not percolate to such unplanned habitations forcing people to avail of private health care through out of pocket expenditure.

Health Research

Over the years, health research activity in the country has been very limited. In the government sector such research has been confined to the research institutions under the Indian Council of Medical Research and other institutions funded by the states and central government. Medical research in the country needs to be focused on the therapeutic drugs and vaccines for tropical diseases, which are normally neglected by international pharmaceutical companies on account of their limited profitability potential. The thrust will need to be in the newly emerging frontier areas of research based on genetics, genome based drug and vaccine development, molecular biology, etc.

Mental Health

Mental health disorders are actually much more prevalent than is apparent on the surface. While such disorders do not contribute significantly to mortality, they have a serious bearing on the quality of life of the affected persons and their families. Sometimes based on religious faith, mental disorders are treated as spiritual affliction. This has led to establishment of unlicensed mental institutions as an adjunct to religious institutions where reliance is placed on faith cure. Serious conditions of mental disorder require hospitalization and treatment under trained supervision.

Information, Education and Communication

A substantial component of primary health care consists of initiatives for disseminating to the citizenry, public health related information. Public health programs particularly, need high visibility at the decentralized level in order to have an impact. This task is difficult as 35 percent of our country's population is illiterate. The present IEC strategy is too fragmented, relies too heavily on the mass media and does not address the needs of this segment of the population. It is widely accepted that school and college students are the most impressionable targets for imparting information relating to the basic principles of preventive health care. The policy will attempt to target this group to improve the general level of awareness in regard to health promoting behavior. Currently, non-governmental service providers are treating a large number of patients at the primary level for major diseases. However the treatment regimens followed are diverse and not scientifically optimal, leading to an increase in the incidence of drug resistance. This policy will address itself to recommending arrangements, which will eliminate the risks arising from inappropriate treatment.

Health Statistics

The absence of a systematic and scie4ntific health statistics database is a major deficiency in the current scenario. The health statistics collected are not the product of a rigorous methodology. Statistics available from different parts of the county, in respect of major diseases, are often not obtained in a manner, which make aggregation possible or meaningful. NHP, 2002 address itself to the program for putting in place a modern and scientific health statistics database as well as a system of national health accounts.

Women's Health

Social, cultural and economic factors continue to inhibit women from gaining adequate access even to the existing public health facilities. This handicap does not merely affect women as individuals; it also has an adverse impact on the health, general well being and development of the entire family, particularly children. This policy recognizes the catalytic role of empowered women in improving the overall health standards of the community.

Medical Ethics

Professional medical ethics in the sector is an area, which has not received much attention. Professional practices are perceived to be grossly commercial and the medical profession has lost its elevated position as a provider of basic services to fellow human beings. In the past, medical research has been conducted within the ethical guidelines notified by the Indian Council of Medical Research. The first document containing these guidelines was released in 1960 and was comprehensively revised in 2001 With the rapid developments in the approach to medical research, a periodic revision will no doubt be more frequently required in future. Also the new frontier areas of research impinge on visceral issues relating to the sanctity of human life and the moral dilemma of human intervention in the designing of life forms. Besides this, in the emerging areas of research, there is the uncharted risk of creating new life forms, which may irreversibly damage the environment, as it exists today.

Enforcement of Quality Standards for Food and Drugs

There is an increasing expectation and need of the citizenry for efficient enforcement of reasonable quality standards for food and drugs. Recognizing this the policy will make an appropriate policy recommendation on this issue.

Regulation of Standards of Standards in Para Medical Disciplines

It has been observed that a large number of training institutions have mushroomed, particularly in the private sector, for Para medical personnel with various skills, e.g. lab technicians, radio diagnostic technicians, Physiotherapists, etc. Currently, there is no regulation or monitoring, either of the curricula of these institutions, of the performance of the practitioners in these disciplines. This policy will make recommendations to ensure the standardization of such training and the monitoring of actual performance.

Environmental and Occupational Health

The ambient environmental conditions are a significant determinant of the health risks to which a community is exposed. Unsafe drinking water, unhygienic sanitation and air pollution significantly contribute to the burden of disease, particularly in urban settings. The participants conventionally undertake the initiatives in respect of these environmental factors, whether private or public, in the other development sectors. Work conditions in several sectors of employment in the country are sub standard. As a resist, workers engaged in such employment become particularly vulnerable to occupation-linked ailments. The long-term risk of chronic morbidity is particularly marked in the case of child labor.

Providing Medical Facilities to Users from Overseas

The secondary and tertiary facilities available in the country are of good quality and cost effective compared to international medical facilities. This is true not only of facilities in the allopathic disciplines, but also of those belonging to the alternative systems of medicine, particularly Ayurveda.

There are some apprehensions about the possible adverse impact of economic globalization on the health sector. Pharmaceutical drugs and other health services have always been available in the country at extremely inexpensive prices. India has established a reputation around the globe for the innovative development of original process patents for the manufacture of a wide range of drugs and vaccines within the ambit of the existing patent laws. The addressal to the future imperatives of health security in the country will be looked after.

Sectoral policy documents are meant to serve as a guide to action for institutions and individual participants operating in that sector. Consistent with this role, NHP, 2002 limits itself to making recommendations for the participants operating within the health sector.

Population Growth and Health Standards

Government has separately announced the National population policy-2000. The principal common features covered under the National population policy 2000 and NHP, 2002 relate to the prevention and control of communicable diseases, giving priority to the containment of HIV/Aids infection, the universal immunization of children against all major preventable diseases addressing the unmet need.

Alternative System of Medicine

Under the overarching umbrella of the national health framework the alternative systems of medicine, e.g. Ayurveda, Unani, Siddha and Homeopathy. Because of the inherent advantages such as diversity, modest cost, low level of technological input and the growing popularity of natural plant based products, these systems are attractive, particularly in the underserved, remote and tribal areas. The alternative systems will draw upon the substantial potential of India as one of the eight important global centers for plant diversity in medicinal and aromatic plants

BIBLIOGRAPHY

1. Creasia JL, Parker B. Conceptual Framework of Professional Practice (2nd edn.) Mosby; St. Loius, 1996.
2. Danasu R. Standard nursing care: An Asset. The Nursing Journal of India 2007. VOL. XCVIII No. 6.
3. Hall JK. Nursing ethics and law. W.B Saunders company; Philadelphia., 1996.
4. Kockrow EO, Christensen BL. Foundations of Nursing (4th edn.) Mosby, 2003.
5. Lillies C, Taylor C et al. Fundamentals of Nursing: The art and science of nursing care. Lippincott publications; Philadelphia, 2005.
6. Potter PA, Perry AG. Basic Nursing; Essentials for Practice (6th edn.) Mosby; St Louis, 2007.
7. Potter PA, Perry AG. Fundamentals of Nursing (6th edn.) Mosby; St. Louis. 2005.

Index